Brain Control of Behaviour

Contents

10 Concluding Remarks

Appendix

Preface

This book represents the development of a previous (1992) Italian general review [Pinelli and Ceriani, 1992] dealing with theoretical and experimental aspects of neural motor control of speech. Preliminary results obtained with reading reactions from normal subjects and neuropsychiatric patients were also reported. The basic experiments consisted of reading aloud some verbal tasks presented at random with choice reaction modalities and with different pre-executive foreperiods. Thus, we measured the time taken by the brain to generate the innervation patterns we recorded by means of electromyography and the time taken by the executors shaping the vocal tract and producing the air vibrations requested for speech and recorded as acousticogram.

The previous research has now been extended with more systematic investigations including different tasks and multiple delays in reading reactions: a new methodology (MDRV, multiple-delayed-reaction verbochronometry) was so set up. New collaborations have been commenced.

Some meetings were held in Nijmegen and Veruno with experts in the field, including psychologists, neurologists, neuropsychologists and bio-engineers from Denmark, the UK, Italy and the Netherlands. Thus, it was possible to co-operate in a way that could yield a large amount of data, promote new investigations and methodological refinements and stimulate various speculations and experiments.

In spite of a large number of still unsolved problems, the application of MDRV yielded new issues in psychophysiology, and MDRV appeared to be a reliable methodology able to provide quantitative information on brain functionality at the level of clinical routine assessment.

Systematic results obtained in many specialized laboratories were integrated to form a body of information worth compiling in a book developing the line of study of the previous basic works of Levelt and of Peters and collaborators.

Although the general issues including the conceptualization and the motivation of speaking have not been ignored by us, the neurolinguist or the theorist of behaviourals neurology looking at this book must be warned that the main contents of our work concern a limited part of man's ability to speak: speech rather than language has been the principal target of our study.

Nevertheless, even if restricted to the brain processes involved in reading aloud some phonemes, syllables, words and simple sentences, and in two-alternative picture naming, our research covered a complicated series of neural events: active and restorative processes in the cyclic succession of central programmers and distal executors. Multiple interchangeable strategies and intermediary adaptations of detailed final patterns of innervation were also taken into consideration.

The application of MDRV in the study of stuttering is universally accepted and its value as an indicator in mental diseases like schizophrenia has recently been demonstrated [Pinelli et al., in press; Pinelli, in press], but its extension in other neuropsychiatric fields, particularly in childhood, is reasonably predictable.

MDRV is in fact a legitimate candidate among the biological methodologies capable of assessing dyslexia and the phonological deficits linked to primary learning disabilities. If we keep the high frequency of learning disabilities in mind, which affect more than half of all schoolchildren classified as disabled, and the fact that until now we have no specific diagnosis for learning disabilities [Rugg, 1995], we can easily see that it is worthwhile making a note of the biological and diagnostic validity of MDRV for the investigation of learning disabilities.

As for the foundation of MDRV, a General Introduction seems to be helpful to analyse the main questions we faced in the search for the neurophysiological substrates of the processes involved in the production and the motor execution of phonological and grammatical tasks. The data obtained concern the temporal parameters of reading reactions performed under different experimental conditions. They yielded new data not only on the activation of the visuomotor representations in the brain but also on the dynamic intermediary processes implying mental transfer operations.

We expect these premises and their related definitions, covering a mixed psychological and neurophysiological area, to arouse the reader's interest and orient him towards the 'glimmers of light' that MDRV can offer in the study of brain functionality.

Acknowledgements

My pupil Dr. Fiorenzo Ceriani helped me 4 years ago to publish the Italian preliminary text *Processi e rappresentazioni della parola* and later followed my advice and encouragement to apply and extend the methodology to paediatrics.

Bio-engineer Roberto Colombo kindly offered me consistent advice and accomplished the technical realization of the devices requested by the continuously evolving methodology. My friend Dr. Carlo Pasetti offered me his precious help for the organization of this research. Dr. Roberto Conti and the technician Danilo Pianca carried out carefully thousands of investigations and recordings of multiple-delayed-reaction verbochronometry. To the patience and skill of Anna Colombo, Dr. Marco Danioni and Stefania Bicelli I owe the transformation of my handwritten manuscript into the final typescript, the change of my drawings into the final figures and the elaboration of my data into well-defined diagrams.

The cultural atmosphere of the Institute of Research and Care of the Fondazione Salvatore Maugeri Clinica del Lavoro e della Riabilitazione in Veruno with the collaboration of Dr. Cinzia Miscio and Fabrizio Pisano provided the intellectual tuning.

Perkell's demonstrations and suggestions in the MIT laboratory during the 1991 Congress of the American Academy of Neurology in Boston, Levelt's participation at the 'Gargnano' workshop on Speech Control at Milano University in 1992 and the 1994 Meeting at Nijmegen University with Peters and his collaborators acted as catalysts.

Eventually I express my gratitude to Prof. Detlev Van Zerssen who, with Dr. Dieter Wildenauer (Max-Planck-Institut für Psychiatrie in Munich) and Prof. Wolfgang Maier of the University of Mainz, discussed my results on schizophrenia and provided useful suggestions for the definition of the brain intermediary processes and for the development of further research with multiple-delayed-reaction verbochronometry in populations with an increased risk of schizophrenia.

Grants were provided by the International Center for Studies and Research in Biomedicine, Luxembourg, which also supported the organization of the research, and by the CNR group of research directed by Carlo Loeb. The research on amyotrophic lateral sclerosis was supported by Theleton.

General Introduction:
The Core Subject

The mysterious cognitive disorder related to functional impairment in frontogangliobasal circuitry remains shrouded by the newly arising questions open by the most recent neuropsychological studies.

[Spicer et al., 1994]

Unconscious mnemonic and motor set functions of specific pyramidal neurons in the prefrontal cortex seem to lay the bridge from perception to action across time. [Fuster, 1993]

The study of brain representations and processes implied in purposeful complex sequential actions has benefited in the last 10 years from sophisticated brain imaging techniques like functional magnetic resonance imaging (MRI) and positron emission tomography (PET) [Heiss, 1995]. However, a functional test of cerebral processes is still needed and has recently been developed in several institutes with a shift from the neuro-psychologically oriented investigation of *reaction* times (where the response of the subject is aspecific with respect to the task stimulus) to the neurophysiologically oriented investigation of *action* times (where the response of the subject specifically corresponds to the task stimulus). Thus, unconscious brain activities in their succession and development with a correspondent modelling of multiple parallel and serial internal processes, buffer coding and decoding, and execution circuits become the core target of research. The hidden brain function related to the mental activity in the elaboration and control of behaviour becomes accessible to the examinations that the neurologist can carry out in clinical laboratories. Performances, like attention with its multiple aspects, perceptive-motor transfers, operative memory and the most subtle processes of adaptation and internal error correction, can then be restudied in their relationship with actual neural functions. The classical psychological terms are in this way better analysed, revised and clarified. To the neuroscientists, their links with the real brain activities appear in fact to become progressively looser, and new models of neural networks are worked out allowing a better understanding of the mechanisms involved in the control of human behaviour.

An analysis of the normal physiological processes of psychomotility and its different alterations in neural diseases was carried out by Serratrice and Habib [1993] in relation with the processes of writing. 'Since the language is not an organ in itself', says F. Lhermitte in the Introduction to their book, 'but it is rather a modality of information processing, and an organization able to produce an infinite number of creations, this function must be integrated into the ensemble of mental functions, that means also the ensemble of brain functions.'

A fundamental step in the methodological approach was achieved by us with the acknowledgement that speech represents the most powerful 'temporal visualization' of these highest-level brain functions in human beings. Abbs and Gracco [Abbs et al., 1984; Gracco, 1987, 1991; Gracco and Abbs, 1986, 1988] in Haskins' laboratories, Perkell [1991] at the MIT and Honda [1994] at the International Institute of Advanced Telecommunication Research created a basic substantial theoretical and experimental background to record and evaluate all vocal tract muscular activities.

The goal of this review is to outline a set of tests with a view to investigate and measure the time taken by the brain to accomplish multiple phonological and grammatical tasks included in reading reactions. Two-alternative tests of picture naming were also carried out.

Latency times and acousticogram (ACG) durations of immediate and delayed reactions were measured with different, short and long, intervals. Mean values and standard deviations were obtained from normal subjects of various ages and conditions. Their reliability and constancy in repeated examinations at long time intervals were statistically evaluated. Corresponding models for the interpretation of the basic structural and functional substrates were proposed and discussed.

Several pathological disorders in the neurological and psychiatric fields were also investigated and evaluated. Specific patterns of slowed functions were identified. Moreover, upward repercussions from impaired distal executors (equivalent to mechanical constraints) on the central programmers were detected and evaluated.

The leading motif of our research was the identification of the parallel and successive operations of the brain in speech production, control and execution. The theoretical background could be indicated in a revised modular interpretation.

As reference points in the analysis of our findings, three main operative processes were taken into consideration: (1) programmation, (2) intermediary processes and (3) executive mechanisms.

However, possible subassemblies were pointed out as: initiation versus hierarchical and temporal (timing) programmation in operation 1; active memory, specific working memories, non-mnemic temporal bridging, adaptation of invariants to variants and pre-executive facilitatory processes in operation 2; triggering of the servo-mechanism, final adaptation, coordination and sequential setting of myo-articular movements (diadochokinesis) in operation 3.

In intimate connection with the elaboration of the neural commands, we analysed the anatomofunctional constraints represented by the biomechanical properties of the vocal tract with its muscular structures.

Whenever the organization of the speech control by the brain and the repercussion that changes in one assembly or subassembly exert on the central brain machinery were to be reconstructed, an integrative holistic theoretical frame was adopted.

The relatively narrow range of tests facilitated their application to a wide field of normal and pathological conditions. During pattern researches, the identification of an impairment in intermediary processes of delayed mental transfer in schizophrenics, with a statistically highly significant score, represented a successful achievement.

However, many issues remain still unsolved and new ones arose. When delineating the different topics, we had to face the task of homogenizing the different terminologies previously used by various specialists to describe partly overlapping facts or models of neural networks. For this purpose, our choice was guided by the principle that the search for objective quantitative investigations should prevail over speculations and indirect evidence.

Taking into account the great complexity and the extensive connections even within the confined topic of our research, the reader should not undervalue our results and speculations. We are sure indeed that he will grasp the strict link between speech production and speech perception as well as between speech and language formulation processes.

When setting up a valid and reliable *clinical* methodology, we took into account the general theories of brain motor control and more specifically those of motor action in speech. Several artificial procedures and tricks, engaging the individual subject not only in immediate but also in delayed complex performances, have been worked out: brain processes related to intermediary functions including working or dynamic memory and buffer retrieval could thus be explored.

An ambitious aim was to set up quantitative tests able to detect *subclinical* changes in the brain machinery considered as a general system of psychomotor control. In this context, some 'functional probes' have been applied in the course of brain parallel diffuse processes (PDP) producing speech.

Many results are reported under both normal and paranormal conditions: they did not only improve the identification of the corresponding functional state, but they also provided new insights into the programmation and execution processes of speech. Thus, new laws of these functions were defined and new principles of interpretation were proposed; new issues emerged at both theoretical and experimental levels.

We are hopeful that the reader, as a physiological psychologist, will profit by some deeper insights into the neurobiological mechanisms and, as a neurologist, will acquire a more available and, at the same time, reliable way of following up investigations of brain functions and related executive constraints.

There is still a long way to go to interpret the new acquisitions in the light of behavioural neurology, but we can begin by just knowing the temporal parameters of some modules making the machine really work and by comprehending the logic according to which the *representations* are organized (coded and decoded) in stores and *process* flows in internal circuits. Some blueprints were drawn, some models elaborated.

No doubt the core of this book consists in the tests that, in routine clinical application, from childhood to old age, derive from the most advanced knowledge and which are consistent with the artificial neural network models of speech motor control. This is indeed the first fundamental step in the progress of science: once we better know the functional potentialities and the functional and structural limits of the individual human brain, we can try to better define the most suitable information and programme society must provide to improve individually organized neural networks. This should be done particularly in the learning period of life, when neuroplastic processes are particularly efficient and formative.

However important these acquisitions may appear, the majority of people reading the title and maybe the Preface might wonder whether these investigations and lucubrations are of immediate clinical usefulness. Our answer is based on the experience with these speech tests in the assessment of brain function in neurorehabilitation. The following advantages can be listed: (1) the neural speech tests are particularly sensitive to detect and quantify mental deterioration; (2) with these tests, a more reliable early evaluation of the functional consequences of major psychotic mental impairments, like manic-depressive disorders and schizophrenia, can be carried out; (3) backward effects on attention efficiency due to impairment of executive processes can be detected and assessed; (4) the effects of drugs and neurotoxic substances on brain functions can be measured; (5) alterations in the programming (timing) and executive processes can be detected, providing a fundamental criterion for the temporal accomplishment of neurorehabilitative treatments; (6) the use of artificial feedbacks to correct topic and temporal discoordinations can be better chosen and planned for selected patients.

The work will continue, but I hope this book will not only provide the essential technical and theoretical information to basic scientists and clinicians engaged in this effort but will also allow the reader to spend some hours immersed in what can be regarded as the most fascinating and intriguing field of human sciences: the brain trying to understand itself, its wonderful creative processes but also its *intrinsic liability to errors*.

Reading these pages and looking at the amount of data collected, the students will become aware of a paradoxical dissociation between the degree of subjective efforts of everybody involved in an action and the complexity of the processes producing the actions. Reading simple words or sentences seems to be a very simple action because it is elaborated unconsciously in our brain, thanks to 'mental organs' that have genetically been developed in tens of thousands of years. In contrast, they are extremely intricate, even if not beyond the reach of our knowledge. We must mind the brain, respect and treasure it as the most powerfully ambivalent phylogenetic and epigenetic creation. Moreover: 'To have forgotten that some severe mental disorders are brain diseases will go down as the great aberration of the twentieth-century medicine' [Ron and Harvey, 1990; Raja, 1995].

Neuropsychology, psychophysiology and functional neuro-imaging fulfil common scientific goals but differ in their individual methodologies. The objects of these three branches of neuroscience are the physiological mechanisms of the high cognitive functions, emotions, affectivity and more generally of the complex capacities subserving intelligence and human thought.

The specific neuropsychological methodology developed by Broca, Wernicke and their followers is essentially based on mental tests that have been progressively elaborated to differentiate the subfunctions and factors implied in human language and the capacity of problem solving. Its main procedure is the anatomoclinical correlation.

Psychophysiology has its pioneers in Pavlov, McCulloch and Pitts for the mathematical elaboration of the analogous neural three-level networks, Kornmüller and Zappoli for the cognitive and event-related evoked brain potentials, and Gastaut and Moruzzi for the fundamental investigations of the brain processes related to vigilance and consciousness. Even with multiple technological approaches, the methodologies that are specifically used by psychophysiologists might be identified by a differential chronometry of the neural processes of behavioural performances. The measurement can rely directly on cognitive evoked potentials or indirectly on reaction times of purposeful complex sequential actions. Speaking is the most complex, uniquely human, action: Kutas et al. [1988] have systematically studied the event-related potentials of speaking; we have developed the multiple-delayed-reaction verbochronometry (MDRV).

Functional neuro-imaging, with PET [Petersen, 1988], functional MRI and spectral single-photon emission computed tomography, detects the metabolic changes that occur in different brain regions during well-defined performances.

The application of the three methodologies, in both normal and pathological conditions, can often overlap and can be associated, the resulting data being profitably correlated with each other. The knowledge of the brain machinery can thus be greatly enhanced.

However, each methodology requires qualified experts and scholars. Psychophysiology comprises in fact different schools and laboratories, and it is just one of the most recent – namely the last developments concerning delayed reactions and recordings of verbal articulators and the resulting ACG – that this book will deal with. The general *principles* that led to the elaboration of the most reliable and fruitful methodology and to the evaluation of the results will be particularly considered and explained.

The paths we followed to disclose some processes of speech control by the brain will now be expanded to the reader in the Outline of the sections and chapters into which it seemed convenient to subdivide the book.

An Outline of the Principles and Investigations with Multiple-Delayed-Reaction Verbochronometry

The subject of this book concerns the representations inherited and acquired in the brain and the neural processes able to produce speech, that is the most specialized purposeful human performance. We have developed a methodology (MDRV) that enables us to measure differentially the time taken by the neural processes of programmation and execution as well as the time of the successive movements in the action expressed by the duration of the responses.

The search for the most convenient verbal tasks and responses to be recorded in order to develop the most fruitful analysis of the underlying brain processes in normal and pathological conditions has always been the main goal which engaged the neurologists and the psychologists aiming to examine the functionality of the brain in the single subject with quantitative, reliable tests.

A rational development of the methodology and a correct exhaustive interpretation of the results require also a comprehensive knowledge of the data acquired with other methodologies and of the theoretical models elaborated in brain behavioural science.

These being the premises, we will list now the 10 sections of the book.

Section 1 describes the fundamental role the motor control has acquired in the phylogenetic organization of the human brain and particularly of the 'mental organ' of speech. The origin of vocalization in children is analysed and the underlying neuro-anatomical substrates are outlined.

The temporal parameters related to the neural processes of speech production are reported in *Section 2*. Particular emphasis is given to the latency time of the ACG and to its duration in response to verbal tasks to be read aloud in delayed reactions. Brain formulation processes are found to be specific for phonological (in contrast to grammatical) tasks in verbal choice reactions but also in picture naming. A preliminary diagram of MDRV is reported. Records of oromandibular muscle electromyograms (EMG) allowing a measurement of preparatory tuning processes are presented.

In *Section 3*, simple reaction times are evaluated as a complementary investigation into the executive processes.

Since the main functions are of a stochastic kind, a certain number of repeated trials is requested to obtain a reliable mean value: this is specified in *Section 4*. An analysis of the origin of the time needed to produce the ACG and of the causes producing ACG variability in a 12-trial sequence is carried out with reference to the whole chain of speech control and execution processes.

Section 5 deals with the methodology of MDRV and the general criteria for the evaluation of the results. Very short (100 ms) foreperiods are introduced in the delayed reactions to check the condition of PDP occurring in the early and central visuomotor and computational activities of the nervous system. Longer foreperiods (500–4,000 ms) in delayed reactions are adopted to investigate particularly intermediary processes occurring between programmation and execution processes. The intermediary process is the subject matter of analyses and discussions, with drawings of theoretical schemas and methodological adaptations, and examples illustrated throughout the whole Section. It is pointed out how many terms are not clearly defined in the literature and overlap in their meaning. The delimitations in the methodological approach to conscious, intentional, active short-term memory in contrast to the more automatic working memory are particularly confusing. This topic is specifically treated in *Section 6*.

In our investigations, we analyse how the intermediary processes are related to active afteractivity with reverberatory circuits and triggering of internal feedbacks. Short-term delayed intentional processes can be investigated with MDRV: one set of trials presents the word stimuli that remain on the screen until the 'go' signal appears above and below the word stimuli; otherwise, in the second set of trials, the presentation of the word stimuli lasts only 1.5 ms with a foreperiod of 4 s between the presentation of the word stimulus and the 'go' stimulus.

Because of their central role in our study, with particular reference to the original findings obtained from schizophrenic patients, it seems appropriate to further discuss in this general Outline the use and misuse of some terms included in the classification of intermediary processes and mental delayed tasks.

Some authors [Zipser et al., 1993], focusing on short-term active memory assumed to last for a period of many seconds, developed a corresponding network model and showed that the behaviour of many real cortical memory neurons is consistent with an active storage mechanism based on recurrent activity in networks with fixed synaptic strengths. This model concerns an animal performing a short-term memory task and substantially differs from the procedure adopted in our methodology where the subject perceives a task stimulus maintained until the appearance of the 'go' signal 1.5–4 s later. In our investigation, we deal with an *unconscious activity of a prepared action* that does not imply – as a memory process does – a coding and decoding or a storing and retrieval mechanism, since the task to be performed is actually under continuous perception. Just after the presentation of the task, the subject has performed the sensorimotor transfer with a cortical-subcortical pattern of impulses that, in the case of a delayed reaction, continue as an afteractivity of recurrent circuits in a loop connected to a neural assembly. This remains at a subthreshold level for the executive process until it is triggered by a decisional act of the subject when he perceives the 'go' signal.

With these premises, the kind of recurrent activity in our test of delayed reaction can hardly be equalled to the more complex series of processes implied in the term 'memory'. The above-mentioned afteractivity rather corresponds to the recurrent internal feedbacks in the loop with clean-up units of the model of reading elaborated by Hinton and Shallice [1991] and reported by us in Section 2.

The relationship and possible interferences between this afteractivity that occurs in the pretriggering phase and short-term memory processes will be a matter of specific analyses in Sections 2 and 5, but it seems worthwhile giving already some preliminary definitions in this introduction.

As far as our investigations are concerned, we prefer to avoid the generalized use of the terms 'working', 'dynamic' and 'active memory'. There is no doubt that the term 'process' means that some active event is in progress: to define a process as an active event is simply a tautology. Moreover, adjectives like 'dynamic' and 'working' represent analogous translations that are too far from their meanings in physics: they originally relate to forces and weights that have nothing to do with the brain intermediary processes we are dealing with. These are in fact ongoing processes integrating the invariant preprogrammed patterns with the pre-executive processes and may then be qualified as teleological transfer events. One could object that the term 'weight' is used in neural network models to indicate the equivalent of synaptic threshold, but this refers only to levels of excitability and synaptic strength. Forces and weights are really implied in the myo-articular movements of the vocal tract, from the vocal folds to the velum, tongue, lips and jaw: the brain computes the related forces, weights, stiffness and position by the proprioceptive afferences that converge in the body scheme of the parietal cortex. But this series of processes occurs in the early programming phase and in the associated correcting and adjusting phases: the physiological executive work represents the substrate and not the qualifying essence of these processes.

On the other hand, the term 'memory' is applied to the afteractivities of the pretriggering phase on the grounds of the observation that the afteractivity appears as an event that just persists after the end of sensorimotor transfer and programmation. However, mnemonic events imply something to be stored, a memorization in some magazine that is conceived as a static phenomenon. Therefore the scientist using the term 'memory' to indicate intermediary processes, being aware of its passive-static implication, corrects this label with the adjectives 'active' and more improperly 'dynamic' or 'working'.

We will limit our terminology to the concrete targets of our tests for delayed reactions on one side and short-term memory performances on the other: 'afteractivity' of recurrent internal circuits and 'short-term active memory'. With relation to the latter term, a more precise specification would be 'a short-term delayed intentional process', a definition that indicates a remembering process so that the implication of the word 'memory' seems to be justified in the general diction 'short-term active memory'. This term can be accepted as far as, on the other hand, the word 'memory' is avoided in the specification of the afteractivity of recurrent internal circuits of the delayed reactions tested with our methodology: otherwise a confusing overlapping indication would ensue for the two different processes.

Section 7 has been reserved to the effects that different factors, either genetic or acquired, biological like aging or environmental and cultural like the degree of education, exert on the ACG and its duration. The changes occurring in the central cerebral computing processes (CCP) during normal and abnormal aging are discussed in detail.

A landmark in the semiological area of this study was the identification of two ratios, related to the early programming processes and to the intermediary processes of the brain, respectively. The reliability and semiological meaning of these ratios are discussed in *Section 8*.

The results of the investigations with foreperiod reactions, carried out under pathological conditions, including multiple sclerosis, amyotrophic lateral sclerosis, Parkinson disease, schizophrenia and mental deterioration, will also be reported.

The recourse to early and intermediary processes makes it possible to eliminate the interference of individual psychomotor traits in our MDRV, on one condition: changes in the intermediary process ratio (that is ACG latency at foreperiod = 1,500 ms, i.e. $FP_{1.5}$, divided by ACG latency at foreperiod = 0, i.e. FP_0) must not primarily depend on a decrease in ACG latency at FP_0, that is on immediate reactions.

The results of the investigations with MDRV carried out under pathological conditions, including multiple sclerosis, amyotrophic lateral sclerosis, Parkinson disease, schizophrenia, mental deterioration, depressive and obsessive-compulsive disorders, beside spastic dysphonia and stuttering, are reported in *Section 9*. The most original discovery in the pathological field was a statistically significant specific increase in intermediary process ratios in schizophrenics, a change that could be related to a failure in the control exerted by prefrontal neurons on delayed activities.

On the opposite side, obsessive-compulsive disorders (and, with different patterns, stuttering) were found to be characterized by a marked decrease in intermediary process ratios.

Section 10 deals with the main issues of the previous theoretical and experimental data. Some diagrams of MDRV results are presented with the diagnostic value of the most significant changes and their importance in functional longitudinal assessments. The organization of related brain systems is drawn in blueprints showing the chain of representations and processes implied in speech control under normal and pathological conditions.

Criteria of evaluation of what can be primary and what secondary slowing are outlined together with some general principles of psychophysiology.

The results in schizophrenia are particularly stressed: the impairment of intermediary processes represents a specific marker to identify subjects at risk of schizophrenia.

Five appendices are added:

In *Appendix 1*, a summary of the main semiological results is given.

Appendix 2 evaluates the results obtained from schizophrenic and non-schizophrenic patients.

Appendix 3 presents a printed form to be filled in for recording the findings of MDRV in research and clinical routine work.

Appendix 4 describes the equipment and criteria of measurements.

Appendix 5 summarizes the origin of MDRV, its areas of application and practical benefits.

1

Speech as a Sequence of Purposeful Actions

Brain Control of Psychomotility

Motor control of speech
is not equivalent to word articulations. Its pathological counterpart
is not represented simply by dysarthria. It implies also task-independent processes.

Psychomotility represents the main ultimate function of the brain. Adhering to a bi-
ological-evolutionistic philosophical view, Patricia Churchland [1986] states that the right
subject matter of the scientific research on human behaviour should be centred on the
brain processes producing the most efficient psychomotor performances. The motor control develops on the grounds of selected ongoing information, but the related sensory activity is to be regarded as an essential contribution and not as an autonomous or prevalent function.

A goal-directed approach is at present privileged also in linguistic (the pragmatic
linguistic) experimental neuropsychology and even cognitive psychology [Shallice, 1988;
Simone, 1990; Edelman, 1992; Bertucelli Papi, 1993; Magno Caldonetto and Tonelli,
1993].

An important point to be stressed is that most brain processes of motor control occur at an unconscious level, and this is the reason why they can be detected and analysed
only by objective biological methods.

We are indebted to Bernstein [1984], who initiated the analysis of the intrinsic characteristic features of purposeful motor actions and identified the main variables upon
which the brain computes its control [Arbib and Caplan, 1979]. This approach led to the
formulation of the principles and mathematical psychophysical laws that allow the student to understand the cerebral processes governing our behaviour [MacKay, 1965]. On
this ground, an increasing amount of work was carried out in both experimental and clinical research under normal and pathological conditions. Moreover, in the last 10 years, associated teams of bio-engineers, neurophysiologists and neurologists devised new models
of connected PDP networks. The neuroscientists, enlightened by these models, started a
critical revision of the previous interpretations of the functional meaning of the associative cortical areas and their connections with the subcortical nuclei.

These are some of the principles that seem to govern the 'logic of the living brain'
[Sommerhoff, 1974; Pinelli, 1977]. For a more detailed approach, we must delineate the
different kinds of purposeful actions that men can perform: (1) oculomotion; (2) gait;
(3) manual performance; (4) speaking.

One assumes that a common set of programming and organizing processes is structured to steer all these complex motor sequences (fig. 1). This structure is represented by
two main stages:

(A) *a starting process* including a conceptualizer and a driving impulse generator – in the
psychological sense, they correspond to the concepts of motor will and emotional initiation [Posner and Mitchell, 1967; Joseph, 1993];

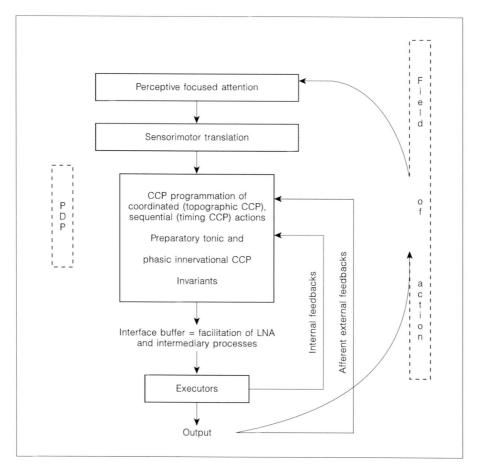

Fig. 1. A general blueprint of brain psychomotor control for reactive reactions. The reactive action corresponds to only a part of the spontaneous action which implies 'higher-level' systems of the conceptualizer and driving generation. Intermediary processes include working memory. LNA = Low-threshold neural assembly; CCP = central computing processes.

(B) *a translation* of the sensorial, mainly visual signals in a computational process providing the pattern of impulses producing the muscular contractions and then the movements requested to reach the target or more generally to carry out the task, that is the sensorimotor transformation studied by Flanders et al. [1992]. To fulfil this operation, the brain has to calculate the number and the distribution of the nervous impulses that must be sent to specific motor units of agonist and antagonist muscles in due temporal succession. This corresponds to a feedforward operation that gives rise to descending patterns of impulses that, in the earliest phase, are related to rather abstract, absolute and simplified schemes of action. Since they are not yet diversified to fit all ongoing contingent events and factors, they appear as a sort of *invariants* [Bernstein, 1984; Bizzi, 1984; Gracco and Abbs, 1986].

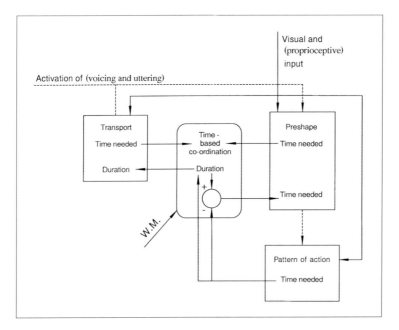

Fig. 2. An overview of a model of motor schemas and their coordination by timing, for reaching and grasping, with analogies for voicing and uttering (in parentheses). W.M. = Working memory. From Jeannerod et al. [1995].

Some blueprints, more specific for speaking, are reported in figures 2 (according to Jeannerod et al. [1995]) and 3 (according to Levelt [1989]).

The forward processes imply a series of three-step developments. Firstly (first level or L1), there are (1) preparatory processes associated with (2) programming processes. The preparatory processes lead to a *tuning* (fig. 4, at the level of the phonological operator) of mechanisms acting on the stiffness of the muscles of the coordinated action. These in turn are selected by the programming process we will analyse in the second stage. In fact, there is not only a horizontal reciprocal association but also a vertical one between different stages, i.e. levels. This kind of multiple connection represents a basic structure also in artificial neural networks [Banks, 1991].

The second step of the first stage corresponds to a *phasic* mechanism (fig. 4, 2/L1) producing the instantaneous changes in neuromuscular innervation requested to reach the target. The tuning allows a better muscular reactivity to the successive stream of air in the vocal tract; the phasic innervation produces the necessary expiratory contraction and the following shaping of the vocal tract.

Secondly, there is a *topographical* distribution of the innervation in the programming phase associated with a *temporal* sequential ordering (fig. 4, 2/L2) of the innervation. The topographical distribution concerns the muscles of the coordinated action, whilst the temporal sequential ordering concerns the cyclic operations for the single elements of the action, i.e. the utterance in the case of speaking. These phases develop within the programming processes occurring in two stages: There is a general plan of action (the *grammar* formulator) that should be associated with the stage of the detailed plan of action (the *phonological* formulator).

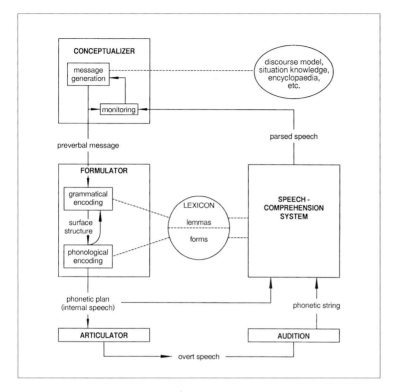

Fig. 3. Levelt's [1989] model of speech.

At the third stage, the resulting invariants are conjugated to the *executors* where the invariants (fig. 4, 1/L3) undergo a process of *adaptation* (fig. 4, 2/L3). This stage corresponds to the final or distal order of processes.

There is more than one internal system acting as feedback. The control systems assure the adjustment between the intended operations expressed by the invariants and the ongoing operations in the executors.

Besides the internal feedbacks (autogenic recording, according to Gracco [1991]), there are final externally generated feedbacks, mainly visual and acoustic, operating at the open output.

Altogether, brain production and control of behaviour develop clearly with a *trial-and-error* modality, at variance with the algorithmic manner the engineer conceives for this architectural model [Alexander and Crutcher, 1991]. The relationship between this kind of operations and the stochastic way of functioning represents a core problem in the theory of action [Folkins and Brown, 1987; Perkell, 1991].

The set of processes exercising motor control operates in the four previously named fields of motility. However, with a view to approach a more detailed and exhaustive analysis, the student is required to consider the different conditions and constraints of each specific field that create different problems to be solved by the brain each time.

The gravity factor plays a dominant role in locomotion during the translation phase of gait, while it is quite *negligible* in oculomotion and *speaking*. On the other hand, in this

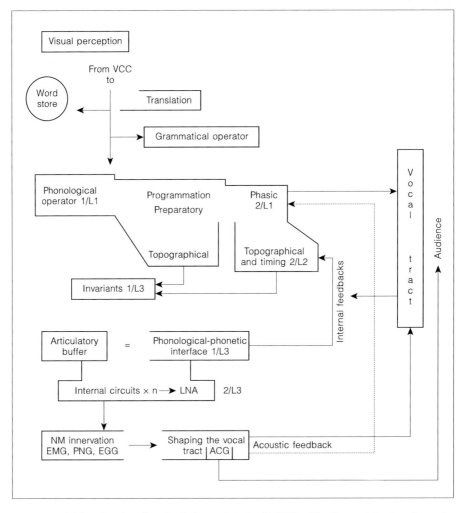

Fig. 4. A blueprint of reading aloud visuoverbal stimuli. VCC = Visual central circuitry; figures indicate first the step and then the level (L) of development; n = number of recurrent CCP; LNA = low-threshold neural assembly; NM = neuromotor; PNG = pneumogram; EGG = electroglottogram.

last field, even the spatial external environment has a low impact as a variable to be included in the computational processes performed by the brain. In fact, the speaker does neither reach a precise point in space nor act on an object, as it happens in manipulation. What he does is to shape the vocal tract and activate the respiratory, glottal and epiglottal muscles in order to produce the requested series of vibrations in the expiratory air flow. Then the train of air vibrations reaches the listener's ears in space. But this represents a passive effect, whilst the speaker computes his program only on his *internal environment,* that is on his own instruments in his body executing the changes that create the voice and speech. Computing the distance with respect to the listener represents an extra request that he fulfils simply to regulate the amplitude of the voice without any precise relationship with factors included in the original programming process.

Production and Control of Speech: Phylogenetic and Ontogenetic Remarks

> Misunderstanding the area of speech control as a simple executive task rather than a *cerebral processing of sequential purposeful coordinated actions* depends on the fact that speech is produced by a 'mental organ' which is organized operatively since early infancy, develops unconsciously and does not require a great subjective effort.

1.2.1
The Origin of *Homo loquens*

The opinion that speech and language appeared in the course of phylogenesis with the development of related brain centres as the main creative condition and the idea that it corresponds to a gap in the evolution of animals and men were abandoned on the grounds of new palaeo-neuro-anthropological discoveries and comparative neuro-anatomophysiological evidence since 1971 [Lieberman and Crelin, 1991; Tobias, 1980; Johnson, 1983].

What appears to an external observer as a gap between animal and human behaviour is the amazing boost produced in intelligence and creativity by the logic tools forged by the spoken language [Joseph, 1993]. But in a more thorough investigation of structural neural and biomechanical changes, the evolution appears to have unfolded as gradually as the genetic-darwinian factors and the environmental extrinsic influences required.

It was recognized that a precise time-localized origin of *Homo loquens* still seems to remain an unsolved problem [Johnson, 1983]. The palaeo-anthropological discoveries identified some points that allow us to delineate the slow and intermittent formation of *Homo loquens*. The correct question is not about instantaneous creation but rather about a progressive multistep moulding.[1]

The emergence of spoken language does not represent an unexpected mental capacity creating, since its origin, a specific and unique attribute of *Homo loquens*. In fact, the brain structure and particularly the cortical area corresponding to Broca's centre proved to have been highly developed already in primates and in *Homo habilis* [Lieberman, 1991; Pivetau, 1986; Eccles, 1990].

The change, consisting in a series of mutations that provided the substrates for a *tachyphemic performance* [Gigley, 1983; Lieberman, 1991; Pinelli and Ceriani, 1992], did not take place primarily in the brain but at the level of peripheral executive organs. The critical change consisted in the descent of the glottis from the second to the sixth cervical vertebra. A cue for this anatomotopographical change was searched in a modification of the basal cranium which became more arched. In fact, an arching line of the basal cranium was found in *Homo erectus* and *Homo habilis*, i.e. about 300,000 years ago. Only in-

---

[1] In the analysis of continuously developing processes that lead to the shaping and organization of newly arising behaviours, like bipedal gait and speaking itself, the identification of the 'moment of its appearance' is accomplished only by conventional-formal criteria related to the definition of that behaviour and the time of discovery of the corresponding documents.

complete signs of glottis descent were found in the Neanderthal man (who lived 50,000 years ago), a finding that led the anthropologists to consider the Neanderthal man as a collateral branch in the evolution of man. According to Lieberman [1991] and Lieberman and Crelin [1991], he never reached a stage of complete human speech.

Therefore we should admit the existence of a long period of about 200,000 years during which the new increased efficiency of the vocal tract and the corresponding great number of sounds produced by it could be linked to single motor sensory representations able to induce, by a countless number of repetitions, the neuroplastic changes of the neural networks of speech control. This slow re-organization and new formation of a 'speech system' provided the biological fundamentals for the development of the spoken language. The specialists have not yet reached an agreement as to when *Homo loquens* made his appearance in the world: it should be between 100,000 and 40,000 years ago. A reconstruction of human evolution was attempted by Cavalli Sforza et al. [1988], bringing together genetic, archaeological and linguistic data.

Pinker [1995] advanced the opinion that the brain of *Homo sapiens* was endowed with a universal grammar [Chomsky, 1965] 200,000 years ago. His argument is that '*Homo sapiens* is *us* and all modern humans have language'. 'The major branches of humanity', he writes, 'diverged well before the age of the gorgeous cave art and decorated artifacts of Cro-Magnon humans in the Upper Paleolithic. Their descendants have identical language abilities; therefore the language instinct was probably in place well before the cultural fads of the Upper Paleolithic emerged in Europe.' Pinker minimizes the importance of the larynx descent, as it was emphasized by Lieberman [1991], and he claims that, even if *Homo sapiens* had a standard airway with a reduced space for possible vowels, 'we cannot conclude that hominids with restricted vowel space had little language'. Evidently the pupil of Chomsky does not analyse more thoroughly the other anatomical features of the vocal tract that are modified as secondary effects of the glottal descent and that have relevant repercussions also on the utterance of consonants and first of all on the velocity of speech required for a comprehensible sequence of sentences.

Rejecting the idea of a 'microcreation' of the universal grammar, Pinker tries to explain how it derives, by natural selection, from an intermediary grammar. This hypothetical grammar could have symbols with a narrower range, rules that are applied less reliably and modules with fewer rules. Some support for this hypothesis seemed to come from the research of Dereck Bickerton [1992] on the 'protolanguage'. This might be represented by the child language in the *two-word stage* but also by the unsuccessful partial language observed, after the critical period, in *wolf children;* other heterogeneous partial languages, like pidgin and even chimp signing, are taken into consideration under the common label of protolanguage. According to Bickerton [1992], *Homo erectus* spoke in protolanguage. 'A single mutation', he writes, 'in a single woman, African Eve, simultaneously wired in syntax, resized and reshaped the skull and *reworked the vocal tract.*' Thus, at this point, Bickerton corrects a too simplified application of acoustics to the constraints of the anatomical structures of the vocal tract.

1.2.1.1
Changes in the Vocal Tract

Most neuro-anthropologists agree that the whole phylogenetic history started with the modification of the vocal tract. A long series of studies demonstrated how the conformation of the vocal tract, and particularly of its length, plays an important role in the amplification and the modulation of vocalic and consonantal sounds; very sophisticated investigations [Saito, 1992] defined how the muscular articulatory movements modify the shape of the vocal tract and the corresponding resonance effects.

The factors governing the formation of the frequency in the ACG, and particularly of the formants (f), can be analysed with the voice spectrogram. The following equation allows the calculation of the respective ratios:

$$f = \frac{v}{z \cdot L},$$

where v is the velocity of the sound in the air, z the area of the tube (the vocal tract) and L its length. Of course, the measurement of the area of a multiform tube like the vocal tract requires very complex calculations. A great accumulation of data and of mathematical formulas has recently been obtained from experimental research particularly in Japan and in the USA [Saito, 1992; Tokhura et al., 1992]. The emerging knowledge allowed the development of very good instrumental models, which however do not yet include the related central neural mechanisms. Anyway, the import of the elongation and volume increase of the vocal tract as a preliminary step in the development of speech has been confirmed.

In the human pharyngeal-palatal-nasal resonance compartment, there are about 100 muscles able to change its shape. The respiratory muscles provide the expiratory air stream. The vocal cords produce the first formants, while the uvula and tongue, acting along 13 vectors [Saito, 1992], together with the oromandibular muscles, produce a very broad range of finely modulated changes in the area of the vocal tract along its length [Saito, 1992].

It pertains to the central nervous system to elaborate the descending commands representing the innervation formulas of each muscle in the proper temporal order. On the other hand, the neural reflex servo-mechanisms are immediately engaged to provide the appropriate changes of distribution and gain, in relation to the peripheral constraints and occasional obstacles.

1.2.2
Early Utterances in Human and Primate Children and the Development of Speech Production

> The way how the human brain acquires the language is too complex
> for the human brain itself to conceptualize it.   [Hacking, 1975]

1.2.2.1
The Motor Control of Vocalization

Prelinguistic communication, expressed by vocalization, implies an apparently automatic kind of programmation in relation to a rather stereotyped utterance. The correspondent articulations require the subject to open the mouth, to position the tongue even if with rather little modulation, to adduct the vocal cords and, to a relevant degree, to modify the respiration, each movement being exactly coordinated.

A primitive, more stereotyped expression is crying; it could be considered as a more elaborate way of communication compared to weeping. Laughing presents a greater variability of modulations: smile, smirk, beam and grin. How these expressions may be integrated in the listener's oriented attitude was studied in a particular situation: vocalization under conditions of isolation. The observations were carried out not only in children but also in an anthropomorphic monkey, the chimpanzee *(Pan troglodytes)*. It was found that the vocalizations were differentiated implying a reference to abstract concepts. In fact, in his early months of life, the child, placed far from the baby-sitter whom he can neither see nor hear, starts crying in an aspecific manner as he is reacting to endogenous affective impulses [Joseph, 1993] rather than producing a sort of communication to somebody. On the contrary, in a later period of his life, he cries turning his head towards the direction where he *supposes* his interlocutor should be.

Moreover, when he begins to pronounce his first protowords, he is able to utter different intonations according to the circumstances, in relation to the help he needs and the person he thinks he is addressing. This presupposes internal models of an even simple linear spatial mapping and indicates that the vocalizations and protowords are integrated in the sensory cognitive processes.

1.2.2.2
Phonetic Mechanisms

Phonetic analyses showed that in prelinguistic utterances only fundamental vocal frequencies (F_0) are modulated, known to depend on a purely laryngeal function.

A main issue concerns the role played by the emotional components characterizing the prelinguistic phase. They are the prosodic factors that integrate the descriptive or colloquial communications with pitch and accent processes, which remain still active in adult speech.

Besides laryngeal movements, the prelinguistic vocalization implies tongue and mouth movements, however in a moderate range, whilst the frequency and harmonic structuralization begins to involve also the pharynx.

One further performance of great interest in the vocalization phase is represented by non-organized repetitions, implying temporal sequences. There are redundant series in which just the same vocalization is repeated so many times with small changes in intensity, frequency and sometimes also in rhythm.

Thus, already at this early stage of speech development, we have to face an issue of paramount importance for the study of the brain processes that are the origin and cause of the variability that produces a stochastic kind of function.

One wonders whether this stochastic output is related to affective changes or rather to vigilance or attention oscillations at any moment. This matter will be analysed more thoroughly in the following chapters with reference to adult variability in repetitive performances, as an expression of a trial-and-error behaviour and of flexibility in strategies of trajectories [Lacquaniti and Soetching, 1982; Lacquaniti et al., 1986].

But even in a preliminary orientating interpretation, we must underline once again that this variability in spontaneous utterances seems to evidence primarily a non-algorithmic kind of functioning of the brain central computing processes. Edelman's [1991] theory of a neural selection able to produce a more efficiently operating and restricted system is particularly pertinent to understand the biological meaning of these redundant series of repetitions: the 12 reactions requested for each task of MDRV still represent a preliminary phase in a possible learning process. Likewise a learned reaction time is revealed by a diminution in immediate reaction time and in its standard deviation.

In a similar but independent way, the analysis of the investigations carried out with delayed reactions revalued the concept of hebbian neural assemblies and facilitated neural assemblies (or low-threshold neural assemblies), which is treated in the following parts of this Section (1.2.2.3.2) and in 2.4.

1.2.2.3
From Prelinguistic to Linguistic Communication

We analysed in the previous chapter how the appearance of language does not correspond to a gap in phylogenesis. The first man of Jebel-Kalsah endowed with a descended larynx, at variance with *Homo habilis* and *Homo erectus* and the Neanderthal man, represents the issue of a rather continuous evolution. The acquisition of the powerful phonetic instrument of the human vocal tract produced in its turn a sort of loop with neuroplastic effects on the frontotemporal-cortical areas.

An alternative opinion that formerly acquired some popularity maintains that the passage from the emotional-instinctive prelinguistic phase to the logical-cognitive linguistic phase implied a hierarchical predominance of the second over the first. It is not venturesome to assume a certain connection between this view and freudian mythology, hinged on the conception that the development of the language-linked culture hindered the instinctive emotional components of our personality. A rough extension of this line of thought was accomplished with the popularized idea of three anatomofunctional brain levels: reptile, lower mammal and man. These opinions were revisited on the grounds of several lines of research [Sperry, 1984].

Quite a different matter is the investigation of the final output of emotionally driven and logical-cognitive linguistic expressions. The experiment consisted in the request to speak while laughing. The analysis, carried out in adults, showed that a certain opposition occurs when the two expressive processes are in progress. Certainly, an emotional overt vocalization like laughing implies more stereotyped and fixed articulations that disturb or even prevent the more ductile and dynamic speech articulations of a communicative utterance.

A dualistic alternative, with emotional expressions maintaining their own autonomy even in adults, corresponds to an extreme condition that is far from reflecting the usual control of speech. The real issue concerns a 'vocal tract that must respond to the different choices of the brain programmer': emotional, cognitive-communicative functions and, for the oromandibular sector, also the masticatory function. One should then evaluate the anatomofunctional constraints and reconstruct how the vocal tract is dynamically shaped in relation to functional hierarchies and multiple arrangements, in a chronological order established by centrally computed preparatory and executive innervations.

On the other hand, in the mature linguistic processing, emotion-dependent drives and cognition-dependent wants become simultaneously integrated into the fluent progress of speech.

1.2.2.3.1
The Dualistic View of R. Joseph

R. Joseph [1993] shares the alluring freudian view that the 'human organism is a veritable living museum' since 'our modern human ancestor, the Cro-Magnon, 130,000 years ago, completed the brain evolution from the limbic system shrouded by the neocortex progressively expanded to cover the forebrain and the olfactory bulbs, from two-layered cortical motor centres to a seven-layer-thick neocortex'. These ancestors first possessed the necessary neural tissue to issue forth temporal sequential grammatically complex spoken language with the frontal lobes reaching their greatest size conferring the powers of foresight, cunning and planning. 'These accumulated different parts of the brain independently struggle over and produce solutions: these different brain regions act at cross-purposes, each according to their agent and perceptions, with consequent misleadings and confusion.'

An opposite view is assumed by philosophers of science like Cotteril [1989] and Sperry [1984] who, according to the anthropic principles, are of the opinion that the actual brain organization of *Homo sapiens* would be the same even if one creates it ex novo just now: 'The project of the human brain accomplished at the end of the phylogenesis was in fact foreseen since the origin of life, with the birth of the earliest genes.' The misleadings and confusion foreseen by the dualistic or accumulation theory of Joseph are in fact contradicted also by the observation of the neuromotor systems with double competing functions, 'accumulating' along the phylogenetic evolution. One example is represented by the oromandibular system that serves two quite different functions, with mastication and deglutition for feeding and with coordinated tongue, jaw and lip movement for spoken language. (According to Joseph's view, we would bit our tongue while speaking and utter some vocalizations while eating.) Other examples can be found in metabolic respiration versus dynamic expiration for speech in the vocal tract.

In fact, Joseph himself states that important connecting systems, like the corpus callosum, functionally join the different centres. Joseph admits that the right and left frontal regions of the two brain halves – called by him 'two brains, two minds'– co-operate in producing speech and melody; the left frontal region (Broca) and the melodic-emotional speech area, located in the right frontal lobe, act in concert 'like the two wheels joined together by an axle'. It is true that 'if we squeezed our fingers into the interhemispheric fissure, our progress would soon be interrupted by a large strand of nerve fibres, the corpus callosum', but it is equally true, even at a microscopic level, that also between the limbic system and the neocortex there are many interconnecting fibres which allow information to be transferred between the two systems.

The differentiation of the performances of the two hemispheres has been studied with reference to abstract and concrete words (see Section 8), particularly in depressive psychoses [Rizzolati et al., 1981; Pinelli et al., 1994] and in schizophrenia [Gruzelier et al., 1995].

1.2.2.3.2
The Descent of the Glottis in Children and the 'Maturation of Speech'

Certainly the descent – first occurring in our modern human ancestor, the Cro-Magnon, and now in human infants at the tenth month of age – of the glottis to the level of the sixth cervical vertebra and the re-organization and amplification of the supraglottic tract have produced an enormous increase in freedom of the executive machinery. A large series of phonemes, vowels and consonants were thus available to match the requests the conceptualizer makes for speech communication [Levelt, 1993]. The voice nasality was reduced with a better differentiation of the patterns of formant frequencies. The tongue could be better rounded with production of more marked spectral peaks in the quantile (a term used in statistics and acoustics to indicate differentiated groups of data and sounds) sounds i, u, a, k, g and greater acoustic stability, in as much as the length of the oral cavity equalled the pharyngeal one. On this ground, one could obtain spectral peaks without a difficult, precise timing of tongue positioning. Moreover, the verbal codification in the transition of the formant frequency could be effected with a 3–10 times quicker data transmission. Therefore this first stage of efficiency corresponds to the acquisition of the tachyphemic threshold, that is the threshold of speech production velocity requested for a comprehensible communication of sentences.

In this period, the child acquires the ability of speech changes from vocalization to monosyllabic combinations – consonant (C) + vowel (V) – and bisyllabic ones – Cx, V1 + Cy, V1 and C1, Vx + C1, Vy.

Shifting again our attention from ontogenesis to phylogenesis, one must stress that the brain processes of language-independent conceptualization precede the changes occurring in the vocal tract [Edelman, 1992]. In their turn, the improved peripheral phonological performances co-operate to form new synaptic connections and other neuroplastic modifications with memorizing processes: the resulting neural assemblies correspond to the cortical areas identified as Wernicke's and Broca's centres with the corresponding associative pathways. These neurophysiological events represent the basis for speculations on neurodarwinism and internal cerebral re-entry processes [Edelman, 1992; Tononi, 1995].

Greenfield [1991] put forward many arguments against the opinion that the neural circuit organization of the prelinguistic phase had been wiped out by the new organization specific for the linguistic phase. On the contrary, it is true that the prelinguistic neural organization became integrated by the new neuroplastic developments leading to the spoken linguistic phase. This statement is in agreement with the fact that, after birth, increased neuronal maturation exceeds neuronal death (apoptosis) due to natural selective processes.

The development of the previously described redundancy phase suggests that in this period of life the selection process corresponds to a sort of learning-dependent facilitation of specific neural assemblies with the formation of facilitated neural assemblies producing low-threshold neural assemblies inside a cerebrocortical system that increases in size with newly proliferating connections and encoding processes.

In parallel with these crucial biological events, one observes that, at both phylogenetic and ontogenetic levels, the production of speech, in its early phase, evolves progressively or in a small-step gradual way: the child becomes able to pronounce single incomplete words and elementary sentences with associated words composed for the greatest part by differently modulated vowels and pronounced at a slow, sometimes intermittent rate.

The continuity between the prelinguistic and the linguistic phase was proved by manifold arguments. Categorizations are created in the prelinguistic phase by explorations and data collections determined by emotional-ludic impulses [Eccles, 1990]. They become greatly amplified with the acquisition of speech: previous categorizations provide the abstract representations that are translated in the *verbal motor units,* while these represent symbolic elements that increase the development of categorizations.

On the other hand, in the inventory of the multimodal features that allow to recognize whether a certain sequence of sounds can be defined as language, some have an emotional connotation: among the 21 features in the inventory of Hockett and Altman [1968], the ninth and the twenty-first are of specific emotional nature. In adults the prosodic analysis reveals, at the highest degree, manifold intonations occurring since early childhood. Pitch, acoustic formant frequencies, rhythms and pauses in speaking are continuously modified so that, in association with gesticulations, they make the speech abundant in emotional qualities.

The engagement of the speaker, the emphasis he wishes to impose on some enunciations – or vice versa the lowering of intonation for relatively dubious, less important or more delicate assertions – and again drawing the attention of the listeners, stressing the importance and urgency of some information are a few of the prosodic connotations of the spoken language.

An Introduction to the Organization of Speech

> All these actions are apparently very simple. Yet, this is not so.
> [Jeannerod et al., 1995]

1.3.1
The Structure of Prelinguistic Communications and the Passage to the Linguistic Phase

In neurophysiology, the cerebral structures involved in speaking have been investigated with many methods: cortical electrical stimulation, anatomoclinical verifications and more recently coherent electro-encephalography (EEG) and electro-encephalographic mapping [Murri, 1991], brain blood flow imaging, functional MRI and PET. Many data were so collected and interpreted in line with phylogenetic and ontogenetic knowledge.

The development of neural circuits follows three mechanisms: genetic endowment, critical early neonatal maturation and further acquisition during the whole life-span. The genesis of vocalizations and the passage to speech follow the first two mechanisms. The main acquisition of this period is the attainment of the *tachyphemic threshold* with an utterance velocity allowing to produce olophrases and eventually some complete phrases efficiently.

The ability of rapid speech is intimately related to the hierarchization of strategies for purposeful sequential acts. The hierarchical planning develops in the first-year child in parallel with speech control and hand control. Greenfield [1991] studied whether these two orders of organizations proceed at the same pace in the earliest phases following the prelinguistic period.

The issue faced by Greenfield was the following: if the development of both abilities depended upon a common cerebral system, the ability of object handling and that of the first utterances would be found to become manifest simultaneously. This comparative investigation was carried out in the vocalization phases not only of human children but also of the most highly developed anthropomorphic monkeys.

1.3.2
Are Object Handling and Early Speech Control, in 1- to 2-Year-Old Babies, Produced by Common Neural Circuits?

Relying on some researches carried out in primates and in human children, Chomsky [1965] hypothesized that the human new-born is endowed on a genetic basis with a mental organ specific for language. Even if it remains true that this statement is reasonably convincing at a functional level [Pinker, 1995], it appears hazardous and debatable when we try to identify its anatomofunctional development. Some neuropaediatrists share the opinion that, in the earliest phase of life, there is a common module for different purposeful sequential actions like hand use and speech. The solution of this issue required:

(1) a careful thorough study of the *analogies* among the progressively more complex actions the subject becomes able to carry out;

(2) the passage from simple analogies to *homologies,* that is to extend the evaluation of the parallel developments from the behavioural level to the biological neural level, with a precise relation to the corresponding cerebral operations; this evaluation required a preliminary clear definition of modularity;

(3) the application of the neurophysiological knowledge of the functional organization of the brain not only to the cortical better defined areas like Broca's and Wernicke's but also to the *subcortical loops* and to the coordination of the *executive systems.*

In fact, the inclusion of primates besides human children in this research yielded essential information on the comparative functional anatomy of the brain.

First of all, it was shown that the communicative capacities of primates during their first year of life are quite similar to those of humans. Moreover, the cerebral structures are also similar but with a greater size of the frontal lobes in men and, at a lower degree, also of the limbic lobe.

The study of communication in children, compared with that of anthropomorphic monkeys reared in a human environment, showed that the appearance of speech is the result of a gradual development with some periodical remaking [Zovato, 1994]. Only few authors [Wind et al., 1992] noticed that some increments in speech production seem to occur rather abruptly in a stepwise manner. In fact Andersen [1980], Lieberman [1991], Jacobs [1977], MacNeilage [1983], Gardner and Gardner [1992] and Masataka and Symmes [1986] demonstrated that the primates, who can acquire a certain number of inputs in the early evolutive phase and in a suitable environment, become able to formulate descriptive words. During the first year, the anthropomorphic monkeys perform purposeful organized actions and, in the same period of time, utter some sentences; this behaviour is observed to occur some weeks before the analogous performances of the human children. In contrast, the human ability to speak more complex sentences surpasses that of monkeys in the second year of life.

Taking into account all the previously reported observations and analyses, one can assume that there is not a prelinguistic-linguistic gap. Moreover, convincing evidence was produced that, in the first year of life, hand hierarchical performances, implying a kinetic praxic centre or system, and sequential articulatory speech, implying a verbal praxic centre or system [Pinelli and Ceriani, 1992], show a parallel course of development. These data substantiated the issue about a common cerebral structure for handling and speaking in this early phase.

In order to prove this, Greenfield [1991] carried out a systematic series of researches in children during the first 2 years of life. The leading idea was formulated according to the rules to detect *homologies.* If the two orders of *hierarchically organized sequential purposeful actions* (HOSPA), like handling and speaking, showed an identical rate of formation and development, one should infer a common cerebral structure without separate modules. It is interesting to mention here that, in a quite independent research carried out at a superficial semiological level, Gracco [1987, 1991] identified, in analogy to HOSPA, what he called *characteristic neural patterns.*

A preliminary point to be ascertained in this line of research regards the definition of *modularity*. For this definition Greenfield relies on Fodor's analyses [1983], who proposed a list or precise criteria for the identification of different modules: (1) domain specificity; (2) there are innate specified structures; (3) they are not assembled by a combination of more elementary processes; (4) they are associated with specific neural systems localized and structured in an elaborate manner; (5) these are autonomous at a computational level.

In our case, the domain is represented by the hierarchization process for the production of motor performances. The identification of the field of action or task in which the process takes place represents a critical intriguing issue.

The essential point regards the choice of the two units of HOSPA for kinetic and for verbal HOSPA, respectively, that should appear as outputs of the hypothesized common cerebral praxic centre responsible for a general brain computational process elaborating a certain hierarchization. The choice of the kinetic HOSPA relating to the use of objects could be made rather easily: the experiment consisted in handling a spoon to eat something from a bowl, analysed and represented with the rules of generative grammar.

The choice had been more doubtful as for the unit of HOSPA relating to speech generative grammar. One should decide whether the unit consisted in the word with its constituent subunits (the syllable) or rather the sentence with its constituent subunits (the words or lemmas). To find the right answer required suitable experiments and new theoretical views.

1.3.2.1
Homologies between Single-Word Production and Object Handling

Greenfield's research starts with 1-year-old children, when they begin to combine intentionally two objects. Parallel examinations of hierarchical combining organization of phonemes and spoon handling in the first 20 months of life allowed her to distinguish five phases.

During this early period, Broca's area guides the hierarchical organization with circuits originated from orofacial and hand motor areas, while specific prefrontal circuits with active modalities have not yet been differentiated.

1.3.2.2
Development Phases of Manual and Verbal Praxic Functions

First phase (9th month); combination-repetition of two units at random. The infant says /dada/, /mama/. He touches one object with another repetitively.

Second phase (12th–13th month): associative denominative combination. He says /no/; he says /pa/ for /pap/. He is able to put the spoon into the bowl.

Third phase (13th–15th month): harmonizing consonants. He says /biba/, /tato/ (C1, V1, C1, V2 and C2, V2, C2, V3), that is identifying a consonant and using it. On the handling side, the child is able to put the spoon into the bowl with one hand and to bring up the food to his mouth with the other.

Fourth phase (15th–16th month): harmonizing vowels. He says /tafa/ (C1, V1, C2, V1), that is identifying a vowel and using it. In this period of time, previous handling performances are perfected.

Fifth phase (17th–20th month): subassembly combination. He says /hand/, /mouth/. He takes the food from the bowl, with the spoon, and brings it to his mouth.

Greenfield [1991] tried also to identify, in a rather simplistic way, the cerebral substrates of these performances. In fact, for the first operative stages, the whole brain is implied from the visual centres to the associative areas up to the frontal lobe, and, in the case of the idiokinetic praxic functions, also the parietal lobe is activated where the body scheme is represented.

Greenfield [1991] focused her attention on the intermediary and final stages, i.e. essentially on the *formulator*. In Greenfield's blueprint, the common neural substrates for handling and speaking correspond to Broca's centre and the connected prerolandic gyrus. However, the neurophysiologist [Alexander and Crutcher, 1990] considers the cortical functions to be closely linked with the basal ganglia. Thus, the role played by the subcortical coordinating system of both hemispheres is to be related to both right and left parts of the vocal tract that must be considered as a unitary organ. The cyclopic eye is a clear point of reference in the visuomotor system. Hence, we must be aware of an essential difference between speaking and handling, since (at variance with the unique median location of the vocal tract) handling concerns mainly one contralateral hand, innervated by the dominant cerebral hemisphere. A prevailing involvement of a dominant hemisphere occurs also in speaking, particularly in the case of abstract words, but the difference regards the organization of the final pathways to the articulatory median vocal tract.

Anyway, apart from her neurofunctional interpretation, the analysis carried out by Greenfield [1991] with Fodor's criteria [1983] for the identification of modular function still supports an interesting line of thought.

1.3.2.3
Some Inferences from Homologies to Specific Language Organization

On the grounds of the previously reported investigations, Greenfield [1991] states that children in the first 2 years of life present some *homologies* between speaking and handling. Each domain has an inborn base of neural circuits and the analysis of homologies seems to prove that it is neither modular since birth nor at the onset of the early development of language.

Only after 2 years of age do language and object combination start developing more autonomously so that each eventually generates its own special forms of structural complexity. Then, language might become increasingly modular with aging and neural differentiation, with the formation of what Fodor [1983] calls a 'modularly structured neural system'. Greenfield [1991] however proposes a partly different model with developing circuits that add, by a maturational process, elementary cortical subprocesses. Hence, Broca's area, after 2 years of age, differentiates itself creating two neural networks, one for verbal and the other for non-verbal performances, which separate in the most anterior parts of the prefrontal cortex.

1.3.3
The Grammar Explosion at the Age of Three and a Half Years

It is just after the second year of life that the neural network for verbal performances completes its own specific organization. And this is just the period when Chomsky's mental organ specific for language reveals its capacities.

Pinker [1995] observed that by the age of three and a half or earlier, English-speaking children use the -s agreement suffix in more than 90% of the sentences requiring it and virtually never use it in the sentences that forbid it. This mastery – in agreement with Chomsky's theory of the universal grammar – is part of their *grammar explosion*, a period of several months in the third year of life, during which children suddenly begin to speak in fluent sentences, respecting most of the fine points of their community's spoken language. They could have been simply imitating their parents, memorizing verbs with the -s attached. They can utter word forms that they could not possibly have heard from their parents. They must then – concludes the author – have created these forms themselves using an uncommon version of the English agreement rule: 'Language is a specific instinct.'

The following pages provide essential information for a better understanding of the corresponding brain architecture.

The Brain Machinery and the Intermediary Processes Including Psychomotor Working Memory

A Premise on Delayed Reactions and the Intermediary Processes Including Psychomotor Working Memory

If we ask the subject to look at a word appearing on a PC screen and to get ready to pronounce it aloud (fig. 5), immediately after the successive appearance of some asterisks below and above the word (the 'go' stimulus), we establish a *delayed* reading task (fig. 6). If we then measure the reaction time from the appearance of the asterisks to the onset of the ACG (fig. 7b) and subtract it from the total reaction time of the *immediate* reaction (measured from the appearance of the word stimulus; fig. 7a), we obtain the time taken by the visual-verbal processes, the translation to the formulators for the grammatical and phonetic plans and the programmation of the commands to the executors (fig. 8). There is a rather high variability of reaction times to the same task, under the same conditions, in successive series (see Chapter 4). Reliable parameters are mean values of 12 reactions (see 3.2.2 and Chapter 4).

The working time of the delayed reaction should be shorter than the time of the immediate reaction. But this is true only under certain conditions that are of both methodological and functional nature. We must be aware of these conditions if we intend to include the delayed reactions in our methodology with a correct application and the most reliable criteria of evaluation. Their analysis requires a specific theoretical background and a series of experimental data on both normal subjects and patients, which we will expound in the following Sections.

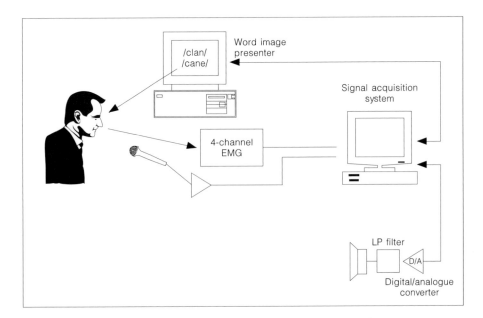

Fig. 5. Testing reading reactions. LP = Low-pass filter at 4,000 Hz.

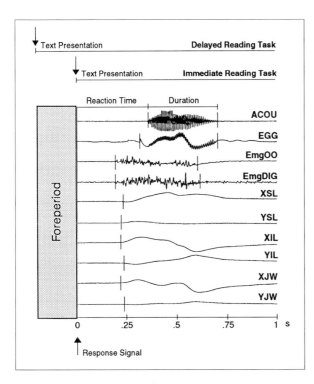

Fig. 6. Acoustic signal (ACOU), electroglottographic signal (EGG), EMG signals of orbicularis oris (OO) and digastric (DIG) muscles, and signals related to displacements of the upper lip (XSL, YSL), lower lip (XIL, YIL) and jaw (XJW, YJW) in a normal subject reading the word /muro/ and pronouncing it after the foreperiod; the y-axis reports arbitrary units.

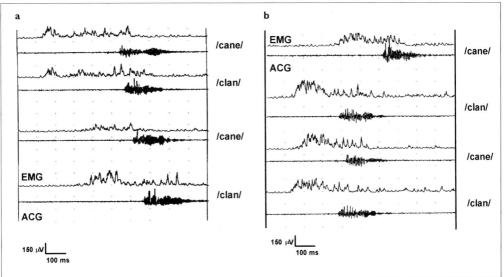

Fig. 7. Subject Z.G., male, 69 years old. Immediate (**a**) and delayed reactions at FP$_3$ (**b**) to /clan/ and /cane/ with EMG of the orbicularis oris muscle (filtered and rectified). Four consecutive recordings. It can be seen that most latency times are shorter in delayed reactions, i.e. the second, third and fourth reactions in **b**.

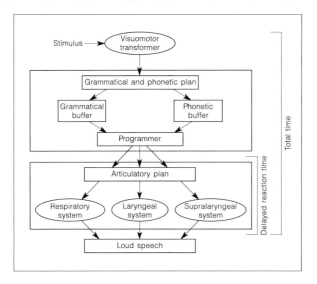

Fig. 8. Levelt's [1989] simplified model.

2.1.1
Rules for the Parameters of Delayed Reactions

As it will be better specified in the following chapters, the foreperiod must last until the end of the previously described processes of visuomotor and programming operations and is to be measured as the difference total time – delayed reaction time. Secondly, the foreperiod must be longer than the duration of the ACG to avoid a busy-line condition blocking the execution of the commands.

2.1.2
Criteria of Evaluation: Task-Dependent and Task-Independent Processes

The subject carrying out a delayed reaction must be able to pay attention to the 'internal task'. This is the psychological definition of what we will call, in more functional terms, his ability to perform a 'working memory' task that, in the specified test, is of psychomotor nature.

Within these conditions the delayed reactions seem indeed to represent a substantially valid tool to investigate an area of paramount importance, not only for the speech control by the brain *(task-dependent processes)* but more generally for its functionality *(task-independent processes)*. How this aim may be technically pursued and what the complex heterogeneous processes and representation activations are, taking place during the foreperiod, will be analysed progressively and more thoroughly in the chapters of this section and the following. This represents an intricate task indeed that we must perform thoroughly in order to know the possibilities and the limits of our research with MDRV, in both normal and neuropsychiatric populations.

....

Neurophysiological Substrates of Speech Control: Comparative and Developmental Data

> Actually we deal with *the brain activity which creates speech,* i.e. a *specific mental activity* when we measure the operative times of the related processes. Its pathological counterpart includes the impairments of the cortical-subcortical systems with reference not only to task-dependent processes, i.e. speech, but also to task-independent processes, i.e. *general abstract, panmodal mental activities.*

2.2.1
Inside the Black Box

It is a long way from perception to the utterance of the word stimulus. The processes and the representations that must be activated are so many that with the average 25 m/s conduction velocity of our brain, we could not speak in the quick sequence allowing our sentences to be understood by listeners. PDP overcome this obstacle.

In order to identify the intermediary processes occurring between programmation and execution in these complex and partly overlapping speech activities, we must perform a detailed analysis of the neural substrates involved in the whole sequence of the operations, of the modalities of the generated impulse patterns and of the time taken by the impulse conduction and transmission. This analysis alone, as complete as it is, leads to the measurement of the psychomotor working memory, which had its pioneers in Plum [1993 a, b].

The preliminary results of comparative and developmental studies of language, reported in the previous Section 1, will now be completed in order to provide an outline of the brain machinery of speech control.

2.2.2
Brain Anatomofunctional Bases of Vocalization

The elaboration of vocalization (fig. 9) depends on the activity of two systems: the limbic (cingulate cortex) and the frontal prerolandic (fig. 10).

The limbic system is formed by the cingulate cortex that sends fibres to the central periaqueductal grey of the brainstem and hence to the bilateral relay nuclei of the pons and medulla; eventually it reaches the motor nuclei of the cranial nerves V and VII (for the oromandibular muscles), XI (pharyngeal canal and glottis), XII (tongue) and also the spinal cord motor nuclei (diaphragmatic and intercostal respiratory muscles).

On the other hand, the prefrontal and prerolandic (pyramidal) cranial and spinal systems play an important role in fast executive commands. The corticocranial and spinal motor system is not yet myelinated in the first year of life; therefore, the essential executive functions are carried out by the prefrontal (area 6, extrapyramidal or parapyramidal, according to Kuypers' terminology) gangliobasal system that plays a fundamental role also in sequential organization.

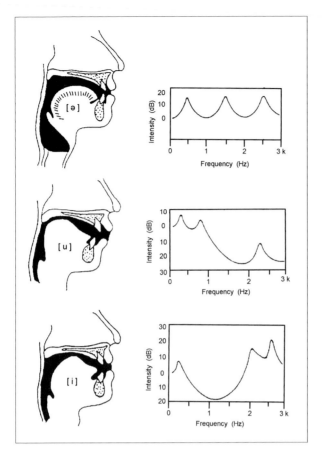

Fig. 9. Shaping of the vocal tract and acoustic transfer function for the vowels [ə], [u] and [i]. k = x 1,000.

The patterns of impulses delivered by the system of the basal ganglia-premotor cortex and cerebellum are transmitted to the peripheral motor nuclei in the brainstem and spinal cord through the intermediary connecting thalamus and mesencephalic coordinating nuclei (in the previously explained homology with the cyclopic eye system; see 2.3.1.1).

There is anatomofunctional evidence of direct and fast connecting pathways only to the oromandibular and lingual nuclei but not to the laryngopharyngeal and diaphragmatic-intercostal sectors. An indirect inference of fast pathways connected to the vocal cords (cranial nerve X) has been advanced on the evidence of the ability of singers to modulate their voice very quickly.

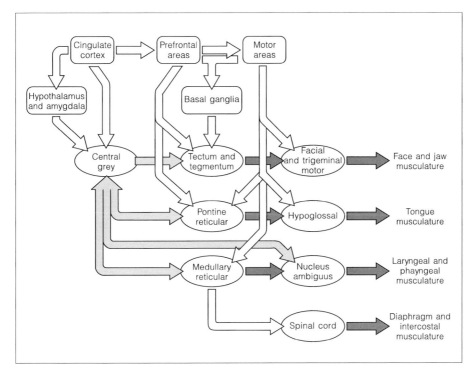

Fig. 10. Activity of the limbic and frontal prerolandic systems. Modified from T.W. Deacon, in Wind et al. [1992].

2.2.3
The Formation of the Most Specifically and Basically Active Neural Systems in Speaking

After the second year of life, at the onset of a more specific organization of brain structures for speech, the prefrontal cortex and the cortex-brainstem-spine system play a primary role: they become able to modulate finely the whole vocal tract in its whole width and extension reached by the anatomical descent of the glottis.

The limbic cortex, more specifically acting on the laryngeal sector, may thus be partly hindered in its previous prevalent role in vocalization, to the advantage of the fast corticomotor system: this innervates the tongue and the oromandibular executors enabling a quicker and more subtle word articulation and more complex motor melodies.

However, the role played by the limbic system is not abandoned. In fact, it maintains an active part in the final expression of language, in relation to its prosodic aspects. The comparison between the human brain and that of anthropomorphic primates shows that the human limbic brain is not at all 'reappraised negatively' [Wind et al., 1992], i.e. reduced. Efferent limbic pathways reach the prefrontal cortex and supplementary motor area that receives an afferent pathway from the aspecific brainstem ascending systems. These last systems provide selective arousal and motor anticipation. By means of averaging techniques one can record the cortical premotor potential that appears 800 ms before

Walter's [1953] expectancy wave, an event that is associated with a conscious secondary mental activity [Plum, 1993a, b].

On the other hand, the preparatory processes are associated with tuning effects on the brainstem and spinal servo-mechanisms. With reference to the study of the development of the linguistic brain, Greenfield's findings [1991] appear to be particularly relevant as a proof of the existence of a neural assembly for a hierarchical organization in the pre-linguistic brain that is not yet endowed with a specific verbal praxic centre separated from the kinetic praxic one. The formation of the neural assembly for grammatical-syntactic organization corresponds to the following step of the linguistic phase starting in the second year of life.

This study and the comparative investigations in monkeys contributed to define better several other issues: (a) word versus sentence processing; (b) tachyphemic threshold and cyclic time; (c) the brain structural systems and the connections activated in the motor control.

2.2.4
Word versus Sentence Processing

One main question to be answered for a correct interpretation of how and in which temporal order Levelt's formulator [1989] works is whether the phonological-phonetic processing appears earlier than the grammatical processing and which is the respective order of the two functions with regard to the degree of availability of the corresponding representations (fig. 3). (This availability is indicated, in artificial networks, as threshold of decoding and expressed by the weight value W.)

The spontaneous speech of adults in Levelt's blueprint [1989] requires the following series of phases: (1) activation of the conceptualizer processes; (2) a formulator provides the grammatical operations, and (3) a formulator provides the more specific phonetic articulatory processing.

In agreement with this blueprint, the linguist considers the enunciation of the sentence as representing the essential language unit, whilst the word – as lexical function – might represent the constituent element to be planned in its syntactic location. This requires syntagmatic and metonymic lexical processes that allow the proper use of the word in the language. These considerations suggest that a primary organization exists for the enunciations that could lead to a more facilitated neural assembly with corresponding easier decoding of the sentences during speech. The existence of a specifically enhanced facilitated neural assembly for the grammar formulator, which has been asserted particularly by Chomsky [1965] and Pinker [1995], suggests a valid neurophysiological interpretation to answer some questions about the more complex task of formulating sentences with respect to pronouncing a word: one should in fact differentiate what we do automatically from what we try to explain logically.

(1) There is no doubt that the intrinsic brain processes implied in sentence enunciation develop in a more intricate series of phases than those required for the production and control of a single word.

(2) The brain spends a longer time to perform more complex tasks.

(3) Then, the time taken by the brain processes should be longer for the sentence than for the word. But, as we report later on, *this assertion is far from being proved.*

(4) Ordinary man, when involved at school in the logical analysis of sentences, experiences a hard task. In contrast, when speaking spontaneously, he automatically applies the grammatical rules, thanks to the grammatical formulator: this in fact develops a large part of unconscious operations without any subjective experience of actual effort.

On the other hand, the situation of the earliest periods of life, when the child utters only words and later on, in a second phase, enunciates sentences, cannot at all be called in support of the idea that enunciating sentences is more complicated for the brain than pronouncing words. The issue is indeed much more complex. First of all, as we have previously explained, the vocal tract cannot be shaped in the early period of life as it is needed for the enunciation in speech of categorizations that already exist in the child's brain. Secondly, the protoword and particularly the oloword of the child contain a syncratic semantic information related to categorizations.

Moreover, the studies of Lieberman [1991] and of Greenfield [1991] proved that the cerebral processes involved in the production and control of a single word are far from being simpler than those required for the enunciation of a sentence.

2.2.5
The Complexity of the Cerebral Control of Words and Some Inferences for Sentence Organization

Lieberman [1991] underlined the great complexity of representations and processes required for the neural control of the single word and made also clear how the intrinsic word-related processes present many analogies with the intrinsic sentence-related processes: 'The brain mechanisms implied in the word control provide in their turn the preadaptive background for a rule-guided syntax.' In fact, the organization processes required for the syntax are comparatively simpler than those required for the complex sequential operations of single words. Thus Lieberman develops the analysis of the four operations implied in the motor control of the apparently simple task of brain control of the word:

(1) Brain evaluation of word length including all letters and syllables. It develops in parallel with the lung expiratory preparatory processes. A disorder in these processes would cause articulatory pauses, dysarthria or dysfluencies (like stuttering).

(2) Organizing and timing processes for the phonological sequence. (Neuroradiologists, in their study of 'ideation' processes with functional MRI, use the terms of 'temporal orchestration' and 'chronometry' for brain programming and intermediary processes in visuomotor activities.)

(3) Computing the air pressure values that produce the prosodic aspects in word intonation (pitch).

(4) Computing the additional vectors depending on the body position (standing up or lying down) and the variants related to serious or joking intentions, emphasis and accentuation.

Greenfield [1991] considers Broca's area as the site of both phonological and grammatical programming. The development of the action grammar (equivalent to ideomotor praxic use of objects) and that of speaking can be compared, starting from a study of the phonological rules of sound combination. The grammatical planning implies – according to Greenfield – a prefrontal control of Broca's centre.

On the other hand, the objective analyses of the outputs of spontaneous and experimental speech and of verbal reading reactions, as thoroughly and systematically as they were interpreted in relation to the underlying neural processes, have not yet provided a reliable reconstruction according to which the different activities of the formulators develop in children, as well as they follow one another in the mature language of adults. Also the occurrence of parallel functions must be taken into consideration in analogy with models of the artificial PDP neural networks.

Some enlightening lines of interpretation might be drawn from the brain's logic models mathematically elaborated by the outstanding neuro-anatomist and neuro-cybernetist Gerd Sommerhoff [1974] or from the more fashionable speculations of the Nobel prize winner Gerd Edelman [1991, 1992].

A rational hypothesis, which we will develop in successive chapters from a methodological and semiological point of view, can be expressed as follows: (a) as far as the formulators are concerned, that is the whole central brain programme, the sentence should be considered as the more easily available unit in the neural assembly; (b) at the level of the executive phonological-phonetic processes, the word assumes the main role.

2.2.6
Domains of Brain Organization: Word versus Grammar

The differentiation of two domains corresponds to Chomsky's theory of the *innate grammar*. Two main tasks are therefore to be taken into consideration when studying the neural events of speech control: (1) to acknowledge a dualism in processes, neural networks, recurrent loops, buffers and stores of words versus grammar; (2) to envisage suitable methodologies and objective biological experiments to test the two orders of neural events separately, in as much as each of them reflects different rules and principles of processing.

2.2.6.1
Speech Motor Control: A Four-Phase General Theory

Levelt [1989], when describing speech motor control processes, clearly indicated that in the first stage (assembling the programme, that is the plan of phonological encoding), the phonetic plan at the output is a detailed motor programme delivering phonological word by phonological word. When the task requires it, the phonetic plan can be stored in the articulatory buffer. The preferred units of storage are phonological phrases.

In the second stage (retrieving the motor programme), when the speaker decides to start a prepared utterance, the verbal motor units (according to the phonetic plan for the phonological phrases) are retrieved from the articulatory buffer. A specific law of a relationship between task utterance and brain operative time emerges at this stage: the time needed to retrieve each verbal motor unit depends on their total number in the buffer.

In the third phase (unpacking the subprogrammes), the phonetic plan for a phonological phrase, once retrieved, has to be unpacked, making available the whole hierarchy of motor commands. The more complex the verbal motor units are, the longer the unpacking will last.

In the fourth stage (executing the motor commands), the motor commands are issued to the neuromotor circuits and executed by the musculature. Retrieval latencies occur, and they can be absorbed by drawling some syllables.

2.2.6.2
Does the Law Relating Time Latency to Length of Utterance Follow Different Correlation Coefficients in the Word versus Grammar Domain?

It was ascertained that, in the previously mentioned phase and particularly in the third phase, at the level of syllables and words, a specific law seems to regulate the relationship between task utterance and brain operative time; the time needed to execute the motor commands depends on the *frequency of use of the word* [Oldfield and Wingfield, 1965] and the *length of utterance* [Klapp, 1974; Sternberg et al., 1978].

As far as the length of utterance is concerned, it was found that the law is valid in the field of words, disyllabic words requiring a shorter latency time (ACG latency) than 3- and, respectively, 4-syllabic words. Yet it is contradicted when a sentence (of 10 letters) is compared to a 4-letter word: *ACG latency is not longer for the sentence than for the word* (see later in this Section and in Section 3).

2.2.6.3
Can the Law Relating Time Latency to Frequency of Use of the Verbal Task Be a Common Factor for the Two Domains Prevailing over the Knapp-Sternberg Law?

We wonder if the law of Oldfield and Wingfield [1965] may cover the two domains: is the ACG latency for the disyllabic word of the above-mentioned study equal to or even longer than the ACG latency for a 10-letter sentence – in opposition to the law of the word length – as the frequency use of the word is equal to or lower than that of the sentence? The answer to this question implies an analysis of the load that word length and word frequency, respectively, require from the brain work.

An increase in utterance length corresponds to a proportionally longer working time, one syllable requiring about 10 ms to be produced. A higher frequency of use corresponds to a lower neural assembly threshold (or of the neural network weight value) as a function of the facilitation exerted by repeated activations. However, as convincing as this fact may be, there are other variables that one must take into consideration when we proceed from the *superficial* level of performances to the level of the *underlying* brain processes.

Besides word frequency – and in a somehow complex relationship with it – genetic factors, specifically or preferentially influential on sentences rather than on syllables or isolated words, can facilitate the brain processes with a lower weight and possibly other related structural modifications.

2.2.6.3.1
Grammar Formulation Is Generated Genetically and Requires a Shorter Working Time
According to Chomsky's innate grammar theory, one may infer that the neural assembly of the grammar formulator is endowed with a lower threshold than that of the phonetic formulator. The subsumption [Hawkins, 1983] can be thus inferred that the

---

grammar neural assembly is more responsive in its input and internal connections than the phonological neural assembly.

2.2.6.3.2
The Extent of Facilitated Neural Assembly Mass Can Offer Alternative Pathways for Sentence Utterance and Thus Shorten Its Latency Time

Lashley's principle [1951, 1980] on equipotentiality of assembled neurons at the level of associative functions makes us infer that the greater the neural assembly – and particularly the greater the facilitated neural assemblies[1] of a certain performance requiring more than one phase of processes – the shorter the corresponding operative brain time. The propositions contained in this statement are the following:

(1) A grammar-syntactic formulation implied in sentences, at variance with syllables and single words, corresponds to larger neuronal networks in relation to both genetic and epigenetic factors.

(2) In a very exhaustive and detailed analysis of the structure of the lexical system, Schriefers et al. [1990] demonstrated: (a) how different steps are involved in the temporal organization of the speech signal and the articulatory programme; (b) how some central assembling and integrating processing units correspond to sequential operations; (c) how other matching processes, including verbalization mapping, *create extensive parallel processing* (i.e. PDP).

(3) In a model with multiple pathways, a larger selection of alternatives is available in more automatic processing through a lower number of synapses and more intentional complex multisynaptic processing with some components representing non-mandatory stages.

All these considerations concern not only the entry access to formulators but also the development of the intermediary processes at the interface with the executors.

2.2.7
The Dualistic Concept of Levelt, and of Dell and Juliano, and the Task Dynamic Model of Saltzman

Both Levelt [1991] and Dell and Juliano [1991] brought evidence in favour of a clear-cut distinction between abstract phonological representation and articulatory programme, and between phonological frames (linguistic structure) and phonological segments (linguistic contents), respectively. Saltzman and Munhall [1989] recognized a significant gap in a dynamic framework between phonemic and gestural representation, but they argued that these separate models can be joined together, offering the existing possibilities of a seamless union of 'higher-level' linguistic-phonological and 'lower-level' sensorimotor-phonetic processes. This concept is also intended to capture the variable and invariant aspects of skilled actions in a single framework.

These statements require further experimental investigations and more detailed analyses: we will develop them in successive chapters. At the semiological level, with reference to MDRV, a main topic of this review will be the demonstration of how the adoption of foreperiods with different delays in verbal reactions represent a reliable way to test

---

[1] This concept represents the neurophysiological side of what is defined *attractor* in neural networks according to McClelland [1994] (see 5.3).

these hypotheses with experimental objective trials in human beings and to develop the theoretical interpretations with corresponding blueprints and models.

Just following this line of thought and with reference to the development of spoken language, we must address our rationale to a fundamental conditioning parameter of speech production, that is the *velocity of word processing*. We are indebted to Lieberman [1991] who made an issue of it in the course of his neuropalaeo-anthropological studies.

2.2.8
Tachyphemic Threshold, Overloading Effects and Cyclic Time

The tachyphemic threshold was applied first of all to the utterance of the single word. The requested rapidity – as Lieberman [1991] writes – is the fruit of cerebral mechanisms able to produce extremely precise and complex muscular manoeuvres. With a view to understand fully the meaning of this parameter for speech production, we must enter into a rather detailed comparative analysis in the field of the HOSPA (see 1.3.2).

A first kind of HOSPA we can take into consideration concerns gait and handling. The individual subject can choose among various HOSPA velocities each time, according to what he wants. You can run or walk slowly. Likewise, you can suddenly grasp an object or pick it up carefully. All these velocity regulations could offer an apparent analogy with the fact that I can utter a word like /muro/ quickly or I can spell it out.

However, there is a great difference between the first two examples and the last one. The whole range of velocities, according to which you can walk or grasp, is determined by a quite suitable, perfect relation to what is required by the situation and the subject's intentional process.

The arrangement is completely different in speech. Spelling or very slow uttering are outside the natural spontaneous kind of performances developing automatically. They require an intentional conscious act that is at variance with the decision to use a communicative language. Spelling and slow utterances imply a change of the most suitable temporal course of speaking. Instead of the usual interpersonal information, a new purpose has to be realized: it is a matter of an artificial modality to teach a language or check some isolated elements of unclear communication. These modes of expression are quite different from the production of communicative speech. In this case, the subject pronouncing a certain word in the sentence will utter it with a determined velocity that is below the minimal value of current speaking, the lowest value of the tachyphemic threshold.

The speaker can also accelerate his speaking above this value, within the range of normal tachyphemic performances according to the requests of environmental conditions and psychological states. Experiments were also carried out [Peters et al., 1989] with explicit instructions of different speech velocities but never below a certain value. When, in a *neutral* experiment of reading reactions, we ask the subject to utter the task words aloud in a *rapid but still normal way*, we only instruct him to engage in the trial to avoid artificial unnatural performances like spelling or, at the other extreme limit, a precipitated utterance with distorted words.

Each individual subject has his own spontaneous usual speech velocity, but the interindividual variations remain within a precise limited range.

A fundamental importance of the tachyphemic threshold in relation to the mental efficiency is verified by the results achieved by Gigley [1983] and Salthouse [1985]. They studied some neural alterations characterized by abnormal slowing of the brain processes and formulated the 'cycle time theory' according to which a slowing below the tachyphemic threshold of the central processes of spatial programmation and timing of speech causes severe syndromes of impairment in speaking. These syndromes are analogous to aphasic dysfluencies: their origin has been attributed by Gigley [1983] and Salthouse [1985] to secondary *overloading effects* produced by abnormal slowing of the brain processes. In psychological terms, the mechanism of impairment was defined as *divided attention*. When we try to analyse it at a neurobiological level, that is along the whole chain of the underlying brain processes, one realizes immediately that we are dealing with a mean value of velocity which represents the result of a series of velocities specific to each single phase of the brain processes. In fact the condition 'divided attention' might depend, in neurophysiological terms, on a dissociation of the component velocities.

We can sketch a preliminary calculation of the time taken by each of the different phases of the speech control, following the path of Levelt's blueprint [1989], but preliminarily we must expound some essential definitions.

The definition of the terms 'velocity at the phonological level' and 'velocity at the neural level' has a great relevance also in relation to the parameter tachyphemic threshold. 'Speech velocity' indicates the number of phonemes (or syllables, words, sentences, according to the task requested in the experiment) pronounced in the unit of time (seconds).

'Neural velocity' indicates the length of the circuit (path between neural assemblies, loops and different systems) covered in the unit of time (seconds). The neurophysiologist teaches us that even the velocity value of each phase is a mean value resulting from different events, like fibre conduction and synaptic transmission including the value of *weight* and the corresponding number of impulses needed to decode the signal. However, these components are not relevant to compute the basal values of operating time.

On the contrary, a factor interfering greatly with the criteria of adding up the single-component neural velocities to compute the mean neural velocity is represented by the *'parallel functions'* (the PDP of the artificial neural networks) that *significantly increase speech velocity.*

Our analysis of the neural velocity, along the path of Levelt's blueprints [1989], starts from (1) the preverbal conceptualization, going (2) to the central computational sensorimotor processes and eventually (3) to the final executors.

We will now deal with some calculations concerning the processes related to point 1, while those of points 2 and 3 will be discussed later in Section 3, after the description of the underlying cerebral structures. A detailed mathematical formula of the retrieval time [Roelofs, 1992] will be reported in 5.2.

The calculation of the time taken in the conceptualizer may rely on previous reviews of Libet [1965a, b, 1985] on neurophysiological data that have recently been analysed by Plum [1993b]. The activation of mental representation during the course of thought implies a flow of impulses [MacKay 1987; Pinelli, 1970, 1992] that have a spatial rather than temporal configuration, i.e. they are simultaneous, in agreement with parallel functions. Some data have been reported [Levelt, 1991] in favour of an initial 'visual feature' of these representations that could be activated with a gestalt modality of processing. This leads to a high velocity of development in the corresponding mental operations.

Following these propositions we can face now three other points: (a) to give some examples that could help to better understand the processing of Levelt's [1989] first phase and the passage to the second phase of translation from the conceptualizer to the sensorimotor processes and then to the motor performances in a chronological sequence; (b) the need for a tachyphemic threshold; (c) the period of early childhood with slow speech control.

As rough but possibly enlightening examples of visual synchronously activated abstract representations, we may consider a picture, a photograph or any painted or sculptured piece of work. On the other hand, in analogy with the sequential processes, we may take into consideration a sequence of notes or phrases of a musical composition. Likewise the brain is endowed with extremely stratified but *spatially mapped representations* (like the picture), but it can also be activated by a series of processes producing successive instructing commands or invariants developing one after the other (like a musical sequence): it is the *temporal orchestration* according to neuroradiologist terminology.

To complete the exemplification, we can now compare two different purposeful actions, body and limb movements on one side and communicative speech on the other. If a mother saw her son run over by a car, she would rush to shield him. In an analogous situation, if you saw an imminent risk and wanted to alert the unaware potential victim, you would shout a warning promptly, with the most concise and clear utterance. To do it, talking man is endowed with a *sufficiently rapid* cerebroneuromuscular coordinated system: otherwise the subject would utter only a syllable or an indistinct word. This would be meaningless and confusing: moreover, if the subject pronounced sentences, the utterance would be so long and slow that he could hardly follow the thread of his own argument and the listener could not associate the meaning of the last word with the first.

The very young infant can utter only single syllables or words when his cerebral and neuromotor coordinated systems are activated too slowly, as they conduct and transmit too slowly. Moreover, since also the sequence of articulatory movements is too slow, he cannot produce a current complete pattern of formant frequencies, and the accuracy of pronunciation remains rather poor.

Stuttering, occurring in the third year of life, could partly depend upon an insufficiently modulated velocity of speech motor control and coordination of the executors. If the velocity of some processes remained below the minimal tachyphemic threshold, some negative effects might arise with consequent syndromes of divided attention. Since the brain works as a self-correcting machine, the abnormally low phases could be corrected with tentatively compensating accelerations in other phases; however, overloading and oscillating effects could not be avoided.

···

The Brain Architecture of Speech Production

> Hierarchical representations, once evolved, rapidly proliferated
> into diverse areas, resulting in common functional representations,
> but disparate anatomical representations.   [Keele, 1981]

2.3.1
The Brain Systems and Their Connections in the Motor Control Machinery

The comparative study of the development of communicative capacities that primates show in the first year of life and of the corresponding brain structures yielded some
useful issues about the neural systems involved in the production of speech since the
earliest phases of development in human children.

On the grounds of these findings, we will further develop the previous comprehensive
reconstructions of the brain architecture involved in speech production (fig. 3, 4, 8 and 10).

2.3.1.1
The Executive Processes

As far as the executive processes are concerned, a main issue regards the involvement of the intermediate stations, represented by the intrinsic thalamus and brainstem relay centres (fig. 10). From them, the neural pathways to the 'pyramidal' corticogeniculate
and corticospinal systems originate. On the other hand, the frontomotor system interrupts, at the proper centres of the brainstem, with direct and indirect connections to the
lower motoneurons. De Long [1990, 1994] identified these centres as *mesencephalic extrapyramidal area* and *pontine proper nuclei*. Whilst the former can contribute to the afferent
aspecific thalamic pathway, the latter could function as effective coordinators for the pairs
of symmetrical muscles of the vocal tract. Thus the pathway to pontine proper nuclei
could be related to the so-called verbophasic system [Pinelli, 1991]. This neural organization presents a strict homology with the neural architecture of the facial mimic expressions and, in another field, with the gaze centres of the oculomotor system: these coordinating proper nuclei were described as the *cyclopic eye*. In our case of speech control, we
could propose the term of *executive neural speaker*. This organization is not yet well defined with specific anatomofunctional investigations and one could ask whether it might
be in some way connected with the corresponding structure of the articulatory buffer. In
fact, the exact anatomoneurophysiological structure and pattern organization in the chain
of speech control and mainly intermediary pre-executive mechanisms is still an open field
of research. We will discuss them fully in the following chapters.

2.3.1.2
The Intermediary Relay System Is Also Involved in the Bi-Univocal Connection with the Limbic Brain

We have already emphasized that the contribution of this system is essential to the motivational driving [Gray, 1994] in the first preprogramming phase and to the prosodic modulation in the executive articulatory phase.

The limbic brain is not reduced in humans with respect to monkeys, but, as we reported previously, it is actually increased even if this increase occurs at a lower rate than that of the frontal lobe.

2.3.1.3
Mingazzini's Verbophasic System

The coordinating relay system of the *executive neural speaker* carries out a fundamental function, avoiding an independent activity of the two lateral, right and left, series of motor nuclei as it would be the case if they were innervated directly with a consequent increased risk of asynchrony and discoordination. The inadequacy of a direct innervation of the efferent motor cranial nuclei by the hemispheric pyramidal systems was emphasized quite clearly by Mingazzini [1981], who in fact postulated the existence of a *verbophasic system*. In support of this view, he advocated Pierre Marie's findings [1906] concerning the effects of lesions to the quadrilateral region at the level of the basal ganglia on speech control [Pinelli, 1991].

On the other hand, at the level of the executors the muscular fascicles show a continuous path, crossing the middle line in some related parts of the vocal tract as the oral orbicularis muscle and also the tongue to some degree.

2.3.1.4
Broca's and Wernicke's Neural Assemblies, Multiple Representations and Processes

Greenfield [1991] showed that Broca's area develops in humans after the first year of life, with specific language representations. Broca's area performs two types at least of dynamic processes (the square boxes in Levelt's blueprint [1989]), that are organized as stores and buffers (the circles in Levelt's blueprint).

2.3.1.5
Sensorimotor Transformations

Wernicke's and Broca's neural assemblies are activated not only by acoustically perceived images in hearing but also by visual images in reading and by thought representations in spontaneous speech. Language areas are in fact connected to occipitotemporoparietal cortexes and to the frontomotor and supplementary motor areas of both hemispheres.

2.3.1.6
Stores and Buffers

2.3.1.6.1
The Vocal Tract Cortical Representations

Proprioceptive and exteroceptive afferent stimuli are conducted by several afferent feedbacks from the tissues of the vocal tract to Wernicke's and Broca's areas. In fact, the enlargement of Broca's neural assembly in human beings with respect to the kinetopraxic area of handling and voicing in monkeys is due to the much larger extension of the vocal tract in man and the consequent development of progressively broader representations [Lieberman, 1991].

2.3.1.6.2
Verbal Encyclopaedia and Grammar Representations

Wernicke's neural assembly for the perceptive secondary connections and Broca's neural assembly for the motor connections are the sites of encoded abstract generalized 'soft' representations for grammar and speech unit formulation. The quality specified by 'abstract' and similar terms can be understood following the description of Plato's ideas, in contrast with the aesthesic (sensorial) more detailed and concrete qualities of the perceptive images. It must be noticed that, at another level, a differentiation must also be made between *abstract* and *concrete words,* but it must be added that both these qualities refer to an abstract order of neural organization. In fact, the word is already in itself the issue of a symbolic high-order elaboration. Therefore the terms 'concrete' and 'abstract' in this case represent only a secondary qualification indicating the nature of the objects (concrete) or concepts (abstract) that the words signify; but all the words in themselves are actually primarily abstract representations or symbols. We will further analyse these concepts when we discuss the experiments carried out to test the role played by each of the two cerebral hemispheres in processing concrete and abstract words (see 4.4.2.1).

One must also be aware of the fact that both grammatically formulated sentences on one side and single words and syllables on the other are encoded and memorized in separate stores (the circles of Levelt's blueprint [1989], fig. 3). As previously explained, the grammar store is more strictly involved in the processes activated by the primary frontal categorization centres and the vocal tract representations in Broca's area, whilst the phonological store is connected only to Broca's vocal tract representations.

According to the law of direct proportionality between the 'mass' of neural representations and mental efficiency [Lashley, 1980], we may infer that the sentence representations are more easily available for decoding than word and syllable representations (see 2.2.6.3.2).

2.3.1.6.3
The Preparatory Processes

The preparatory innervation is effected in shorter times than the articulatory executive innervation [Peters et al., 1989; Pinelli and Ceriani, 1992]. It corresponds to the tuning of selected muscles, like the oromandibular ones, and does not require a complex computational planning and timing of coordinated muscles. One might then suppose that the invariant descending commands of the spatial and timing processes of preparatory innervation, starting from Broca's neural assembly, could directly reach the premotor and motor area in correspondence with the oroglossomandibular part of the integrated system of the homunculus. The first station is in the dominant (left) hemisphere, whilst the callosal interhemispheric connections allow to reach the corresponding motor areas of the non-dominant (right) hemisphere.

2.3.2
The Evolution of Verbal and Non-Verbal Purposeful Complex Sequential Functions and a Psychometric Methodology for the Analysis of Brain Speech Control

The origin and evolution of vocalizations and language in children were studied with a large involvement of scientists in different fields. The progressive neuromuscular and cerebral changes, from anthropomorphic primates to *Homo loquens,* and the oldest (30,000 years ago) documents of human communicating signs yielded important cues.

From 10- to 20-month-old children, behavioural data were collected by Greenfield [1991], who was particularly concerned with handling and speaking, while Eimas [1974, 1975], Mehler et al. [1981, 1991] and Mehler and Christophe [1992] studied the children's reactions to verbal stimuli from the earliest month of life. The authors aimed to identify the genetic innate speech abilities with respect to those acquired by imitation. Speech prototypes were studied by Kuhl [1985, 1992].

The progressive levels of branching in the sentence organization of children 15, 21 and 23 months old were also identified.

Wejner [1991] recorded the spontaneous speech of 2- to 3-year-old children and measured the proportion of repetitions and errors.

Tests of symmetric picture reconstruction according to Greenfield [1991] were carried out with 6- to 11-year-old children. At the age of 6 years, the child copies the pictures with a chain, non-hierarchical strategy, each element being linked to the previous one. At the age of 7–9 years, the hierarchical organization of the model pictures is used starting from top components to the bottom. Most 11-year-old children use a top-bottom method with passages from one branch to the other; this strategy depends on a process of internalization of the hierarchical organization model. This might correspond to the development of timing processes in the programmation of word production.

2.3.2.1
A Tool for the Analysis of Brain Speech Control: The MDRV

A fruitful methodology to investigate the programming and the executive processes of word production might be developed along the lines of verbal choice reactions (fig. 11). This implies the measurement of the temporal parameters of latency time and duration of word stimulus utterance. In reading reactions we should be able to differentiate the following stages: (1) visual perception time, (2) visual-ideomotor transfer time, (3) sequential programmation time, (4) adaptation of the invariant patterns to constraint-specific conditions (buffers, working memory) and (5) articulatory neuromotor execution time (fig. 4).

The trial-and-error type of functioning implies a certain range of variability for the same task: a series of reactions must be carried out by the subject for each task, giving statistically reliable mean values and standard deviations (SD). Learning and fatigue effects should be avoided or calculated apart.

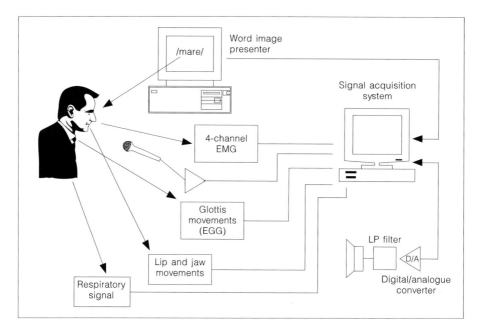

Fig. 11. Word production in verbal choice reactions. EGG = Electroglottogram; LP = Low-pass filter at 4,000 Hz.

Both pictures (for children at preschool age) and word stimuli (di- and trisyllabic) will be shown after an acoustic warning signal (100-ms interval) on a PC screen, while the subject keeps the respiration in the inspiratory phase. The picture must be named and the word read aloud, immediately after the task stimulus presentation or after an interval, at the appearance of a 'go' signal; the intervals were randomly paired and corresponded to 0.1, 0.5, 1.5, 3 or 4 s. As responses, ACG through a microphone, surface oromandibular EMG, electroglottograms and oromandibular kinetograms (fig. 6, 7 and 12), are recorded on an electromyograph screen.

The differences in time of the latencies and durations of the reactions carried out at different foreperiods allow to obtain some cues for the central programming versus executive processes. The ratio of the time of the response (ACG) at $FP_{1.5}$ to the ACG time at FP_0 was found to give a cue for the intermediary processes and it was named intermediary process ratio. Its meaning and evaluation will be analysed at length in a later section dealing with 'delayed reactions': but, from now, we must warn that the intermediary process ratio has that meaning on condition that ACG latency at FP_0 is equal to or greater than the normal mean value.

With aging, at the preschool age, more stereotyped branch operations (chain algorithms) have been found to occur [Pinelli and Ceriani, 1992] implying serial phonological coupling with broader jitters. In the following years of life, an improvement occurs in the transfer of visual-semantic information with acceleration in the modular processes and minimization of information loss in transmodular passages. These changes reduce time latency and duration in the range of adult values. The organization of PDP functioning might also develop with a broader extension and better simultaneity.

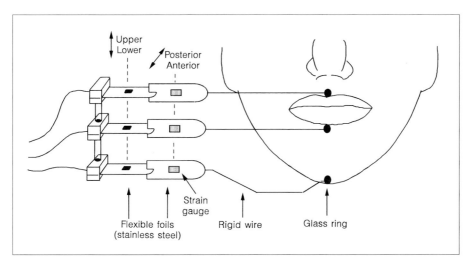

Fig. 12. Transducer for lip and jaw displacements. Modified from Schönle et al. [1992].

2.3.2.2
The Usefulness of the Application of MDRV in Neurology and Neurorehabilitation

It is worthwhile stating in advance, while still explaining its fundaments, the interest for both basic scientists and clinicians to apply MDRV to normal and diseased subjects. Six points can be underlined:

(1) The knowledge of the temporal parameters of speech control in the early phase of development, provided by these tests, might bring important details on the brain organization for speech (task-dependent processes) and more generally for other purposeful complex sequential actions (task-independent processes) [Arbib and Caplan, 1979].

(2) A better evaluation of mental maturation might be achieved, as speech processes develop in relation to well-determined epigenetic factors.

(3) Individual normal patterns of brain maturation and performance strategies might be identified. Clearly defined abnormalities should be statistically ascertained. In both normal and pathological conditions, primary vocal-tract-depending characteristics and changes must be evaluated first, since they can influence intrinsically normal brain functions.

(4) Changes in multiple output articulatory coordinated components and related physiopathological impairments might be assessed in dysfluencies like stuttering, dysarthrias and verbal apraxias [Van Lieshout et al., 1993; Hardcastle, 1994].

(5) Rational criteria of treatment, including well-specified types of artificial feedbacks, might be determined for each subject in the course of the disease.

(6) Natural and treatment-dependent courses of functional alterations and compensative processes might be assessed and measured.

The Production of 'Invariant' Guiding Patterns

2.4.1
The First Phase of Sensorimotor Integration

The first phase of the brain processes involved in production of speech, in both reading and interlocution, is represented by a sensorimotor transformation [Munhall et al., 1992] with a well-defined afferent input and successive transmission to higher-order and more diffuse associative networks (fig. 13): they were named in the neurological literature 'brain motor schemas', in the psychophysiological literature 'hebbian assemblies', while the bio-engineer tried to reproduce them in artificial neural networks.

Current views of brain organization [Pinelli, 1970; Sommerhoff, 1974; Alexander and Crutcher, 1990; Rosenfeld, 1993] suggest that in these neural networks there is a multilayer interposition of synapses in *connective loops,* where internal flows of discharges are activated far from the areas of projection. Here, the afferent discharges arrive from the input, and from there the efferent discharges reach the output. In this architectural frame, multiple-order representations are formed in the brain with more generalized, integrative and abstract formulas.

However, this kind of *abstract* generalization does not mean that the connections between the elementary localized inputs and outputs are lost or become weaker or less precise [Cummings, 1993]. One must admit that spatial and somatosensory representations maintain their exact correspondence also in the *brain scheme.*

A question thus arises about the passage from localized functions to diffuse functions and vice versa [Lashley, 1951, 1980]. A precise answer has not yet been formulated. It was questioned whether the terms of the issue are appropriate. They are indeed reliable terms in the field of a three-dimensional static space but become inadequate for events developing *dynamically* in a certain period of time. The languages of analogous computers, fractal geometry or mathematics of chaotic events have been considered for a better approach to the understanding of the diffuse functions of the brain, but this has been found to be true only in a very limited field of speculation [Cotterill, 1989].

The Boltzman-Shannon probability theory, with Venn diagrams [Sommerhoff, 1974] and Markov's system [Lee, 1960] represent a first-order reliable way of description [Woody, 1982]. In fact, the most consistent 'language' is represented by the artificial neural networks according to Banks [1991]. Having analysed the way these neural networks function, one realizes that, at the level of the inner-unit neural layers, the range of combinations becomes extremely wide with progressively more generalized and abstract representations. At the same time, it must be kept in mind that the relationship between the perceptually derived patterns of impulses and those that elicit the efferent chain of neural events is quite precise and well defined in a sign-to-sign matching: Kelso et al. [1986] found a mathematical relationship between each couple of variables. Proprioceptive impulses reach the neural representations and modify them according to the mechanical properties of the musculo-articulatory structures of the whole vocal tract.

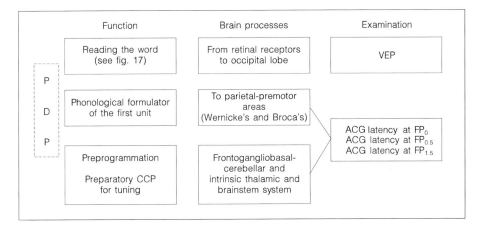

Fig. 13. First phase: computational CCP in reading reactions. VEP = Visual-evoked potential.

These processes require a definite decoding time that – as previously reported – can vary in relation to the frequency of use of the target word: it increases for less usual words. Other factors, like the length of the word and the prosodic changes, influence the time of brain processes in the latest phases. A more detailed analysis of these events will be carried out in Section 5.

2.4.2
The Preparatory Phase

The preparatory processes were well studied by neurophysiologists at the level of the neuromuscular innervation. In contrast, the corresponding CCP have not yet been the object of systematic experimental research.

First of all, one must eliminate any possible misunderstanding over an association of these preparatory processes with the contingent negative variation and the expectancy wave of Walter [1953] or the 'Bereitschaftspotential' [Craggs and Carr, 1992]. These are the EEG signs of later events related to a conscious readiness to react. On the contrary, the processes we are dealing with are the earliest central computing processes involved in programming the tonic innervation of the muscles, making them ready to develop the best contraction when the invariant-to-variant command arrives. The neurophysiologists [Abbs, 1973; Abbs and Cole, 1982; Abbs et al., 1984] investigated a series of mechanisms, including the γ motor systems, operating to modulate muscular stiffness. This chain of modulations produces the best response of coordinated muscles to incoming impulses concerned with the executors. In the specific case of speech control, this preparatory activity produces the best tonic innervation of those particular muscles that will be contacted by the expiratory flow of air. The first complex of muscles is represented by the vocal cords: their changes in stiffness for different phonemes under different conditions were the object of many very precise biomechanical researches [Sutako, 1992].

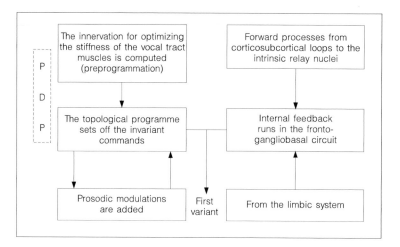

Fig. 14. First and second phases: main functions and CCP. ACG latencies at $FP_{0.5}$ and $FP_{1.5}$.

The link of the γ activity with cortical centres was considered by Granit [1955] and his pupils [Baldissera et al., 1981]. Anyway, the CCP involved in this activity should be defined as 'preprogrammation' (fig. 14).

2.4.3
The Programmation

The second phase of processes was indicated by both neurophysiologists and neurologists as *programmation* [Marsden, 1984; Rothwell, 1987]. One main task of the programmation processes corresponds to a spatial somatotopic realization of the coordinated action: the CCP computes which are the muscles able to produce the vocal-tract changes required to utter the word, starting with its first unit. We might term this programmation the *'spatial or topic programmation'*. It has also been observed more recently that the programmation phase includes also a *timing programmation* (fig. 4). The innervation provided must be chronologically ordered for each phonetic unit inside the combination corresponding to the word.

2.4.4
Making the Point Concerning the Production of Invariants

Summarizing the analysis carried out in this chapter, one can give the following blueprint:
(1) the first phase is represented by the transmission of the perceptual elements to the corresponding neural motor schemes (fig. 13);
(2) the preprogramming CCP performs the tuning operations (fig. 14);
(3) the spatial programmer chooses the paths to the coordinated muscles (fig. 15);
(4) the time-ordering programmer produces the sequence combination of the successive elements in the phonological structure of the word.

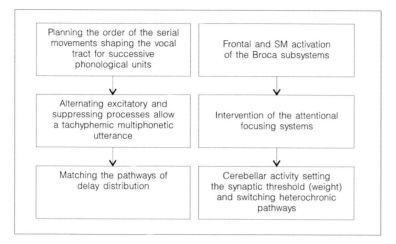

Fig. 15. Third phase: timing computational activity of cyclic processes. SM = Supplementary motor area. ACG latencies at $FP_{0.5}$ and $FP_{1.5}$.

As we will specify later, it is known that these four processes occur partly simultaneously [Cummings, 1993]. This is one of the reasons why, in the current language [Levelt, 1989], they are included in the common term 'programme'. So, in the course of our review, we will use the term 'programme' indicating all these CCP, but we will reserve their proper specific denomination for the four individual processes, when a more detailed analysis is required.

2.4.5
The Phonological Unit and the Pre-Invariant

There is still some doubt about the real elementary phonological unit of speech. Many experiments are in progress to identify the so-called prototype [Sutako, 1992], but from now there is consistent evidence in favour of the syllable being the smallest point of reference in both perception and production of speech, at least in Romance languages.

The organization of patterns of discharges guiding the chronological innervation of the executors for multisyllabic words requires specific computational processes (CCP) in the brain. They must provide the programme for cyclic excitation and inhibition of coordinated muscles with a determined time of pauses and duration of the single phoneme and syllable [Levelt, 1993] (fig. 4).

These guiding patterns of discharges (absolute programmes) are produced in a first stage as first invariants or pre-invariants (fig. 14). Still in the programming phase, they are modified in relation to the information coming from the peripheral constraints, represented by the biomechanical dynamic properties of the muscles that will produce the articulatory movements. We will mention later the co-articulation, a change that occurs in a following phase.

The programmation from pre-invariants to invariants takes place at the level of CCP, well before the adaptation process supervenes. The demonstration of this early occurrence was proved by the experiments of the 'pipe in the mouth' that we will analyse in Section 5.

....

The Intermediary Pre-Executive Processes

> Many of the sequential representations of skill are not dictated by
> higher-order sequential representations; rather they are a conse-
> quence of such things as mechanical properties of the musculoskel-
> etal system that carries out the action.   [Keele, 1981]

2.5.1
A Neurophysiological Analysis of Intermediary Pre-Executive Phases:
The Articulatory Buffer

The central highest-level [Rothwell, 1987] processes develop with a PDP modality
[Alexander and Crutcher, 1991]. In the ensuing stages, the flow of impulses is transmitted
to the relay nuclei of the intrinsic thalamic and brainstem system and then to the executive stations (fig. 16). However, one can hardly conceive that this flow of impulses occurs
with a regular, continuous course in an autoregulated modality, already organized for the
final innervation.

In fact, the impulses created to produce the articulatory movements of speaking are
coming to the adjusting programmers in successive waves, coming out of a sequential cas-
cade of different processes: sensorimotor transmission, computations and timing for the different channels. This causes the produced flow of impulses to occur at a discontinuous heterogeneous rate, even if the cycle of each operation were aligned in similar temporal courses.

Thus, it is clear that the temporal course of the impulse patterns emerging from the
CCP depends on autonomous physiological properties which can hardly match the rules
by which the sequence of phonemes, syllables and words should be phonologically gov-
erned at the level of the vocal tract. These rules relate to structural constraints and complex prosodic modulations that must be accomplished within certain limits of speed. On
the other hand, one could state that the qualification of 'invariant' applies not only to the
pattern constitution but also to its *rhythm of production*.

Shifting our attention to the shaping of the vocal tract, we should try to define the
pattern of innervation, i.e. the number of impulses in a unit of time, which must reach the
muscles in a precise *order*, able to produce the requested contractions [Kelso et al., 1986].

A further range of factors is represented by the prosodic requirements leading to a
structural reshaping of the *pauses* governing the fragmentation of the articulatory movements requested for the necessary 'matching between production and perception of
speech' [Sutako, 1992].

These considerations allow us to better define the problem: how do these pacing
mechanisms operate and prevail over those previously activated in the intrinsic frontosubcortical circuit of speech programmation?

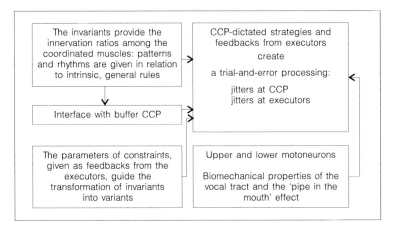

Fig. 16. Fourth phase: adaptive processes at the interface between CCP and executive systems. ACG latencies at $FP_{0.5}$ and $FP_{1.5}$.

2.5.2
The Misleading Proposal of the Abstract Question with Static Implications

One hypothesis was put forward to explain the rearrangements between programmation and formulation on one side and execution on the other: it postulates the *existence* of an intermediate phase during which the first-order invariants are collected and gathered [Levelt, 1989]. The way how this phase can be conceived appears to be of fundamental importance to arrive at a more concrete and neurophysiologically definable model of interpretation of the whole chain of neural events. Particular attention must be given to the meaning of the term 'existence'.

'I assume that an entity is located somewhere in the brain to contain those encoded signs. Then I put a circle in my blueprint.' But we should paraphrase Occam's razor principle: do not add circles (representations) instead of squares (processes)! On the contrary, the anatomically minded neurophysiologist or the hardware-minded bio-engineer is inclined to use easily abstract schematic terms implying static assumptions that might be quite mismatched and distant from the real events; these, in our case, seem indeed to be characterized by a dynamic, continuous flow of activity. The panta rhei of Heraclitus represents an alternative, more pertinent view for the interpretation of the logic of the brain.

In fact, we could ask the following more correctly defined question. Do we have to do with some specific new systems localized in the brain or do we rather refer to an *additional process* of functional intermediary arrangement of the previously activated systems? The present knowledge seems to support the latter view.

We owe it to Levelt that the terms of the issue were set clearly. In fact, he postulated an intermediary stage located after the process of speech formulation. His scientific attitude led him to accumulate an important amount of data helping the neurologist to better define the ambit where the buffer-related functions play a role and what these functions really are. A step towards the solution can be made by taking into account two recent contributions, the 'working memory' and the 'internal feedback' hypotheses, trying to revise them in the light of the previous elucidations.

2.5.3
The Intermediary Processes of Spontaneous Speech, with Reference to
Baddeley's Interpretation

In the General Introduction, we have analysed the improper use of the term 'memory' for the processes involved in the *delayed* reading reactions of our MDRV and the incongruous correction with the term 'working'. In fact, in the intermediary phase occurring between the early end of the programming phase and the onset of the executive phase, we can identify several processes which do not imply a storage or static phase as the usual term 'memory' would suggest. Implied in the delayed reactions are afteractivities with timing and adaptive processes: active internal circuits developing in loops 'coordinate' and adjust the multiple flows of programmed invariants. On the other hand, in our case, it would be incorrect to speak of attentional processes of the central execution, since they occur at a completely unconscious level.

Baddeley [1985, 1992] attributed a duration of about 2,000 ms to the active circuit of the 'working memory'. The relation with our experiments must be analysed with some distinctions. In agreement with our results, a value of 2,000 ms roughly enters the time range required to obtain the shortest reaction time of the examinee in delayed reactions, i.e. to maximize the excitability of the neural assembly responsible for the task execution. However, this time corresponds to a certain number of recurrent internal circuits. In contrast, the single internal circuit of spontaneous speech remains in the order of 250 ms with relatively small variations according to the parameters of the task to be carried out.

Paulesu et al. [1993a, b] tried to identify by PET the underlying anatomofunctional substrate including the slave system or servo-subsystem of the articulatory loop. They concluded that 'Broca's area may represent the rehearsal system, while the parietal lobe may correspond to a phonological buffer'.

2.5.4
A Relevant Neuromodellistic Analysis

An accurate model of short-term memory processes proposed in 1968 was reported in our previous essay on speech control [Pinelli and Ceriani, 1992] with reference to iconic (related to the visual channel) processes. It was a two-component model, including buffers and short-term stores, with two operative conditions. In the simpler condition, corresponding to an immediate reaction, the flow of neural activities ensuring the language operations, develops in line.

In the second condition, the neural flow stops in appropriate stores, where it is unpacked in a following phase of 200–250 ms. In this condition the short-term store has some connection with working memories.

In fact, the short-term store box contains several processes: control, decision revision and recall strategy. Moreover, it is both ways connected to long-term stores related to permanent memory.

In the sensory short-term store records, the codes are closely fitting the physical characteristics of the stimulus, and the traces have a very short duration: according to Curtiss and Tallal [1991], the iconic memory does not last more than 250 ms, but it has a large capacity for verbal stimuli.

The peculiar role of the working memory for the control of the information flow and in relation with consciousness constraints has been underlined. However, at that time, no specific methodological studies were carried out to differentiate short-term-active memory and recall, versus more automatic working memories.

The modal-type model was further developed by Baddeley [1985, 1992; Baddeley et al., 1986] and by Cornoldi [1995] in more complex multicomponential models. In the visuospatial short-term store, Shallice [1988] included a subsystem with specific visual components for verbal stimuli, working for phonological recodification and articulatory rehearsal.

2.5.5
The Internal Feedbacks and the Hebbian Assembly:
A Neurophysiological Interpretation of Focused Attention

Hinton et al. [1993], reproducing a faithful model of dyslexia, developed an integrated concept of internal feedbacks (fig. 17) that greatly improves our interpretation of the processes involved in the intermediary function attributed to some sort of buffer. It is worthwhile stressing that the analysis of Hinton's internal feedbacks is connected with the classical principles of reverberating activity, first advanced more than 50 years ago by Lorente de No [1938] and elaborated by McKay later [1987].

In our blueprint of immediate reading reactions, the internal feedbacks can be thought to represent a process passing immediately from the central sensorimotor computations to the programming PDP phase. In fact the internal recurrent feedbacks will provide a facilitation and possibly a re-organization of the neural assemblies activated in the sensorimotor computations.

With a view to offer a more detailed description, we might envisage a reverberatory activity that, repeating itself in previously activated neurons, can be modified by afferent impulses and exerts a homogeneous facilitation of the synaptic permeability of the neural network. As a consequence of this facilitation, the internal output of the acquired (low-threshold) neural assembly might be promptly and efficiently triggered in the final phase of speech production.

The core of our study has been confined to the actual ongoing processes occurring during the pronunciation of a word, a performance which is thought to require a phase of focused attention. This corresponds to a mental operation [Cohen, 1993], even if at an unconscious level with an underlying process of organization of the hebbian assemblies. Posner and Dehane [1994] speculated about the appearance of the attentional effects generally as a *suppression of unattended information*, early in the processing stream and as an enhancement of relevant information later on. The frontal areas, with the prevalence of the right one, appear to be involved with a network including at least portions of the basal ganglia and of the anterior cingulate gyrus. The anterior portion of the cingulate gyrus appears to develop a wide range of activities termed collectively 'executive autonomous functions'.

In agreement with the neutral conditions maintained in our experiments, we assume that the models adopted by Hinton et al. [1993] are particularly pertinent as a key of interpretation of our investigations. Thus, we will look at the brain processes involved in the control of speech in the light of *internal feedbacks*.

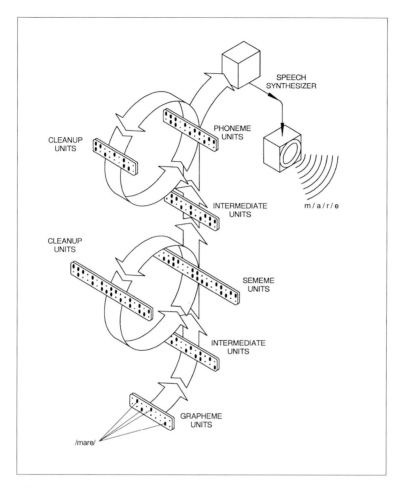

Fig. 17. Network for reading aloud. (1) The neural network for reading contains four layers. The first corresponds to the letters in each word. Connections between input and intermediate units and between intermedate units and 'sememe' units convert the word form to a representation in terms of semantic features, such as size, edibility or aliveness. 'Clean-up' units are connected to sememe units in a feedback loop that adjusts the sememe output to match the meaning of words precisely. (2) The speaking network adds another set of three layers: intermediate units, phoneme units and clean-up units. The sequences of phonemes can then be fed to a speech synthesizer. From Hinton et al. [1993].

This kind of processes can be well reproduced by the most recent models of speech control [Banks, 1991] and fits satisfactorily the sort of reading reactions characterizing our MDRV.

Particularly we refer to the delayed verbal choice reactions that, among other things, afford the possibility of a differential analysis of the sequential chain of cerebral processes in line with the paulesian studies carried out with PET.

In figure 7a and b, a sample of 4 reactions to double random stimuli is reported, with the EMG and voice (ACG) responses. Figure 7a shows EMG and ACG latencies at FP_0. Figure 7b shows the same variables at FP_3. One can easily see the great variability of reaction time and EMG, and of ACG duration and shape. The mean values of ACG latency at FP_0 and at FP_3 were 591 ± 38 and 407 ± 22 ms, respectively.

The heuristic values of the introduction of foreperiods in the execution of reading reactions will be the subject matter of detailed analyses in Section 5. At the moment, to give a preliminary idea of the 'trick' achieved with the delayed reactions, we can anticipate that this experimental setting reproduces in fact a phase of artificial pausing in the development of the executive processes devoted to speech production and control.

2.5.6
Some Observations about Central Cerebral Process Duration and Cyclic Repetitions

In Levelt's blueprint [1989], the above-mentioned articulatory buffer requires an operative time that develops just at the end of the CCP and at the onset of the executive articulatory phase. The classic papers by Libet [1985] and Libet et al. [1991] and the more recent analyses by Markowitsch [1995] and by Plum [1993b] on the operative times of neural processes provide useful references for the interpretation of immediate and delayed reading reactions.

On the grounds of these neurophysiological calculations, we will suggest a preliminary synoptic table, that will be discussed in Section 5 in the light of preliminary measurements. We introduced also a correcting factor in relation to the PDP type of functioning occurring in the first phases of central neural processes: in fact, the time taken in the earliest phase by the sum of the durations of the single individual processes were decreased by roughly calculated 50 %:

(1) The visual perception process can be calculated as approximately 100 ms;
(2) The partly simultaneous transmission from visual centres to frontal areas, supplementary motor area and Broca's area can be reckoned to last about 30 ms (from visual centres to frontal and Broca's areas = 30 ms);
(3) The formulator [Levelt, 1989] process might require a similar lapse of time (30 ms);
(4) The timing process might also last about 30 ms.

On the grounds of these conjectures, however approximate they are, we might now calculate the time that a single cycle of CCP needs to complete one single course and then to facilitate a corresponding neural assembly.

We must take into account the 30 ms of visual centres to frontal and Broca's areas plus 30 ms of the formulator plus 30 ms of the timing processes. We must then add the time of the corticosubcortical loop, which we can assume to correspond to about 100 ms. A cue for this value emerges from the period of the α EEG rhythm, i.e. 10 Hz [Walter, 1953; Woody, 1982]. The total time for the CCP cycle should thus correspond to about 190 ms.

However, a CCP cycle represents a simple instantaneous phasic activity without any consequent dynamic memorization. As we will better analyse later in this review, the production of changes in a neural assembly, leading to a lower threshold, requires a certain number of CCP cycles of internal intrinsic reverberatory feedbacks. Such a repetition could actually secure a facilitating mechanism and could reasonably be identified as the intermediary processes reiterating the programmed patterns of pre-executive impulses. A discriminant point of reference for the request of efficiency of these internal intrinsic reverberatory feedbacks is the value of the neural assembly's *weight,* that is the availability of the corresponding neural assembly representation. An emergent of this availability seems to be the frequency of use of these representations.

The Psychomotor Working Memory – Verbochronometric Expected Results: Differences and Ratios, and Semiological Criteria

2.6.1
Investigation of 'Working Memory' in the Neurological Domain

In spite of its potentially high heuristic value, the assessment of the 'working memories' has been neglected by the neurologists, and it has been accomplished by very few psychiatrists [Thomas et al., 1993; Jerry, 1995]. Moreover, the papers published in this field deal more with deductive inferences than with direct specific measurements. In fact, the latter imply difficult theoretical discriminations and concern still questionable [Cornoldi, 1995] neuropsychological tests. Some of them are quite aspecific, while others imply very sophisticated and complex methodologies [Baddeley, 1992; Baddeley et al., 1984, 1986]. Therefore the caution of the clinicians can hardly be criticized.

Some preliminary trials have been carried out in a few patients, affected by intracranial meningiomas before and after surgery, by a team working in the neurosurgical department of the University of Turin. Asteggiano et al. [1995] defined the working memory as the control processes allowing the subject to keep the information at the level of the short-term memory during a time sufficient to solve the problem, to make a decision or to let the information flow. They measured short-term memory and working memory with the forward and backward digit span tests. In fact, these psychological performances imply attentional and active short-term memory processes: the identification of working memory time among so many interfering factors remains a rather hard task.

The authors indeed associated to the previous tests those for attentional levels in the behavioural field (attentional matrixes). Moreover, in the same patients, they carried out an investigation of event-related potentials and P_{300} acoustic and visual-evoked potentials and studied the correlations between the neuropsychological and the neurophysiological data. The most reliable measured parameter was found to be the latency time of the acoustic and visual P_{300}.

However, the susceptibility of this parameter to the effect of many different factors is so high that its changes can hardly be interpreted as specifically related to only one series of processes like the working memory. The authors claim to have been able to see 'a good trend of correlation between the neuropsychological and the neurophysiological evaluation of the working memory'. They simply found a rather parallel course of the changes occurring in the two different investigations 'before and after the surgical treatment'. It has also to be underlined that very few of their findings were abnormal under basal conditions. Therefore, further research is needed in order to evaluate the actual consistency of these preliminary results.

A more promising methodology with different multiple patterns of acoustic stimuli eliciting the P_{300} has been applied by Jerry [1995] as it will be reported in Section 9 dealing with schizophrenic brain dysfunctions. Anyway, the resort to MDRV seems to be greatly expedient.

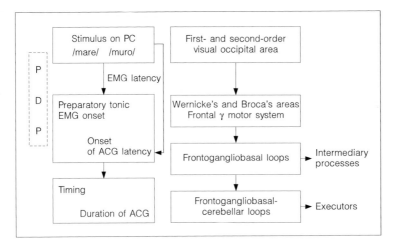

Fig. 18. General blueprint of verbal reading reactions (see also phases 1–4, fig. 13–16). Intermediary processes are prolonged in delayed reactions.

2.6.2
The Heuristic Value of Delayed Reactions

In 2.1., we described the delayed reactions: in comparison to the immediate reactions, the delay (foreperiod) allows the subject to be tested with a prolongation of the period of time during which intermediary processes take place (fig. 18).

The evaluation of the intermediary processes will represent the main issue among the questions related to the principles of psychophysiology emerging from MDRV. The identification of psychomotor working memory among the heterogeneous intermediary processes will represent a leitmotiv in the following sections. It will be discussed from a methodological point of view as a 'trick' to improve the heuristic value of our investigations. The results will be interpreted in relation to the neurophysiological knowledge on the temporal course of the brain processes of psychomotor control.

Their significance will be investigated by screening vast areas of physiological states like old age and many neurological and psychiatric disorders.

However, a careful consideration of inherent pitfalls together with continuous autocriticism are necessary for both the methodological modifications we must consistently adopt and the criteria of evaluation we must propose for the interpretation of the results. In all new methodologies, some artefacts, mistakes and miscalculations may occur, as drifting mines in our path. Therefore it becomes urgent to light the path in its whole course in order to recognize the best accessible ways, the limits for correct inference and its order to make the best use of those findings that seemed to be discriminative among significant alterations of the intermediary processes.

We will now outline the modalities that the intermediary processes may present under different conditions and the alterations that we can identify in the pathological domain.

2.6.3
Measurements and Evaluations of Psychomotor Working Memory

The performance of delayed reactions, with the foreperiod longer than the single CCP, i.e. in the practical application >0.4 s, requires an unconscious mental process that maintains the programmed invariants emerging from the visuomotor early processes active and efficient: these invariants can be conceived in the hebbian terminology as activated neural assembly.

Under normal conditions, the mental process allows a facilitation to occur in the neural assembly that can be triggered when the 'go' signal is shown to the subject. This facilitation results in a shortened reaction time.

However, the processes and factors occurring and interfering during the foreperiod are numerous and heterogeneous. In fact, they correspond to recurrent internal circuits and dynamic biophysical processes concerning the regulation of the facilitated neural assembly threshold at the input and at the internal connections. Consequently, the duration of the single recurrent circuit and the number of recurrent circuits requested for a sufficient facilitation can change with relevant effects on the reaction time.

Moreover, parallel processes take place at the level of invariant-to-variant adaptation.

While these last processes will be analysed in Section 4, we will now discuss the possible methodological approaches to get some cues to these mental intermediary processes. They appear to cause fundamental issues in a functional phase that is undoubtedly linked to the area investigated in cognitive psychology as short memories and working memories. In fact, the recurrent circuit represents an elementary essential brain activity that is common to many mental performances: the results are different according to the hierarchical level where the recurrent circuit occurs and can imply thought, understanding, decision and purposeful actions in delayed tasks.

In our methodology we deal with a process of working memory related to psychomotor performances.

A first way to measure the time taken by the psychomotor working memory could use the differences or/and ratios between the total immediate reaction time (ACG time at FP_0) and the delayed reaction time (ACG time at $FP_{>0.4}$). An obvious condition to be respected for a correct measurement is the foreperiod being longer than the duration of ACG in order to avoid a busy-line effect. This effect will be analysed in Section 8, with relation to a case of marked increase in duration of ACG, due to spastic dysphonia.

2.6.4
A Paradoxical Inversion of the Intermediary Process Ratio and the Resort to Simple Reactions

As we found in systematic researches [Colombo et al., 1993; Pinelli et al., 1995], a lowering in neural assembly threshold or a slowing in reaction time can diminish or even invert the value of the differences and ratios between ACG latency at FP_0 and that at $FP_{>0.4}$.

Inversion of the intermediary process ratio has been found to be pathognomonic for schizophrenia [Pinelli et al., 1995]. This means that the difference between ACG latency at FP_0 and ACG latency at $FP_{1.5}$ can be taken into consideration for an inference on early programming processes only in normals and in non-schizophrenic patients.

Then we turned our interest to simple reactions instead of delayed reactions. The differences and ratios between immediate choice reaction time and simple reaction time may represent a more universal approach to a measurement of the total time taken by intermediary processes (see Section 3).

2.6.5
An Axiomatic Condition Makes Meaningful Heterogeneous Differences and Ratios: Only One Number of the Equation Is Specifically Changed

There is no doubt, as Sternberg [1969] and Peters et al. [1989] observed, that the differences and/or ratios between the reaction times of the same task in different conditions, like immediate and delayed reactions, choice and simple reactions, do not correspond to homogeneous processes, and from this point of view the correspondent products may not indicate a well-defined quantity of whatever process or entity.

With reference to a well-defined factor, these time measurements might be considered as incongruous, but, at the present phase of the research, this is not a sufficient reason, in a diagnostic or physiopathogenetic context, to renounce a priori these 'dirty indices', once one is aware of their limits of informative contents.

In all normal and in most pathological cases, ACG latency at FP_0 – ACG latency at $FP_{>0.4}$ (at the condition foreperiod > duration of ACG) gives a positive result. Its evaluation can be carried out in a mosaic-like context, taking into account an integrated pattern of data.

An axiomatic condition requires that only one member of the equation undergoes a change or that a change of an identical sign affects also the other member. In the difference ACG latency at FP_0 – ACG latency at $FP_{1.5}$ or in the ratio ACG latency at $FP_{1.5}$/ACG latency at FP_0, the second member must remain identical or might increase.

When these criteria are respected, the differences or ratios may be evaluated as indicators of the temporal parameters of the central and intermediary processes. A further differential analysis can be carried out by comparing the different changes of these equations with foreperiods of different duration. Paradigmatic examples will be given in Section 8.

To avoid the interference of specific short-memory impairments in our basal methodology, the task-stimulus is visible on the PC screen until the end of the foreperiod, at the presentation of the 'go' stimulus.

A further justification of these measurements is of semiological nature, i.e. the search for statistically significant differences in the results between well-defined populations. We found in fact an inversion of the ratio ACG latency at $FP_{1.5}$/ACG latency FP_0 (intermediary process; at the condition ACG latency at FP_0 = the normal mean value) to be quite specific for schizophrenics. This finding will be evaluated in more detail in Section 7 in agreement with the principles of psychophysiology previously outlined.

Executive Processes and Simple Reactions

(1)	tACG at FP_0	
(2)	tACG at $FP_{0.1}$	($< tCCP$)
α	(1) – (2) = 0	under normal conditions
β	(1) – (2) < 0	if facilitatory attention occurs
γ	(1) – (2) > 0	if PDP is not available with supplementary open neural channels

Fig. 21. Short foreperiod reactions. t = Latency time.

motoneuron and transmission from brainstem or spinal cord to the muscles and by the muscular processes of transduction activating the contractile mechanisms and producing the muscular twitches. This chain of processes (conduction to spinal cord motoneurons) + (transmission to muscles) + (muscle twitch) will take $5 + 2 + 35 = 42$ ms.

In conclusion, the total event time should be: (occipital lobe to brainstem) + first tuning movement + second phasic movement (ballistic or ramp) + (conduction to spinal cord motoneurons, transmission to muscles, muscle twitch) = $15 + 50 + (20 \text{ or } 30) + 42 = 127$ or 137 ms.

The response considered for the latency time can be indifferently represented by the muscular phasic contraction or *its immediate effect, i.e. the ACG.*

3.1.2
Very Short Foreperiods

It is a rather well-established fact that the sequence of the input (visual) processes takes place in three brain stations: from the retinal bipolar cells to the lateral geniculate nuclei, to the calcarine cortex and to the visual association areas. On the other side, the final motoneural output processes develop in a sequence of three parallel descending systems of 4, 3 and 2 relays, respectively. They are the systems of the motor cortex-brainstem-spinal-interneurons-anterior horn cells, the corticospinal-spinal interneurons-anterior horn cells and the corticospinal-anterior horn cells.

These serial processes develop along 'encapsulated' [Fodor, 1983] pathways of impulses. On the contrary CCP (frontal-brainstem), first tuning and second phasic processes are carried out in PDP networks [Rosenfeld, 1993].

In order to open a window in such PDP networks, we introduced in our tests a very short foreperiod, shorter than the duration of the total CCP (fig. 21). An investigation with five different foreperiods in the range of 0.1–0.2 s showed that the 0.1-second foreperiod could be chosen as the most convenient for our research (see for more details 7.2, fig. 59).

The rationale to adopt this short foreperiod has already been explained in the previous chapters dealing with the general principles of the MDRV. Now, we can analyse the effects that this early 'go' signal might induce in the series of neural CCP and the respective operative times.

The functional condition of a PDP network reaches its best efficiency when there is a high number of available channels for a quasi-simultaneous development of the internal circuits related to CCP1 (preparation or preprogramming) and CCP2 (programming).

In normals, the equilibrium must be maintained particularly at the interface with the final executive pathways that must receive the incoming descending impulses in due time and regular succession. This precise matching is provided by a redundancy of transmitters and receptors. In the long run, biochemical and biophysical molecular feedbacks can induce neuroplastic adaptations that should favour the interface equilibrium. These complex mechanisms allow a determined range of abnormal changes to be compensated within a limit called 'safety factor'.

When these prerequisites are respected during a shortly delayed reaction, the perception of the 'go' signal by the subject will not interfere negatively with the still active internal circuit (condition α in fig. 21) but could even act as a reinforcing stimulus accelerating the ongoing processes (condition β). On the contrary, if the functional basic conditions requested for a PDP network are in some way impaired – as it could happen in case of neuronal or synaptic loss – the time requested to fulfil the reaction could increase significantly (condition γ).

An Analysis of the Word Acousticogram

3.2.1
Zooming in the Word Acousticogram: Its Formation and the Variables of Its Utterance – Importance and Convenience of Its Recording

The ACG appears to be an immediate and reliable objective representation of the whole sequence of kinetic and air pressure changes produced by the coordinated action of respiratory, glottal and supraglottic muscles. This is particularly true for the phasic activity reproducing the phonological sequence of the word but also, even if more indirectly, for the preparatory tuning phase [Abbs, 1973; Gracco, 1987]. As previously stated, the main features of the ACG will be identified by recording its latency time and its duration and by delimiting its frequency spectrogram (fig. 22 and 23a–c).

Before analysing all these variables, we must define the ACG sample recorded in MDRV.

3.2.2
Acousticogram of the Single Word

The heuristic value of the phonological analysis of single words has clearly been demonstrated since 1978 by Sternberg et al.

Following their statement, we adopted pairs of words as stimuli in the choice reactions in the two series of our research. The heuristic value of a comparison of reaction times to word tasks with respect to sentence tasks – as we began to do in our third series of research – is clear in itself. What we wanted to explain in advance, with specific relation to brain motor control, was the great complexity of the neural origin of the pronunciation

(1) Mean tACG and SD of 12 reactions, in *neutral* conditions, with FP_0

(2) Mean tACG and SD of 12 reactions, in *neutral* conditions, with $FP_{0.5-1.5\,s}$
The measured value (2) = the executive time

(1) tACG at FP_0 – (2) tACG at $FP_{1.5}$ = tCCP

(3) Mean DACG with FP_0

(4) Mean DACG with $FP_{0.5-1.5\,s}$
The measured value (4) = the executors' diadochokinetic time

(3) – (4) = time taken by the central timing processes

Fig. 22. Variables in word reading reactions. t = Latency time; D = duration.

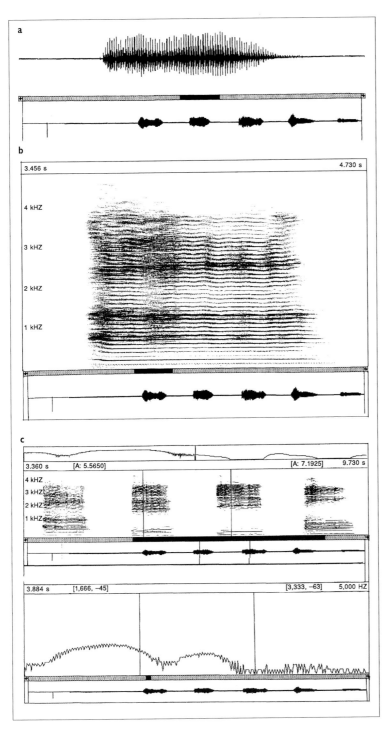

Fig. 23 a–c. ACG recordings of /mare/: one response at high speed of the tracer, five successive responses at low speed of the tracer. A = Analogue conditioning of the signal.

of a word. We have to acknowledge the intricate chain of processes and representations implied in the sensorimotor computational operations requested to utter a word.

If we disregard this essential fact while comparing grammatical to phonological performances, one would be, at first glance, rather attracted by the greater complexity of the grammatical formulation of the sentence. Likewise, the conceptualization from the idea to the sentence [Levelt, 1989], the nearly infinite modifications and modulations produced by the prosodic control in spontaneous speech [Mehler et al., 1991] appear also to the most ingenuous student to require a very complex series of neural events.

On the contrary, the brain processes involved in the production of the articulatory movements to utter a word from a pair could be imagined by an artless student to represent a rather scanty part of the brain control of speech. Against this opinion, in agreement with Lieberman [1991] and Greenfield [1991], we stress again the fact that the complexity of the brain operations involved in the production of the word utterance from its visual image is not inferior to those required for grammatical formulations and prosodic modulations.

We will return now to the preliminary blueprint outlining the main processes and representations involved in spoken language, analyse their original genesis and discuss the findings yielded by the investigations carried out with MDRV of two-word stimuli.

We have already mentioned how one does not yet know exactly which is – in the different languages – the prototypic subword unit with the minimal number of phonemes. If it is true that the syllable seems to be the prototyp in the Latin languages, some cues in Anglo-Saxon languages and – in a different way – in Japanese speak in favour of a subsyllabic unit [Saito, 1992].

Research carried out with 6-month-old children demonstrated that the prototype is learned by imitation from speakers in the environment [Mehler et al., 1991]. But there are *linguistic* factors involved in the perception of infants of 1–2 months of age as it was ascertained with the evaluation of the movements of sucking reactions taken as conditioned responses [Eimas, 1974, 1975].

It was found that there are prototypes which are more quickly perceived and pronounced than others. These results were interpreted to prove that there are graded units with different degrees of goodness [Beckman and Edwards, 1991; Tokhura et al., 1992].

These phonological mechanisms correspond to biomechanical and kinetic requests of pronunciation that can be included in the sector of *constraints* reported in our blueprint. Moreover, the identification of the phonological unit is undoubtedly related to the processes of speech production but, as far as our present research is concerned, they involve a quite specialized field of research: the assumption of the *syllable* as phonetic unit [Levelt, 1993] is an acceptable criterion for a methodology aimed to investigate mainly the neural CCP.

The heuristic value of the word reading tests in MDRV was proven just in the first phase of our research with the confirmation of Sternberg's findings on the time taken by accenting, by multisyllabic words, by unusual words and non-words [Pinelli and Ceriani, 1992]. The word reading tests yielded statistically validated differences in the child's maturation cycle, aging and pathological conditions. These tests are easily accessible also for psychiatric patients. Moreover, comparative and longitudinal investigations with MDRV allow the neurologist to differentiate primary from secondary slow-downs and direct impairments from compensatory readjustments.

In a previous study we reported the theoretical considerations and experimental evidence of the common processes and mechanisms in the production of speech and those of manual purposeful actions: artificial connective networks with an analogous set of

Table 1. Verbal reaction times (ms) for /clock/ and /camel/ (G.J., English-speaking, female, 24 years old)

	ACG latency at FP_0	ACG latency at FP_3	Difference
/clock/			
EMG	265±38 (216–342)	200±52 (127–302)	65
ACG	491±38 (403–547)	315±35 (271–404)	176
/camel/			
EMG	283±56 (226–429)	196±47 (124–290)	87
ACG	500±30 (443–555)	330±78 (213–522)	170

(Boxed values between columns: +18, +9, +15)

FP_0, FP_3 = Foreperiods of 0 and 3 s; difference = ACG latency at FP_0 – ACG latency at FP_3. Results are means ± SD, with ranges in parentheses.

mechanisms and hidden unit layers were envisaged by several authors [Banks, 1991]. If specialized sectors of psychomotility were studied, the principles guiding the MDRV methodology could be applied to set tasks and responses specific for that sector.

3.2.3
MDRV Results of Pairs of Mono- and Disyllabic Tasks, Non-Word Trisyllabic Tasks and Double Disyllabic Tasks

3.2.3.1
Five-Letter Mono- and Disyllabic Words

In table 1, we report the ACG latency values for the 5-letter English words /clock/ and /camel/, read by a young native English-speaking normal subject. These word stimuli are those of the milestone experiment by Sternberg on the accentuation effect.

In table 2, we report the results of reading reactions by native Italian-speaking normal subjects of different ages, for the 4-letter mono- and disyllabic words /clan/ and /cane/.

3.2.3.2
Pairs of Non-Words

In figures 24–27, 8 tracings are shown of a 21-reaction trial of the two non-words /ubavek/ and /ubamek/ presented at random to the subjects. The values of ACG latency, at FP_0 are given in table 3.

Table 2. Reading reaction times (ms) of 34 normal subjects

Age, years		Immediate reaction				Delayed reaction (foreperiod: 3 s)			
range	mean	/clan/		/cane/		/clan/		/cane/	
		EMG	ACG	EMG	ACG	EMG	ACG	EMG	ACG
16–25	21.6	232 ± 44	497 ± 39	225 ± 36	470 ± 36	171 ± 27	377 ± 47	164 ± 32	376 ± 48
(n = 8)		158; 289	417; 550	156; 275	410; 526	131; 202	315; 440	142; 228	309; 449
26–35	29	244 ± 57	449 ± 52	221 ± 31	437 ± 61	158 ± 42	332 ± 66	160 ± 33	335 ± 62
(n = 10)		172; 365	383; 541	185; 265	354; 529	123; 256	266; 459	109; 225	252; 434
36–60	54.3	267 ± 74	551 ± 64	253 ± 61	530 ± 41	169 ± 23	427 ± 56	169 ± 13	436 ± 46
(n = 7)		192; 396	480; 673	200; 357	456; 590	140; 199	322; 479	141; 180	341; 474
61–78	67.7	313 ± 50	585 ± 54	299 ± 39	553 ± 52	184 ± 26	381 ± 49	177 ± 20	385 ± 45
(n = 9)		251; 406	472; 641	240; 354	441; 640	144; 217	308; 455	152; 211	329; 462

n = Number of subjects. For both immediate and delayed reactions, results are means ± SD, with maximum and minimum values indicated below each mean.

3.2.3.3
Pairs of Disyllabic Words

In figures 28–33, a series of 4 tracings is shown out of 80 reactions, to the pair of the disyllabic words /mare/ and /muro/.

In tables 4–6, the 3 original series of 24 successive ACG reactions is reported at FP_0, $FP_{0.1}$ and $FP_{1.5}$ as well as $FP_{0.5}$ and FP_4.

In table 7, we present the results of MDRV in 26 normal subjects in three age groups, examined in 1992. In figure 34, a partial and simplified diagram is given, for a general view of the changes of ACG latency at FP_0, $FP_{0.1}$ and $FP_{1.5}$ in the three different age groups.

3.2.4
The Latency Time of the Acousticogram: Mean Values, Jitter and Standard Deviations in Longitudinal Studies of Normal Subjects and in Investigations of the Same Subject by Various Examiners

The measurements of ACG latency gave quite reliable and constant results. A comparison of the values obtained by different examiners and with manual measurements versus computers [Colombo et al., 1993] did not show differences greater than 1 ms, which is less than 3 %. On the other hand, the SD value of ACG latency mean values measured in the series of 12 reactions of one individual subject is of the order of 7–12 % in young and middle-aged subjects: this is at least +300 % of the value which could be due

Fig. 24–27. The word pair /ubavek/ and /ubamek/ presented at random to subject P.S., male, 30 years old (reaction numbers in parentheses). EGG = Electroglottogram; OS = musculus orbicularis oris superior; OI = m. orbicularis oris inferior; DIG = m. digastricus, pars anterior.

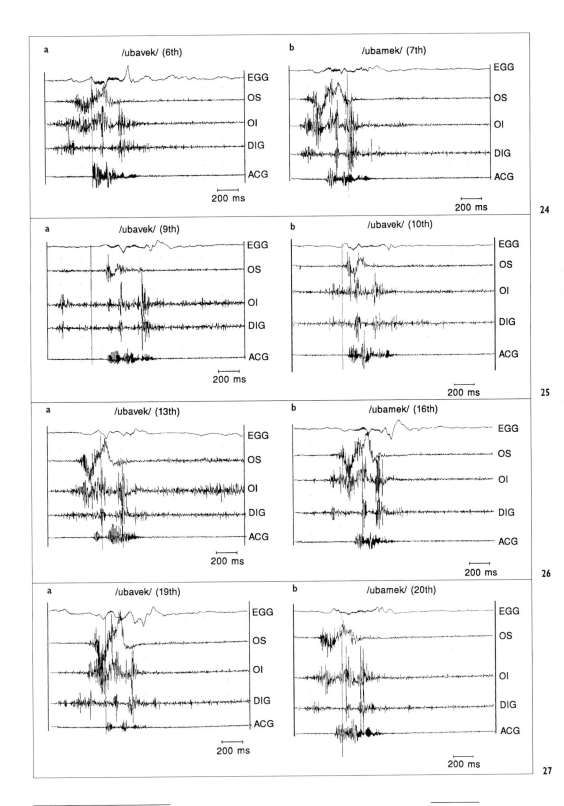

Table 3. ACG latencies (ms) at FP_0

Stimulus	/ubavek/	/ubamek/
1	493	
2		448
3		852
4	476	
5		881
6	412	
7		398
8	426	
9	908	
10	791	
11		583
12		897
13	512	
14		769
15	676	
16		646
17	702	
18	510	
19	598	
20		360
21		600
Mean	591 ± 160 (412 – 908)	613 ± 180 (360 – 881)

Some tracings are reported in figures 24–27.

Table 4. ACG latencies (ms) at FP_0

Stimulus	/mare/	/muro/
1	625	
2		513
3	330	
4	592	
5		493
6		479
7	454	
8		465
9		568
10	441	
11	450	
12		364
13	562	
14		467
15	395	
16	417	
17		509
18		514
19	427	
20		447
21		472
22	379	
23	460	
24		385
Mean	461 ± 88 (330 – 625)	472 ± 56 (364 – 568)

P.S., female, 52 years old, middle school education, IQ = 99. Hand reaction time: 281 ± 25 ms (219 ± 341). Hamilton Rating Scale for Depression: in the normal range.

Some tracings are reported in figures 28 and 29.

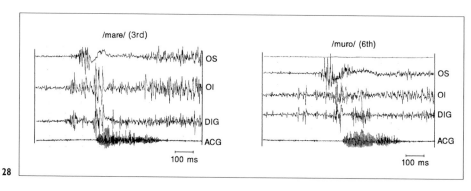

Fig. 28–33. Presentation of the word pair /mare/ and /muro/ to subject P.S., male, 30 years old, at FP_0 (**28, 29**), $FP_{0.1}$ (**30**), $FP_{1.5}$ (**31**), $FP_{0.5}$ (**32**) and FP_4 (**33**). For explanations, see figure 24.

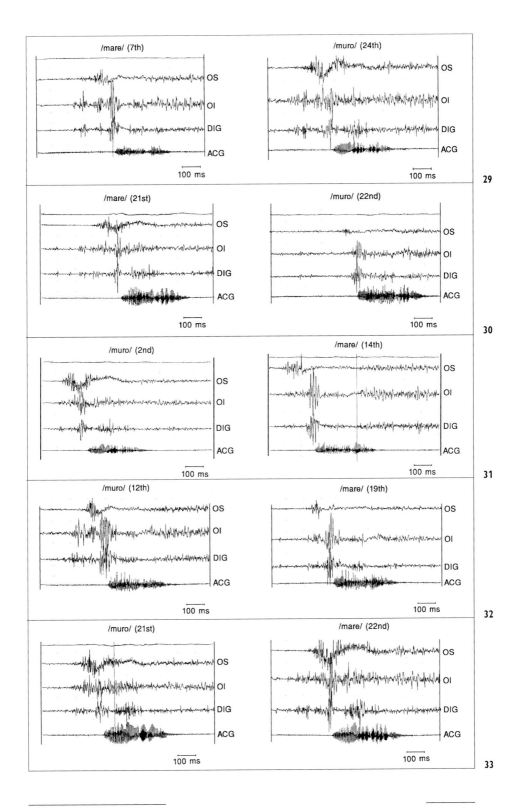

Stimulus	/mare/ FP$_{0.1}$	FP$_{1.5}$	/muro/ FP$_{0.1}$	FP$_{1.5}$
1	691			
2				292
3		322		
4		290		
5			497	
6				447
7			366	
8				400
9		254		
10	685			
11			373	
12	471			
13		346		
14		285		
15			497	
16				556
17	458			
18			446	
19				640
20		373		
21	464			
22			524	
Mean	554 ± 123 (458 – 691)	312 ± 44 (254 – 373)	450 ± 68 (366 – 524)	467 ± 135 (292 – 640)

to technical errors dependent on the accuracy limit of the instruments. In the group of oldest subjects the SD is higher, in a range of 10–30 %.

The SD of ACG latency mean values likely reflects multiple factors of variability. A detailed analysis of these factors will be carried out later, when we will discuss the concept of jitter at both theoretical and applicative levels. On the other hand, we intend to describe here the variability factors with reference to the most correct methodology.

In a rather rough scheme we can classify the variability factors in two main groups: (a) the central neural factors and (b) the biomechanical factors.

The central neural variability is strictly related to what the physicist denominates a *stochastic* kind of function and the biologist observes as a *trial-and-error* kind of functioning.

Which are in fact the processes and the elementary activities recurring in successive cycles with a determined degree of variability? We can identify three levels in this preliminary analysis: (1) the CCP in the corticosubcortical loops; (2) the multiple feedbacks involved in the adaptation processes; (3) the repetitive discharges of the motor units innervating the vocal cords with defined variations in number and frequency of recruitment [Pinelli, 1989].

These variabilities do not occur quite at random but respect a regular range of values within certain limits. In fact, it is a common statement, confirmed by our experience,

Table 6. Complete series of
ACG latencies (ms) at various
foreperiods corresponding to
figures 32 and 33

Stimulus	/mare/		/muro/	
	$FP_{0.5}$	FP_4	$FP_{0.5}$	FP_4
1	508			
2				336
3		290		
4		280		
5			476	
6				316
7	403			
8			370	
9				310
10		293		
11	340			
12			417	
13	365			
14				373
15		334		
16		320		
17			470	
18				328
19	367			
20			363	
21				357
22		365		
23	403			
24			428	
Mean	398 ± 59	314 ± 32	421 ± 48	337 ± 24
	$(340 - 508)$	$(280 - 365)$	$(363 - 476)$	$(310 - 373)$

that a series of 12 trials produces a reliable mean value that might represent a marker of brain functionality of that individual person, i.e. a kind of marker within the limits of stability of the human psychobiological identity [Welford, 1980]. We found that in normal adult subjects, who did not repeat the test in the meantime, the mean latency times do not vary more than $\pm 10\%$ during periods as long as 6 months.

3.2.5
The Duration of the Acousticogram

With reference to a single word, like /mare/ or /muro/, the measurement of the ACG duration by different examiners and manual methods versus computers does not show any variation greater than 3%. On the contrary, the SD of ACG duration amounts to 10% in a series of 12 successive reactions, roughly corresponding to that of ACG latency. As far as the oldest subjects are concerned, no increases in ACG duration as high as those of the SD of ACG latency were found. In conclusion, in individual old subjects, only the SD of the ACG latency increases whilst the SD of the ACG duration does not change in comparison to the young subjects. One should then infer that, at variance with the stochastic factor of the preparatory and programming CCP, the stochastic factor of timing

Table 7. Results of MDRV in 26 normal subjects

Age years	/mare/					/muro/				
	direct	0.1s	0.5s	1.5s	4s	direct	0.1s	0.5s	1.5s	4s
ACG latency										
18–44 (n = 10)	381 ± 54	386 ± 56	325 ± 49	310 ± 70	320 ± 57	371 ± 48	345 ± 50	333 ± 49	306 ± 70	315 ± 78
45–59 (n = 11)	494 ± 75	498 ± 104	420 ± 68	376 ± 93	387 ± 65	499 ± 64	488 ± 100	426 ± 90	385 ± 83	385 ± 76
60–80 (n = 5)	622 ± 156	757 ± 200	517 ± 67	502 ± 122	448 ± 101	616 ± 183	715 ± 136	530 ± 62	509 ± 140	473 ± 113
ACG duration										
18–44 (n = 10)	323 ± 76	287 ± 63	297 ± 63	301 ± 54	304 ± 54	319 ± 81	283 ± 64	284 ± 61	299 ± 62	293 ± 47
45–59 (n = 11)	339 ± 55	329 ± 37	334 ± 39	350 ± 36	347 ± 31	350 ± 54	324 ± 33	340 ± 40	354 ± 48	346 ± 26
60–80 (n = 5)	446 ± 85	441 ± 21	422 ± 36	436 ± 36	425 ± 40	474 ± 94	424 ± 36	419 ± 36	426 ± 44	422 ± 35
ACG latency – EMG latency										
18–44 (n = 10)	122 ± 34			97 ± 47		127 ± 21			105 ± 26	
45–59 (n = 11)	153 ± 56			136 ± 66		183 ± 63			164 ± 37	
60–80 (n = 5)				202 ± 63		228 ± 64			208 ± 86	

n = Number of subjects. Results are means ± SD, indicated in milliseconds.

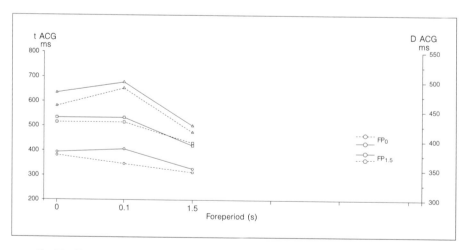

Fig. 34. Changes of ACG latency (t) and duration (D) of /mare/ (———) and /muro/ (-----) in three different age groups: ○ = ACG1, subjects 18–44 years old, n = 10; □ = ACG2, subjects 45–59 years old, n = 11; △ = ACG3, subjects 60–80 years old, n = 5. For standard deviations, see text. Mean ACG durations only for the young group, at FP_0 and $FP_{1.5}$, are given on the right of the figure.

and diadochokinetic processes revealed by SD of ACG duration does not increase in old age or is compensated by some correcting or stabilizing mechanism.

3.2.6
From ACG Latency and Duration to the Formants: Further Specifications How to Instruct the Candidate

In order to obtain reliable results, particular care must be given to homogenize the psychological conditions that could influence the speed and the accuracy of the utterance: the subject must be instructed about the speed and clarity requested for the target word.

In fact, Peters et al. [1989] carried out some experiments requiring the subjects to perform reactions with three different velocities. The examiners paid due attention to the inverted proportionality between reaction speed and accuracy of utterances [Abbs et al., 1984]. It was found that speed affects not only duration but also latency time. Therefore a correct comparative intra-individual and interindividual evaluation of both latency time and duration implies the variable 'accuracy' to be measured exactly. This can be done with voice spectrography. In fact, the spectrographic examination can show the formants of the word according to some principles that we will explain in the next chapter.

The modalities the subject adopts in carrying out the reactions influence the features of the voice spectrograms. As it has been clearly specified in our premises, we refer to a 'neutral' pronunciation and the subject is asked to give an immediate response to the stimulus. This request should automatically imply a high speed of utterance. However, this does not necessarily mean that it corresponds to the highest speed the subject is able to reach. In fact, the examiner does not urge the subject to accelerate during the series of reactions in our methodology. In the experiments carried out by Peters et al. [1989], several encouragements to react as quickly as possible were given to the subject.

Further investigations with higher and lower velocities of utterance and with the request of clear pronunciation represent a development of a more specialized research.

Other important rules concern the choice of the word stimulus to be presented on the PC. The ACG duration can change in relation to the reciprocal position of consonants and vowels. With reference to the simple phonemes, it was found that its duration can change after lexical and accenting factors [Beckman and Edwards, 1991].

As Sternberg has shown since 1978, the ACG duration is increased proportionally to the number of syllables in the word and the rarity of its use. This effect was found to be evident in the immediate reactions but disappears in reactions with foreperiods.

3.2.7
Sound Spectrography

The speech chain, from the physics to the biology of spoken language, has been clearly described by Denes and Puison [1993]. Sound waves generated by our vocal organs are almost never sinusoidal and can be periodic or aperiodic. They all, of whichever kind, can be represented as the sum of a number of sinusoidal waves of different frequencies, amplitudes and phases (Fourier's analysis).

For periodic waves, the frequency of each component is a whole number of one common frequency which corresponds to the period of the whole wave and is called the 'fundamental frequency'; the others are called harmonic.

Aperiodic waves can have components of all frequencies. The vocal cords produce buzz-like sounds which enter the vocal tract. This acts as a resonator: it has certain natural frequencies of vibration and responds more readily to a sound whose frequency is similar to its resonant frequency. The vocal tract can assume many resonant shapes.

Resonances of the vocal tract are called 'formants' and their frequencies the formant frequencies. Every configuration of the vocal tract has its own set of characteristic formant frequencies.

Computer-based digital sound spectrographs allow to obtain frequency-time-intensity displays of the word utterance. The time is indicated along the horizontal axis and the frequency along the vertical axis; the darkness of the traces indicates the intensity level of the spectral components. The vowel pronunciation is characterized by 4 formants; the sound quality is altered during diphthongs with the same vowel and a formant change. The extensive movements of formants and other spectral features are an indication of the rapid movement of the tongue and lips during speech. The movement of these articulators changes the shape of the vocal tract, which in turn changes its resonances and thereby the spectral peaks of formants.

Thus the spectrogram of the voice allows an objective identification of accuracy of the response. If a subject in the verbal reaction time test favours speed of performance at the expense of accuracy, the spectrogram can show the loss of some formants and other changes in amplitude and intensity (fig. 23).

In relation with the variations of the ACG shape, it may be mentioned here that both pitch and loudness of speech are characterized by fluctuations corresponding to the so-called pink or flicker noise [Keele, 1982]. Pitch and loudness carry information and are therefore subject to the constraints that exist generally in communication. Their spectral properties may be due to the fact that flicker noise represents an optimal compromise between efficient transfer of information (maximized by white noise) and immunity to error.

Further factors involved in ACG variations will be discussed later, with reference to the jitter phenomena (see 4.4.5).

3.2.8
The Importance of the Oromandibular Electromyogram

As we have previously stated, word ACG recording remains the fundamental part of MDRV. The ACG response represents the final result of all CCP of speech control. It emerges from the resonances in the different shapes of the vocal tract created by the contraction of a series of muscles of the vocal organs, innervated in a coordinated purposeful action: the utterance of the word. In previous sections, we have underlined the importance of knowing the role played by each single muscular compartment: its stiffness is tuned during the preparatory phase in order to optimize the cycles of shortening and lengthening in the final articulatory phase.

The order of innervation of each, the degree of synchronization and the number and frequency rate of recruited motor units represent precious cues for the way how the whole chain of neural operations develops in producing the correct word utterance [Barlow and Muller, 1991; Titze, 1991].

We should then record the activities and the related effects of the single groups of muscles, beside the word ACG. Muscular contractions elicit *forces* (changes in tension) and *displacements* (changes in length) that can be measured at the level of the muscles themselves or the related organs (chest, glottis, palate, uvula, pharynx, tongue, jaw and lips) or as expiratory flow of air [Bell-Berti and Harris, 1981; McLean, 1991]. Transducers of forces and a series of multiple devices were created and applied in these investigations [Baken, 1987]. However, they are rather complicated and require an intensive collaboration of the subjects to be examined; in fact, they are carried out in laboratories of basic experimental research. *An advantageous alternative for routine investigations has been offered by the EMG.*

Recording muscle action potentials reliably reflects the innervation producing every kind of contraction, both isotonic (with change in length) and isometric (with change in tension). The EMG can be obtained quite easily by means of small surface electrodes. After a preliminary series of researches with simultaneous kinematic and electrographic recordings, we included in our verbal reactions only the EMG associated with the recording of the word ACG.

However, an EMG recording requires a series of rules that must be followed with great care. One must, first of all, identify the muscles which to record the EMG from, then find out which is the optimal site where to apply the recording electrodes [Fromkin and Ladefoged, 1966; Gay and Harris, 1971; Harris, 1981; Kennedy and Abbs, 1979; McLean, 1991].

Moreover in order to compare actual homogeneous events revealed by EMG and by ACG (or kinematic changes), respectively, one must know the temporal delay that normally elapses between the EMG onset and the corresponding kinematic changes. In fact, the air vibrations recorded in the ACG immediately follow the muscular contractions. Therefore, when we compare the onset of EMG with that of myograms (or kinematic recordings), or of ACG, we must add the delay between the EMG and the myogram (or ACG) to the latency time of the EMG as a factor of homologation to the latency time of the ACG.

We recorded simultaneously EMG and myograms (fig. 6) of orbicularis oris, masseter, temporalis and digastric (anterior part) muscles, and of the movements of lips and jaws, respectively. It was found that none of these muscles was activated as primum movens for the /mare/ utterance. The earliest activation occurred in the pterygoideus medialis, the activity of which could be recorded only by means of Adrian's concentric needle electrode.

Saito et al. [1992] recorded both EMG and kinematic changes also of respiratory and glottic muscles and determined the precise order of activation of the different parts of the vocal tract for different phonemes in different contexts.

Some authors [Perkell and Oka, 1980; Schönle and Grone, 1992; Schönle et al., 1992] recorded also the movements produced by the endocavitary muscles of the pharynx, palate and tongue (dorsal body and tip) with a complex instrument producing three-dimensional electromagnetic fields, as it will be better analysed in the next chapter.

Our present research is not specifically concerned with the activity of the speech endocavitary organs; we have adopted only surface EMG recordings that provide the most detailed information on the activity of the oromandibular muscles.

It was shown that the oromandibular muscles are activated very early in /mare/ and /muro/ utterances, immediately after the pterygoideus medialis and just before the onset of the expiratory movement. Thus, for routine reading reactions, we chose the orbicularis oris EMG as a reliable cue for the preparatory innervation [Pinelli and Ceriani, 1992]. A further advantage of this method is that it does not create any discomfort for the subject.

3.2.8.1
Onset and Cessation of Motor Unit Recruitment

We adopted the EMG recording not only to identify the onset of the earliest response in verbal reactions but also with the intention to discriminate its preparatory and phasic executive phases. However, this is a quite difficult task indeed and we can face it only as an attempt to better define the relation between the onset and development of the motor unit recruitment and the course of the ACG. Some interesting cues were found with the analysis of plurisyllabic words and particularly of non-words, like /ubavek/, which is pronounced with a fragmentation of the EMG in relation to each syllable. In the last series of investigations with a triple task, including the sentence /mare è bello/, we focused our measurements on the EMG of this long utterance with well-defined intervals, in order to perform a more detailed comparative analysis of the different phases of the EMG.

For the above-mentioned reasons, we recorded the orbicularis oris surface EMG, but we added the EMG of the digastric muscle to obtain an agonistic-antagonistic simultaneous tracing during cyclic movements of closing and opening the mouth.

3.2.8.2
The Onset of the Electromyogram

There are often a few random motor unit action potentials occurring before the actual onset of the EMG response. They might be due to some 'tonic' or 'tensive' basal activity. If a better relaxation cannot be obtained, we must choose the onset of the EMG response at the beginning of an *intermediary* (i.e. with a 50% decrease in number of recruited motor units) or *interference pattern* of discharges. If the placement of the electrodes is correct, the onset is rather sharp and the localization of the point of measurement for the response onset is accordingly easy; otherwise some attempts to better apply the recording electrodes must be made.

3.2.8.3
The Outline of the Electromyogram with Reference to Tonic and Phasic Innervation

Since the earliest process of speech motor control is devoted to the innervation producing the most suitable neuromuscular stiffness, it seems rational to assume that the first part of the EMG corresponds to this preparatory or tuning phase. One should assume that no clear-cut silent period separates it from the successive phasic activity that develops to shape the vocal tract according to the resonances requested for each phonological unit. In fact, in spite of the marked variations characterizing the series of 12 repetitions of the reaction, a common feature seems to emerge in the EMG, with a diphasic shape.

The variations in EMG latency can be attributed once again to the stochastic kind of functioning in intensity of recruitment.

One should also forecast variations in EMG duration depending on the temporal delay between the tonic and the phasic phases.

In spite of these variations, the intrinsic duality of processes still appears to the electromyographist as a waxing and waning amplitude corresponding to the diphasic shape and creating a sort of 'dromedary outline'. On the grounds of the temporal correlation between the *two* phases and the ACG, we can propose that the onset of the second dome or spindle in the dromedary outline might correspond to the passage from the preparatory to the phasic articulatory innervation.

Even if this seems to be valid at a semiological level for the first phonological unit in the word, it could hardly be extended to the evaluation of the successive units. In such a complex situation, a more detailed comparison of selective single motor unit identification and voice spectrography of the single phonological units in the ACG may yield meaningful results [Titze, 1991].

3.2.8.4
Can We Identify the Cessation of the Electromyogram?

The identification of the end of the EMG is often an intricate task. We can only propose to consider as end point the onset of a silent period lasting at least 300 ms. A few discharges after the intermediary-interfering EMG can be due to reflex tonic activity and may be discarded from the measurement. The occurrence of some EMG activity in the antagonistic muscle can help to localize the cessation of the actual executive performance since it corresponds to a regular modality of stopping an action in the general organization of motor control [Pinelli, 1964; Schieppati et al., 1985].

3.2.9
The Electroglottogram

A small instrument (the electroglottograph) can record the changes in impedance due to the movements of the vocal cords occurring below two electrodes attached to the skin on each side of the larynx. During the word utterance, the electroglottogram shows a slow displacement of the basal line followed by the *glottic* ACG produced by the air vibrations of the vocal cords [Baken, 1987]. A non-invasive EMG measurement of laryngeal muscles has been carried out by Yoshida et al. [1993]. The measurement of the latency of the electroglottogram and particularly of the difference between its latency and that of the ACG was found to be of primary importance to identify glottic dystonia, as it is the case in spastic dysphonia or some iatrogenic dyskinesias.

The search for primary alterations in the executors, like the vocal folds, represents a preliminary requirement in the evaluation of an increase in ACG latency at FP_0. In fact, secondary upwards repercussions can occur: brain processes related to programming and intermediary operations can be altered as a consequence of primary defects in executors.

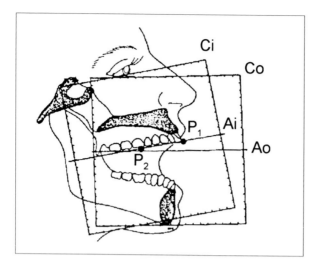

Fig. 35. Selection of a reproducible frame of reference for the definition of a coordinate system. P_1 = Point in front of the embrasure of the upper incisors; P_2 = point at a distance approximately 4 cm from the first point in the midsagittal plane at the level of the occlusional plane; Ao, Co = plane of the open mouth; Ai, Ci = plane of slight occlusion. Modified from Schönle et al. [1992].

Executors can be impaired at the level of either the neural motor systems, the muscles or the articulations themselves.

Upward repercussions and their revertibility can be studied with follow-up investigations of spastic dysphonia treated with botulinum toxin (see 9.2).

3.2.10
Kinematic Recordings

The changes generated by movements of the pharynx, palate, uvula and tongue in three-dimensional electromagnetic fields generated by three sources attached on a stereotaxic helmet are recorded by means of small electrodes placed on the corresponding organs of the vocal tract. The kinematic curves during utterance of letters, syllables, words or phrases are evaluated with reference to a recorded profile of an adjacent part of the vocal tract [Perkell, 1980; Schönle and Grone, 1992] (fig. 35, 36).

Fig. 36. a A normal speaker's production of /kata/, zoomed for the sentence *ich habe Kater gehört* (literally 'I have heard cat'). Plot A: x/y of the trajectories of all five coils; B: zoomed x/y plot of the tongue blade; C: zoomed x/y plot of tongue tip trajectories; D: y(t) (——) and v(t) (velocity, ------) of the tongue blade, the dotted line gives v(t) = 0; E: same presentation as in D for the tongue tip; F: oscillogram of speech output. **b** Plots corresponding to **a** for a patient with multisystem atrophy affecting pyramidal pathways. Modified from Schönle et al. [1992].

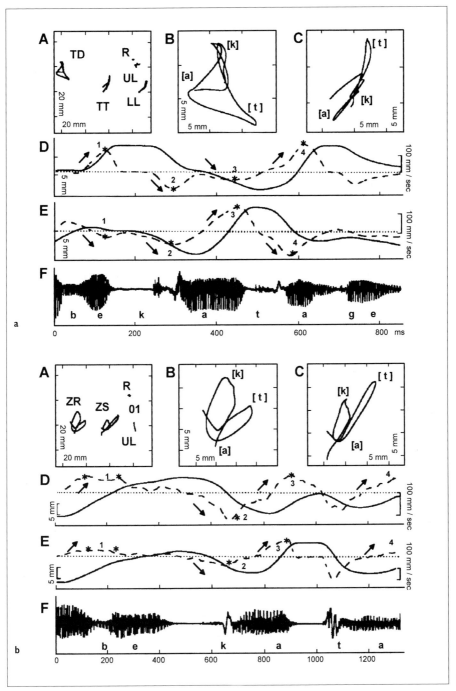

A Critical Issue: The Neural-Assembly-Facilitating Effect of Intermediary Processes and the Resort to Simple Reactions as a Complementary Investigation in Multiple-Delayed-Reaction Verbochronometry

3.3.1
The Intermediary Processes: A Transfer and Matching Step in Normal Speech Control

The processes that occur between programming and executive brain operations in speech control seem to provide the necessary link between the cortical activities, the transfer of invariant patterns to subcortical projections and the adaptation of invariants to variants through corrective internal feedbacks. Their occurrence is proved by the decrease in ACG latency time when a foreperiod occurs between the task stimulus and the 'go' stimulus: ACG latency at $FP_{1.5}$ in normals is shorter than ACG latency at FP_0. The effects of sustained exercises and learning will be analysed in 8.4. A recurrent cortico-gangliobasal activity in internal circuits taking place during the 1.5-second foreperiod maintains the programmed invariants and facilitates the neural assembly that will deliver the commands to the articulators. As previously mentioned, this facilitated neural assembly is represented as 'attractor' in MacClelland's [1994] neural networks, while the recurrent circuits are represented as internal double loops and feedbacks in the reading performance model of Hinton and Shallice [1991].

We assumed that the difference ACG latency at FP_0 – ACG latency at $FP_{1.5}$ includes the initial programmation and the intermediary processes occurring in the foreperiod. We have underlined that in our methodology the task stimulus is continuously shown to the subject in such a way that no memory process is required: the subject unconsciously performs an active temporal transfer of latent commands, a process that corresponds to the 'working memory' concept. Baddeley et al. [1984] promoted a long series of sophisticated investigations in this area, covering different kinds of mnemic and non-mnemic processes of different duration. The complexity of this field has recently been pointed out by Cornoldi [1995] who proposed a more detailed classification of the different processes that are covered by the same label.

At the neurophysiological level, the essence of the process is undoubtedly represented by recurrent loops with impulses transmitted in different layers: internal feedbacks are thus acting from one layer to the next, at short or long polysynaptic stations. Such recurrent internal circuits represent a general functional organization in the whole nervous system. They occur at different hierarchical levels and provide the delivery and refinement of many psychomotor and mental performances. They operate as intermediary loops in reading [Hinton and Shallice, 1991]. They allow us to grasp the meaning of long sentences [Pinker, 1995; Cornoldi, 1995]; moreover, they maintain the connection between the different parts of thinking and language [Pinker, 1995].

These intermediary processes are quite efficient from 4 years of age onwards, but they are rather vulnerable as it is proved, besides other disorders, by the high incidence of dyslexic children. We have also previously mentioned how stuttering occurs particularly at the age of 3–5 years.

The severest impairment of intermediary processes occurs in schizophrenic patients, and it seems to suggest a possible support to the hypothesis of an evolutive alteration, in agreement with the concept identifying the pathogenesis of schizophrenia as a 'static encephalopathy' with an early onset in infancy.

The fact that some schizophrenics have completely lost the ability to shorten the time reaction with a congruent foreperiod may require a revision of the argument about the intermediary processes being the unique, accelerating component of speech control. In other words, one may wonder how far the processes, which are supposed to link the programming patterns to the executive adapted distribution of coordinated impulses, are really a sort of driving belt facilitating the executive system.

An answer to this question could rightly be advanced only after a specific interpretation of the alternative possibilities of psychomotor performances in these patients. If catatonic disorders in the psychomotor area, ideoverbal dissociation and positive and negative symptoms in the perceptive and thinking area determined the whole psychic life of schizophrenics, we could then infer that the impairment of the intermediary processes is a catastrophic event and conclude that the efficiency of the internal circuits is indispensable for the brain functions subserving the mental activity.

However, it seems nearer the reality of the whole behaviour of schizophrenics to recognize that they are still able, in a rather large part, to read, to carry out purposeful actions and to solve complex problems. If these are the facts, the intermediary processes – in the form we have inferred from the delayed reactions – are not necessarily a time-sparing process in delayed reactions.

A detailed analysis of the possible correlation of an inversion of the intermediary process ratio with neuropsychological indications of proneness to schizophrenia [Maier et al., 1992] and with genetic susceptibility to schizophrenia will be reported in 9.4.

In order to avoid confusing interferences of the increase in the intermediary process ratio with the interpretation of choice reaction findings, we relied on the measurement of simple reactions as a necessary complement in routine examinations with MDRV.

3.3.2
A Methodological Issue: How to Measure the Central Cerebral Processes when the Acousticogram Latency at Foreperiod 1.5 s Is Longer than That at Foreperiod 0

In the first period of our research with MDRV, we tacitly assumed that, since reaction time appeared decreased in delayed reactions with $FP_{\geq 0.4}$, we could consider the reaction time at $FP_{\geq 0.4}$ to depend mainly on the executive processes. Therefore reaction time at FP_0 – reaction time at $FP_{\geq 0.4}$ should correspond to the early programming and intermediary processes.

A flat contradiction of this argument struck us during an MDRV study of schizophrenics who were characterized by longer reaction times at $FP_{\geq 0.4}$ than those at FP_0, that is by an inversion of the intermediary process ratio. Thus, we were forced to search for an alternative methodological plan able to differentiate central computing processes from executive operations. The recourse to simple reactions seemed to represent the most consistent procedure. No doubt that simple reaction time mainly concerns the executive and neuromotor processes. The knowledge of reaction time and ACG duration of simple verbal reactions – however plain they may appear – provides the examiner with fundamental and reliable information about the time taken by the brain to perceive the word on the PC, to resort from the visual system to the verbopraxic centres, to transmit and conduct the commands to the upper and lower motor systems and eventually about the time taken by the chain of articulatory movements to utter the word. This series of neural and motor processes represents the simplest functional coordinated set of mechanisms necessary to carry out a reading reaction.

The difference between the total time reaction for choice tests at $FP_{1.5}$ and the simple reaction time, limited to a single word of the pair used in the choice reactions, will give always a positive result, whatever dysfunction affects the patient.

3.3.3
Simple Reaction Times Are Shorter than Choice Reaction Times in Whatever Functional Disorder

If a severe neuromotor disease has completely destroyed the vocal channel neuromotor system, the subject cannot speak at all: as a consequence of different causes, anarthria or different forms of mutism could be observed.

If the vocal channel system is only partially damaged, dyspneumic, dysphonic or dysarthric disorders could result with various degrees of slow-down affecting both simple reaction times and choice reaction times.

If Broca's and Wernicke's centres were the target of damage, dysphasic disorders would ensue. The effects would reach not only the executors, but they would also exert upward repercussions on the central computing processes.

The basic principles to carry out the different measurements in association with choice direct and delayed reactions (the latter under normal conditions and in non-schizophrenic patients) will be outlined in the last chapter of Section 5. They form a complementary methodology that is worth being integrated systematically in psychophysiological studies of speech brain control.

On the other hand, the intermediary processes include the adaptive variations connected to a corrective system of trials and errors. The operations involved in this invariant-to-variant adaptation deserve a specific development that will be carried out in the next Section.

4

From Invariants to Variants

The Neural Substrates from Programmation to Adaptation in Gracco's Model

According to the previously reported blueprints (fig. 3, 4, 10, 17), we agree on a double role of the programmation system with two periods of activity occurring successively in time, the early activation being related to the 'prescription' (in Gracco's terminology) of the invariant patterns and the successive activation being related to the adaptive, pre-executive function that is a part of the intermediary processes.

On the grounds of neurophysiological contributions [Alexander et al., 1990], one should assume that these processes develop in loops including the cortical areas and the basal ganglia.

Gracco [1991], on the other hand, identifies two major brain implementation systems to carry out the 'details' of the speech production process, that is, in our conception, the adaptation process. They are the system of the basal ganglia and the supplementary motor area and the system of the cerebellum and premotor area.

A function of the system of the basal ganglia and supplementory motor area was suggested, starting with research on the motor disorders produced by human diseases [Marsden, 1984] and ending with the behavioural studies carried out in experimentally lesioned primates. This system appeared to have the attributes required for evaluating the hypothesized characteristic neuromotor patterns in Gracco's model [De Long, 1990, 1994; Alexander et al., 1986, 1990; Georgopoulos et al., 1981; Brown, 1987; Horack and Anderson, 1984].

Lesions of the supplementary motor area appear to exaggerate the inability to adapt muscle actions to the task which, in the case of speaking, often results in total speech arrest [Penfield and Roberts, 1959; Caplan, 1987]. Moreover, lesions of the supplementary motor area produce a marked reduction in self-initiated voluntary moments [for a review, see Wiesendanger and Wiesendanger, 1984].

Impairments of speech movement occurring in Parkinson disease reflect a generalized reduction in the speed and extent of articulatory movements resulting in perceptually distorted consonants, a slowed speech rate and a tendency towards monotony. It is suggested that these deficits reflect a generalized reduction in the ability to adapt muscle actions to the specific requirements for speech movement. The basal ganglia functions – which are impaired in Parkinson disease – develop along a loop implying the motor cortex with an indirect upstream current of sensory information. According to Alexander et al. [1990], this system is involved in neuromuscular adaptation, with a predominant control exerted by the supplementary motor area.

Aphasic patients with anterior cortical lesions and ataxic dysarthric patients demonstrate a sequencing difficulty manifest in the timing of voice onset [Baum et al., 1990; Blumstein et al., 1980]. The sequencing difficulty observed in these patients is consistent with damage to the premotor area which receives projections from the cerebellum, a neural structure involved in timing movement sequences [Kent and Rosenbeck, 1982; Gracco and Abbs, 1988; Ito, 1984]. Similarly, neurophysiological investigations in non-human primates showed the premotor area to be involved in the sensory guidance of movements [Goodschalk et al., 1981; Halsband and Passingham, 1982; Rizzolati et al., 1981], a function similar to that proposed for the cerebellum [Ito, 1984; Soetching et al., 1976]. In general, the cerebellar-supplementary motor area system appears to function as an important component in the incorporation of peripheral sensory signals into the central motor commands. Thus, according to this view, the two systems are strictly integrated, being both activated in due time for the two functions, preparatory setting and timing programmation. The final component in Gracco's model is the hypothesized central rhythm generator.

Now, as a preliminary, it is of fundamental importance to distinguish between two different domains of the temporal organization of speech. One is related to the sequential organization of the single articulatory movement for each letter (each vowel and each consonant) in the syllable and then in the word: it is in fact the succession of these movements that create, in their regular coordination, the characteristic patterns of innervation for the action of speech.

Alternative theories (as the logogen theory) suggest rather the retrieval of a word to represent the first process, followed by the phonological extraction of subunits. Anyway, a guided succession of excitation-activation and cessation-inhibition of neural assemblies is common to both models. The complex array of corresponding circuitries and alternative processes is what we called [Pinelli and Ceriani, 1992], following Perkell [1980] and Levelt [1989], the neural substrate of the *central programmation of specific serial timing and the diadochokinetic execution.*

A second domain is related to the cyclic execution of the articulatory movements in general, whichever would be the specific task. The biomechanical executors can carry out a commanded series of movements of a certain length only with a succession of contractions of agonists and antagonists, each group of muscles being activated with peaks of innervation and pauses: these might depend on an active process of inhibition or might be in a resting 'null' condition of inertia and passive aftermovement. It must also be kept in mind that in some cases a non-innervation can be requested, particularly when the stiffness must be increased. This rhythmic cycling activity is a more automatic process than the specific timing process, as Abbs et al. [1987] were able to demonstrate with sophisticated methods; they found that the cycles are of approximately 5–6 Hz.

On the other hand, the mechanism regulating the velocity of speech, which can be slowed or accelerated within a certain limit, has to be conceived to depend on a rather autonomous neural activity. This mechanism was named the 'timing of the rhythmic action'.

Gracco reports Ito's suggestion [1984] that the cerebellum may contribute to the timing of many rhythmic motor behaviours. The changes of speech timing associated with cerebellar damage show that it contributes at least. Other possible sites of a centrally rhythm generator would be the intricate synaptic connections within the brainstem that could possibly be temporarily set into oscillation by a directed input from cortical structures, similar to the central masticatory rhythm generator [Nakamura, 1986].

In line with Martin's hypothesis [1972], Gracco considered the possibility that speech rhythm, timing of rhythmic action and serial timing are intrinsically connected: we might consider them to emerge from a hierarchical organization as a network property. In fact, we have previously reported [Pinelli and Ceriani, 1992, Appendix 3] how Sommerhoff [1974] drew some models (Sommerhoff's λ systems) of these hierarchical organizations.

Gracco [1987] considers the vocal tract to be the smallest functional control structure operated by sensorimotor scaling and timing processes; in fact, no subphonemic speech errors occur [Abbs, et al., 1983]. Only focal nervous system lesions, such as dysphonia or lower motor neuron damage, reproduce speech motor impairments specific to an articulatory subsystem.

The deficits associated with various system damages may result in different degrees of impairment because of the biomechanical or physiological differences of individual articulators. It pertains to the neurologists to identify true reflections of underlying differential neural impairments. For a variety of speech motor disorders due to damaged basal ganglia, cerebellum and anterior and posterior cortical areas, deficits are observed that are consistent with a global rather than focal breakdown. That is, the major neuro-anatomical sensorimotor system involved in speech production – including the systems of the basal ganglia and supplementary motor area, cerebellum and premotor cortex and the inferior parietal cortex – appears to function not in the control of movement per se but in processes from which movement originates.

The Neural Tests of Speech: How to Overcome the Articulation-Dependent Variability

We agree with Gracco that surface differences in speech motor impairments in themselves can hardly truly reflect the underlying focal primary lesion. In fact, a test of speech intended to help identify changes in verbal reactions due to neural disorders can be obtained if we do not rely on absolute values but rather on ratios between two series of different tasks or modalities of performance by the same individual subject. In this way, one can get rid of the response components depending on the biomechanical or physiological differences of individual articulators, since they occur as common denominator in the two different series of performances. This procedure will be useful also to correct the influence of the *kinetic factor* (see Section 8).

On the other hand, the evaluation of the results of MDRV must focus on the level of functional neural impairment rather than on the localization of the primary damage.

4.2.1
The Methodological Procedure

We will test different performance modalities of reading reactions. The intrinsic differences will regard many aspects: (1) different delays between the presentation of the task and the 'go' signal; (2) with pressure and without pressure reactions; (3) performances requested at different velocities.

A second order of performance modalities regards the tasks to be accomplished. They can be varied in complexity (like length of the word), frequency of use and nature (with reference to phonological or grammatical and linguistic connotations).

But it is also necessary, in accordance with the general principles of the neurological procedures, to correlate these findings with those of other areas of investigation, particularly in the field of evoked potentials, in both afferent and efferent domains.

4.2.2
Criteria of Evaluation: Functional Level versus Damage Localization

The neural speech test realized with MDRV is intended to yield information about possible changes in neural function and to identify the level of the functional change: whether it is at the input channels, at the output channels or at the programming and computational central processes (the hidden unit layers). This evaluation is of paramount importance for both the longitudinal assessment of the functional state of the patient and the correct elaboration of the best planning of neurorehabilitation treatments for the single individual patient, in the different specific phases of evolution of the disease.

4.2.3
Towards a Diagnostic Evaluation: The Range of Normal Variations

In order to perform a diagnostic evaluation, we must first know the range of *normal* variations as a basis for a correct statistical computation.

In 4.3 and 4.4, we will deal with this question, taking into account not only the experimental data but also the most relevant correlations. To argue the possible sources of the normal variability we pursued two purposes.

First of all, it seemed reasonable that knowing the causes of data dispersion could help eliminate it as much as possible with appropriate methodological modifications.

Secondly, to penetrate the mystery of brain stochasticity might allow us to understand the intrinsic mechanism of speech brain control and to better define the normal range of variability versus a possible abnormal reduction (stereotypy) or increase (loss of control).

The Adaptation Processes and Stochastic Output

The integration of the descending invariant commands with the adaptation system implies an intervention of multiple extrinsic correcting feedbacks [Perkell, 1991]. The consequence is that, when asked to perform a series of verbal reactions with repetition of the same word presented at random from a pair, a subject shows an evident range of oscillations in ACG latency time and formal ACG structure. Some examples of these oscillations have been given in 3.2.

Taking into account these two statements, we can address the above-mentioned question of the variability of reaction performances. This can be envisaged from many points of view. Does this variability correspond to a stochastic type of functioning [Barto, 1989], depending upon a non-algorithmic and trial-and-error operation? Do the continuous adjustments effected by multiple feedbacks characterize a trial-and-error modality of working? Are they the main causes of the variations of ACG latency and duration in a series of successive neutral performances (see 3.2.6 and 4.4.3.3)?

With these questions in mind, we considered the mean values of ACG latency and duration of a certain number of successive reactions, as a reliable cue for the temporal course of the word control CCP. Likewise the corresponding SD could be assumed to give a measure of the stochastic oscillations.

4.3.1
Improving the Attention Span: Warning Stimulus and Other Methodological Homogenizations

In the first 3 years of our research, we carried out the verbal tests without a warning signal. More recently, in line with the methodology adopted by the Nijmegen team of the voice and speech laboratory, we added an acoustic warning signal occurring 100 ms before the presentation of the word stimulus. In this way, the span of attention is shortened and the range of attention oscillations should be reduced.

In association with this modification, the patient was more carefully placed in a comfortable, adjustable chair to avoid all possible eye and head movements when directing his attention to the word stimuli on the PC screen.

The inclusion of the preliminary acoustic warning stimulus in the reactions seems to significantly reduce the SD of the reaction times. In a group of 42 normal subjects (9 aged 19–34 years, 12 aged 35–49 and 11 aged 50–78) and of 53 patients with neurological diseases (Parkinson disease, motoneuron disease, early mental deterioration or schizophrenic syndromes), compared with matched subjects (41 normals and 96 patients) who carried out the reactions without a warning stimulus, the SD showed a significant decrease of approximately 33%. In contrast, the mean ACG latency showed a lower decrease, of about 3.8%. No significant changes were found in intermediary and executive processes.

It can be thus inferred that the warning stimulus plays a significant role in the elimination of a variability factor that could depend on oscillations of perceptive and motor attention during the series of reactions.

4.3.1.1
Can a Variability Factor Depending on the Respiratory Cycle Be Avoided?

Random differences in the basal spontaneous respiratory cycle at the moment of appearance of the word stimulus on the PC would require some little while to adjust the respiratory phase in order to produce the best expiration needed for the vocal air flow. Thus, a variability in the onset time of the expiratory movement could arise and be reflected in differences of ACG latency.

A 'prepared inspiration' could avoid this variability factor. This is realized with the examiner instructing the subject to maintain the inspiration in the interval between warning signal and stimulus presentation.

However, a previously requested inspiratory tonic movement in the postwarning interval was not easily accomplished by our patients, and it seemed, on the contrary, to disturb their attention to the reactions to be carried out. Consequently, we excluded this request from our routine MDRV methodology.

Alternatively we attempted to eliminate the temporal variations in the intervals randomly occurring between the position of the pulmonary excursion at the moment of the stimulus presentation on the monitor and the inspiration accomplished to produce the best expiratory movement to push the air into the vocal tract. This was realized by making a well-defined and constant phase of the basal respiratory cycle trigger the presentation of the word stimulus on the PC.

4.3.1.2
Recording Eye Movements

We have previously mentioned the possibility to keep the subject in the best, most comfortable line of observation of the stimuli appearing on the PC screen: in this way, eye movements are reduced as much as possible. On the other hand, measuring the eye movements during the different phases of the reactions – from warning to task stimulus, from task stimulus to ACG onset, from task stimulus to 'go' stimulus (asterisks), from 'go' stimulus to ACG onset – is very useful as a complementary indicator of visuomotor factors occurring during the early programmations, intermediary transfers, adaptations and executive phonatory movements.

The oculographic indicator might be particularly indicative of pathological conditions when some of the brain processes previously mentioned are impaired. The case of inversion of the intermediary process ratio in schizophrenia (see 9.5) seems particularly pertinent to be studied in association with the oculograms.

4.3.2
Multiple-Delayed-Reaction Verbochronometry as a Test of Brain Functionality

To apply MDRV measurements profitably to the investigation of brain processes of speech control under normal and pathological conditions, three categories of terms are to be defined: (1) what task the subject must fulfil; (2) the variables of the responses to be measured; (3) the reproducibility of the results.

After extensive experiments with reactions where the subject was asked to read phonemes, syllables, disyllabic words and sentences and to name pictures [Pinelli and Ceriani, 1992], we were able to outline and apply the following schedule:

(a) The tasks were represented, in the first 3 years of investigation with MDRV, by a pair of disyllabic words with the same use frequency and similar phonetic features. Since last year we have adopted a threefold task – a syllable, a disyllabic word, a sentence – in order to investigate not only phonological but also grammatical reading performances. Sometimes three-syllabic non-words were presented (fig. 24–27), particularly when testing an impairment of the timing processes or of the recruitment of motor units in preparatory and phasic stages.

(b) The variables to be measured concern the ACG latency time, the EMG latency time, the ACG duration and the ACG spectrography; the latter examines response accuracy and will be included in future studies.

(c) The reproducibility of these parameters in young normal subjects as 1- to 3-month intervals was found to be within $10\pm5\%$ (see next chapter and Section 5).

···

Variability at Different Levels of Brain Control of Speech

4.4.1
Towards a Comprehensive Interpretation of Stochastic Function and Its Measurement

Over and over again we verified that, when one individual subject, performing verbal reactions under constant conditions, repeats the same word several times (12 successive reactions), the values of the total latency time of ACG, the duration of ACG and the ACG spectrogram show a consistent range of variations. The psychologist might be tempted to explain this phenomenon with oscillations in attention. In fact, the concept of attention was submitted to a radical revision by neuropsychologists and neurophysiologists. If we intend the term 'attention' to indicate a reinforcing and focusing process occurring, at least in its beginning, at a conscious level, then we could state that, in our experiments, it seems to play only a minor role. The engagement of the subject in the series of verbal reactions was obtained after few preliminary trials of learning so that the series of 12 reactions required a rather confined channel of mental application. A failure of this mental application could rarely occur and it was conventionally related to single reactions whose values (particularly ACG latency) show a difference from the mean value greater than 2 SD. It is a usual procedure to exclude these extreme values from the final measurements of the mean values.

Then it seems justified to define the term 'attention' according to the neuropsychological evaluation of Cohen [1993]. We should refer to a neural superimposed activity occurring at both the sensitive and the motor sides of the psychomotor performance and involving the central programmer: this means CCP in the inner circuits that are reproduced in the models of connective networks with the hidden unit layer. The neuropsychologists have also identified a thalamoparietofrontal system in the right hemisphere that plays an important role in eliciting and maintaining the attention to somatic and visual hemifields.

The kind of variations in the succession of verbal reactions studied with our methodology reflects a particular course (see tables 3–6, corresponding to fig. 24–33) that would be only tautologically defined as oscillations in attention; a mixture of immediate learning and transient failure of attention could represent only a preliminary 'impressionistic' description. In fact, an experiment we carried out in normal subjects with rather long series of repetitions of multiple tasks [Pinelli and Ceriani, 1992] showed that the variations occur with a random course including some recurrent signs of improvement (fig. 37 for normal subjects). These last events might be taken into consideration as interfering effects on internal learning. Some experiments have been carried out with subjects affected by chronic fatigue syndrome (fig. 38). Pressing the subject to react as quickly as possible produced different effects in the middle and at the end of the series of reactions.

In MDRV we avoid the preliminary early learning since the subject performs a few reactions freely in order to make himself familiar with reading the different stimuli. Afterwards the subject starts the series of reactions submitted to statistical measurements.

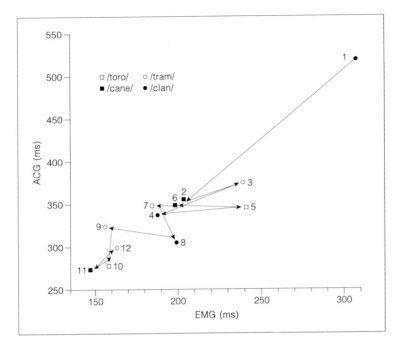

Fig. 37. EMG and ACG reaction times in a sequence of 12 trials presented to a normal subject (male, 37 years old).

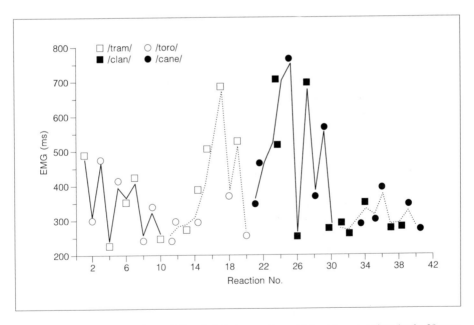

Fig. 38. EMG reaction times of 42 verbal choice reactions obtained from a patient (male, 28 years old) with chronic fatigue syndrome. —— = Neutral reactions; ······ = pressed reactions.

In our current experiments, the course of the reaction variables has always been completely random (tables 3–6, fig. 24–33).

Therefore, in accordance with the interpretation of Perkell [1980, 1991], Abbs et al. [1984] and Kelso et al. [1983], the concept of stochastic functioning seems to be the most objective introduction to a correct biological study on the origin of oscillations in such programmed motor complex performances.

A second type of view might be inspired by studies concerning the degrees of freedom in performance strategy that had led to the concept of 'isogoal multiple trajectories'.

A third order of interpretation might consider variability as an effect of dynamic changes in the peripheral constraints.

These different approaches allow a convergent identification of multiple factors responsible for the resulting stochastic course of the oscillations.

4.4.2
Stochastic Functions

4.4.2.1
A Definition of Stochastic Functions and the Relationship with Attentional Processes

The term 'stochastic function' means that the variations in the neural temporal course of brain speech processes and consequent formant frequencies of utterance, occurring during the repetition of the same task (tables 3–6, fig. 24–33) should not be attributed to extrinsic factors but rather to intrinsic functional mechanisms.

As a general principle, we know from PET investigations that both dominant and non-dominant hemispheres are activated during speaking [Loesner et al., 1993; Paulesu et al., 1993a, b]. Such a widely diffuse activity implies a large number of systems whose processes are known to develop in parallel (PDP), with overlapping, different phases of activity that can hardly recur with rigid intervals of time in succeeding cycles. A hierarchical organization will certainly govern such multilevel systems, and this leads to the existence of an associated brain area that exerts both sustaining and focusing effects on the ongoing diffuse activity. In fact, sustaining effects can be equivalent to excitatory-facilitatory impulses, while focusing should be mediated by lateral inhibition.

These regulating activities can be deemed to be the neurofunctional substrates of what, at the psychological level, is defined by the term 'attention'. As we previously mentioned, there is some evidence that a thalamus-parietal-frontal area of the right (non-dominant) hemisphere can be involved in such a regulation. Shall we conceive it as a sort of pacemaker, acting on the activities of both hemispheres and characterized in itself by a slight degree of variability in its regulation of each cycle?

More likely, the attention system of the right hemisphere is concerned with concrete images and aesthesic representations, just as a corresponding area of the left hemisphere is concerned with abstract representations. The study of verbal reactions proves that uttering concrete words like /mare/ ('sea') and /muro/ ('wall') implies a prevalent activation of the non-dominant hemisphere, while uttering abstract words like /male/ ('evil') and /mito/ ('myth') or /virtù/ ('virtue') and /vizio/ ('vice') involves mainly the dominant hemisphere [Pinelli et al., 1994].

In fact, a general effect resulting in 'attentional shifts' is exerted by the reticular aspecific ascending system of Moruzzi and Magoun [1949] as a general arousal and vigilance system together with the thalamic ascending system that exerts a more 'regional' aspecific activation of the basal function of the cerebrum.

According to the involvement of these complementary systems, we can outline four sources of cycle-to-cycle internal temporal variability of the brain processes of speech control (and more generally of psychomotor complex sequential purposeful actions): (1) oscillations in the upward tuning activity [Bremer, 1936] that take place in the ascending systems of Moruzzi and Magoun [1949]; (2) oscillations in the duration of successive cyclic internal circuits involving thalamoparietofrontal connections; (3) specific variability in the different phonological and grammatical operations; a cue in support of this point is given by the different standard deviations we found for sentence reaction time with respect to a syllable and disyllabic word [a sentence may be /mare è bello/ ('sea is beautiful'), a syllable /ma/ ('but') and a disyllabic word /mare/ ('sea')]; (4) a further source of intrinsic mechanisms of variations could be searched in the adapting processes and particularly in the coupling and matching activities occurring between the descending patterns and the slave executors on the distal side. In this last stage of intermediary processes, one must also take into consideration the processes related to the so-called articulatory buffer [Levelt, 1989]. This kind of adaptation obviously develops with repetitive corrections; this event might be regarded as a trial-and-error modality of functioning.

4.4.2.2
Stochastic Variability and Trial-and-Error Functions

Aiming to better understand the real origin or multiple origins of the stochastic functioning in speech control, we must proceed to analyse the corresponding structural organization of the neural machinery. This leads us to consider a mechanism of internal feedbacks. In accordance with a trial-and-error function, they intervene firstly to adjust the invariant CCP internal outputs in relation to executive constraints and secondly to match the final output to the commanded programme. It was inferred that the central nervous system operates in a trial-and-error way, rather than in an algorithmic sequence of stages, by comparing the results of psychometric measurements [Plum, 1993b] to the operations effected by the inner unit layer in artificial neural networks [Banks, 1991]. The time measured for the most complex reactions is too short with reference to modular sequential operations.

A reconstruction of primary oscillations of impulse generators and/or oscillating phase displacements occurring between different interfering impulse generators requires a detailed analysis of the whole nervous system implied in speech control.

4.4.2.2.1
The Central Programmation Processes and the Invariant Commands
The CCP involved in the programming phase of the speech production give rise to well-defined, precise patterns of descending commands signalling the degree and timing of movements to be performed by coordinated groups of muscles.

These commands include both preparatory and phasic innervation of articulatory muscles. The CCP however cannot specify a more differentiated distribution of innervation for each muscle and even less for each motor unit inside the single muscle. Henneman et al. [1965] have calculated that for more elementary tasks an amount of n^{12} signals would be needed. Such a high performance, with the multiple of similar processes the speech control requires, clearly appears to exceed the abilities of our brain.

In fact, the brain motor control theory assumes that a fine on-line adaptation of the descending invariant commands is implemented by servo-mechanisms of both upper and lower motor systems. The notion that the CCP elaborate the indication of an action to be performed rather than a more specific sequence of impulses for each muscle is based on two considerations.

In line with the remarks of Henneman et al. [1965] we must admit that the central nervous system – in spite of the large population of neurons and PDP functioning – cannot produce, in the available associative areas and output channels, the extremely numerous series of trains of spikes with a determined proper frequency, duration and distribution to thousands of motor units that must be activated in due time for the pronunciation of each syllable.

Moreover, it is well known that the same movement can be effected with differently distributed activations of motor units in agonist and antagonist muscles with one group of synergists rather than others in alternative cycles of recruitment and in a more or less high degree of co-innervation [Arbib and Caplan, 1979]. The ultimate choice of the actual instantaneous distribution is highly dependent upon distal constraints and contingent conditions.

4.4.2.2.2
A Dualistic Organization and Upward Repercussions from Constraints

It follows from the previous outline of the central brain processes that we deal with at least two main systems and an interface between the two. One is the generator of a forward activity that elaborates goal-directed patterns of impulses. The second corresponds to the executive system which is formed by the corticospinal system with the gangliobasal cerebellar loop. This translates the invariant impulses into specific innervations to the most suitable muscles. This translation in its turn requires the co-operation of feedback servo-mechanisms that produce eventually a trial-and-error process. In this way, the goal-directed output from the CCP becomes adapted to the final overt output.

A process of on-line adaptation implies a range of oscillations in the variables of the final performance. They possibly originate from obstacles on the executors and dynamic changes in their functional properties during repeated performances.

4.4.2.3
The Basic Primary Genesis of Stochastic Variability

A trial-and-error modality can cause in itself different effects on the operative time and first of all on ACG latency. When a balance is reached between the characteristics of the patterns of the invariant descending commands and the excitability of the 'prepared coordinated motor units' involved in the utterance of the phonological unit, then we find the shortest time of performance.

If on the contrary a correction is needed to match the invariant with a mislined executive system, this requires a certain additional time and the total ACG latency increases. This increase in time can oscillate according to the degree of misalignment.

We have devised some experimental conditions aiming to test this hypothesis. External stimuli have been applied during the development of verbal reactions: this interference will modify the excitability of the executive neuromuscular system; the consequences for the latency time of the responses could be measured. The results will be reported in 4.4.4.

4.4.2.4
Have Physicochemical Cyclic Events Something to Do with Stochasticity?

A certain degree of variability occurs in the intrinsic neural processes at the molecular level of physicochemical, biochemical and electrophysiological cyclic events of impulse generation and energy restoration [Woody, 1982]. These oscillations are known in neurophysiology as jitter. However, the magnitude of these oscillations, of the order of microseconds, can hardly be called upon to explain the variability we are dealing with in our study. Moreover, the passage from the molecular to the neurophysiological and behavioural level implies a series of averaging processes that compensate for the basal small oscillations.

Some pathological conditions, which may occur in demyelinating diseases, can amplify the instability so much that it reflects at the behavioural level. The consequences can be studied as neural fatigue, pathological pauses and errors [Pinelli, 1993]; this topic will be analysed again in more details in Section 6.

4.4.3
Variability in Strategy of Performance

This field of research embraces a series of experiments carried out particularly by Feldman [1966] and Bizzi [1984]. They examine the different trajectories performed by an animal to reach a certain target. The degree of freedom in human performances translating the invariant commands into the variant executions might represent an analogous functional behaviour, as we will analyse in the next paragraph.

4.4.3.1
Isogoals with Heterogeneous Trajectories and the Variability of Motor Strategies: The Principle of Lacquaniti and Soetching

A lot of observations in animals [Feldman, 1966] proved that an individual can reach the same target by executing different trajectories. One could argue that this fact does not strictly depend on changing constraints, but it rather corresponds to the more general principle of trial-and-error functioning.

Do the intrinsic variability of the CCP machinery and the trial-and-error operations represent two different levels of the same phenomenon? The fact that the CCP intrinsic variability represents the underlying function of what appears at the behavioural level as trials and errors can be considered as a fundament that could be defined and discussed more thoroughly when sufficient data are collected from the two levels of investigations. The study and evaluation of the high degree of freedom in reaching one goal along different trajectories could represent a first test.

On the other hand, the trial-and-error operation could be envisaged as a tendency by the individual subject to perform a certain final task within a wide range of possibilities.

A purposeful action – as speech – is composed of a coordinate sequence of movements. The unfolding of a repetitive series of actions may be represented in the following way.

The pattern innervation of the first trial corresponds to a tentative command with a still incomplete and raw plan of action. Internal and proprioceptive feedbacks help to improve the matching with the executors. However, the series of successive corrections does not correspond to progressive learning processes leading to a more precise action on the target. The information itself reflects erratic events that give rise to an irregular, in some way bizarre, zig-zagging. To grasp better the meaning of this assertion it may be necessary to make a more detailed analysis of the classical example of scratching. Then it would be possible to discuss the analogy with the case of the articulatory movements of speech [Gentil, 1992].

4.4.3.2
The Performance of Isopurposeful Different Trajectories Analysed in the Light of the Motor Control Theory

First of all, we must try to define the field of our observations under all conditions in the best possible objective way. We can identify four conditions in the action of reaching a target.

(1) An individual subject must repetitively reach a target on his body with his hand (or limb). (2) He does not know exactly the position of the target. Therefore he cannot adapt the theoretically ideal shortest trajectory along a stereotyped line of action. (3) In fact, he performs his task with different trajectories. Thus, with a certain number of trials, he has explored a wide space and a large part of that region of his body between the starting position of his limb and the target on his body (more exactly his trunk). (4) As an alternative situation to point 2, perceptually the subject has well localized the target. As a consequence, when this individual subject carries out the task for the first time, he performs fewer different trajectories than the subject of point 2.

It is worthwhile analysing these differences, taking into account the situation at the level of the executors. It should also be discussed whether they represent a variability that must be distinguished from stochastic functions. In fact, the subject changes every time the groups of muscles or compartments of muscles [Feldman, 1966] involved in the coordinated action. In this way, he certainly avoids a possible effect of fatigue adopting a sort of rotatory muscle activity [Pinelli, 1989].

Moreover, he has a broad range of alternative combinations of muscles and related temporal orders of recruitment: the most suitable could later be learned and facilitated at the anatomofunctional level, with functional and, in the end, neuroplastic changes. This is the same as saying that the subject does not immediately adopt the behaviour that would be the most efficient and least energy expensive with a minimal degree of freedom, corresponding to the shortest trajectory. The theoretically best programmed behaviour is not given at the beginning and the subject develops a trial-and-error series of performances that in fact allow him to explore a broad range of abilities. This represents an important phase to create actual definitive specialized abilities in a constant environmental situation requiring such a kind of learning.

An analogous analysis was carried out by Fioretti et al. [1990] and Leo [1993] on the manual prehension of an object. In this case, the first phase corresponds to an exploration of the sliding space until the subject identifies a sliding subspace where he can adopt the most convenient, precise, quick and economical trajectory.

4.4.3.3
Degrees of Freedom in Speech Control

In the field of speaking, the target is not localized, neither in the external environment nor in one point of the body. The spatial relations take form at a more abstract level as *schemas of the environment space* and as *body schemas*. These schemas can be analysed at the level of the brain organization.

The target is an abstract image, a pattern of syllables, and it is realized by a series of processes, from visual perceptive information and translation into corresponding motor patterns. The trajectory is then totally internal. It is equivalent to a path leading from the neuronal assembly of CCP to the motor cortical centres of the coordinated muscular activity producing the utterance of the word.

There are several intermediate stations that in algorithmic models would be represented as boxes in series while it could partly overlap in PDP models. They can be activated or bypassed: the activation might be simply instantaneous or could be reinforced by reverberating feedbacks. In fact, one could repeat the task automatically or understand also its meaning through the semantic box, or even memorize it.

On the other hand, the series of operations is much more stereotyped in the executive systems than in CCP: in fact the executive final channels are ordered algorithmically. The coordinated muscles are activated in a well-defined temporal succession from the glottic to the supraglottic organs. An inverted order in some executors can in fact be recorded exceptionally in paraphysiological conditions or in speech dysfluencies.

Of course, as we have mentioned in the explanation of the great complexity of the brain CCP for a word utterance, the prosodic requests and factors related to the relationships with the listeners exert a great influence on the shaping of the final output with particular impact on the phonological modulation.

As we previously stressed, other extrinsic factors of variability in the strategy of performance are represented by the accuracy and the speed of pronunciation.

It results clearly from all these considerations that a rather large portion of variations is not at all spontaneous or intrinsic. On the contrary, a focused analysis can detect a large series of extrinsic causal factors. Only when they are eliminated or stabilized in a routine well-defined performance, could one face the problem of a trial-and-error functioning and define a stochastic kind of repetitive operations. The elimination of all extrinsic factors with stabilized conditions of reactions becomes then an absolute prerequisite for this kind of research: we propose to call the resultant performance in our test a 'neutral' utterance.

A conclusive evaluation of the role that the variability of performance strategy plays in the production of speech variable oscillations could only be speculative at the present stage of research. However, with reference to our simplified methodology and according to the neutral conditions adopted in the word reading reaction trials, it seems not to be the main factor responsible for the genesis of oscillations in ACG latency.

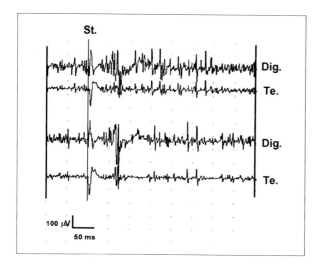

Fig. 39. Exteroceptive suppression during slight to moderate jaw contraction (without speaking). St. = Moment at which the stimulus is delivered (see text); Dig. = EMG of the digastric muscle; Te. = temporal muscle.

On the other hand, we may wonder whether the trial-and-error function implies some variability in the initial planning of the strategy of action. It could be a matter of a low-magnitude choice of action, that is of tactics rather than strategy. Certainly, the analogies with scratching cannot be extended beyond a certain limit: speech production appears to be a much more centrally programmed performance than the relatively more automatic scratching.

4.4.4
A Protecting Gate and Counteracting Mechanisms

Cyclic jaw movements are primarily organized for chewing, i.e. the behaviour basically connected with nourishment. Within this elementary sensorimotor structure, several regulating mechanisms are inserted to modulate the final chewing action and protect its purposeful accomplishment from occasional danger. The exteroceptive-suppression mono- and polyphasic reflex of Desmedt and Borenstein [1973], mediated by the trigeminal arc [Pinelli and Ceriani, 1992], is a powerful defence against nociceptive interferences (fig. 39, 40a, b).

On the other hand, the cyclic jaw movements occurring in the context of characteristic neural patterns of speech prevailed in man over the primitive organization of chewing: this phylogenetic evolution is in fact due to the superior efficiency of an immediate and precise communication on impending dangers [Lieberman, 1991]. We have thus investigated whether the exteroceptive-suppression trigeminal reflex is overbearing if excited during speaking, as it is known to occur during chewing. In agreement with the laws of its phylogenetic development, one might reasonably suppose that it has a minor negative interfering effect: at least with slight- or moderate-intensity trigeminal stimulation, it might only modify ongoing speech movements, without a complete functional block.

The word stimulus adopted was /sas/. The electrical stimulation was applied to the second-branch trigeminal emergency point with just subpainful intensity. The EMG response was recorded from the digastric and temporal muscles. The electrical stimulus was

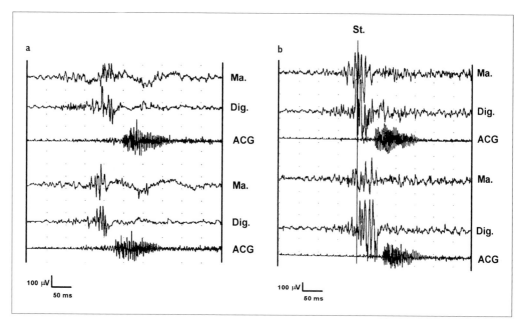

Fig. 40. Reaction to /sas/ under normal conditions (**a**) and with an exteroceptive stimulation 200 ms after the presentation of /sas/ (**b**). St. = Moment at which the stimulus is delivered; Ma. = EMG of the masseter muscle; Dig. = digastric muscle.

delivered at different intervals from the /sas/ presentation: 100, 150, 250 and 350 ms, that is well before and just after the ACG onset.

Normal values of /sas/ EMG and ACG under basal conditions, without trigeminal stimulation, were onset EMG latency time = 45±18 ms and ACG latency = 235±31 ms. The difference ACG latency – EMG latency was 195±68 ms. The ACG duration was 140 ms.

With trigeminal stimulation, a significant delay in ACG latency was observed when the electrical trigeminal stimulation occurred inside the EMG response (fig. 40a, b). A suitable indication of this delaying effect was represented by ACG latency – EMG latency. As it is reported in figures 41 and 42 and table 8, the delay in ACG latency is produced when the electrical stimulus comes within the first part of the EMG corresponding to the tonic-adaptive innervation.

The exteroceptive suppression, observed with analogous mild voluntary recruitment of alternative jaw opening and closing movements similar to chewing, did never occur during speaking. In two other cases, only when higher-intensity trigeminal electrical stimuli were applied, was a suppression reflex actually elicited at intervals of 250 ms between the /sas/ presentation and the electrical stimulation, 20 ms before the ACG onset.

If we now compare the trigeminal excitation effects in chewing movements and speaking, one might infer that a protecting gate is operating during speaking with respect to the trigeminal reflex and diminishing the suppression effect. One might argue that the descending commands for speech articulators enhance the threshold of inhibitory interneurons leaving the speech motor control undisturbed as much as possible. This functional organization seems to correspond once again to the biological teleological predominance of the communicating behaviour.

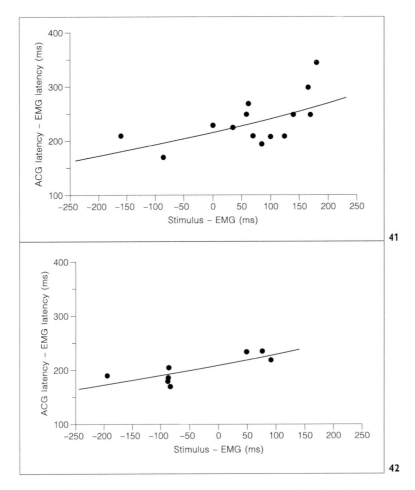

Fig. 41, 42. Delaying effect of trigeminal stimulation. **41** Subject C.I., female, 23 years old. **42** Subject M.L., male, 29 years old.

In fact, the delaying effects that we found to occur during interfering stimulations seem to imply correcting and re-adjusting mechanisms of the ongoing movements of speech.

In contrast, during chewing, swallowing dangerous substances or biting oral mucosas must be avoided and then the trigeminal reflex and suppression effects reach their peak.

4.4.5
Variability in the Peripheral Executors: The Voice Jitter

The variability in the ACG shape was investigated by means of voice spectrography by Baer [1979] and by Titze [1991]. They found that marked differences in the F_0 contour occurred during a series of utterances of the same word. This is the recent conclusion of a

Table 8. Latency time (ms) between the moment of the electrical stimulation and the EMG onset (ST – EMG) and the difference (ms) between ACG latency and EMG latency (ACG – EMG) in 6 normal subjects (initials indicated at the top)

C.I.[1]		M.L.[2]		R.L.		N.C.		C.M.		B.B.	
ST – EMG	ACG – EMG	ST – EMG	ACG – EMG	ST – EMG	ACG – EMG	ST – EMG	ACG – EMG	ST – EMG	ACG – EMG	ST – EMG	ACG – EMG
−165	210	−195	195	−105	204	0	270	−60	195	−210	120
−84	183	−90	210	−75	225	0	270	0	186	−150	120
0	240	−90	195	−60	280	0	285	0	225	−150	114
27	237	−90	195	−39	255	0	315	0	225	−150	120
60	255	−90	186	−24	255	45	255	15	210	−135	114
60	273	−84	180	39	270	60	300	30	240	−90	114
75	240	45	240	60	204	120	255	60	255	−30	105
90	216	75	240	90	270			90	210	−30	120
99	240	90	225	150	321			90	240	0	105
120	240			195	210			105	210	0	105
132	270							114	246	0	135
156	309							135	195	15	114
168	270										
180	345										

[1] See figure 41.
[2] See figure 42.

systemic study begun by Simon [1927], Lieberman [1961], Beckett [1969], Iwata and von Leden [1970] and Horiui [1985].

Frequency (or period) perturbation, called jitter, is defined as the variability of the F_0 or, reciprocally, of the fundamental period. When measured during running speech, variability is reflected in pitch SD.

Jitter measurements however are concerned with short-term variations, i.e. jitter is a measurement of how much a given period differs from the period that immediately follows it and not how much it differs from a cycle at the other end of the utterance. Jitter then is a measure of the frequency variability not accounted for by the voluntary changes in F_0. According to Baken [1987], perturbation is an acoustic correlate of erratic vibratory patterns that result from diminished control over the phonatory system.

Over 50 years ago, Simon [1927] concluded that there are no tones of constant pitch in either vocal or instrumental sounds. The phonatory system is not a perfect machine and every speaker's vibratory cycles are erratic to some extent. But, on the face of it, one would guess that an abnormal larynx would produce a more erratic voice than a healthy one.

Period perturbation measures that ignore the speaker's F_0 can be said to be absolute [Lieberman, 1961].

A different kind of perturbation measure was proposed by Hecker and Kreul [1971]. Their 'directional perturbation factor' ignores the magnitude of period perturbation; it is concerned only with the number of times that the frequency change shifts direction.

On the other hand, the magnitude of frequency perturbation shows a considerable correlation with mean F_0. A number of researches noted that larger cycle-to-cycle differences are associated with longer fundamental periods [Sorensen and Ord, 1984].

The simplest form of F_0-adjusted perturbation index is the mean perturbation divided by the mean waveform duration. When done in terms of period, the measure is called the 'jitter ratio' [Horiui, 1985]. By definition,

$$\text{jitter ratio} = \frac{\frac{1}{n-1}\left[\sum_{i=1}^{n-1}(P_i - P_{i-1})\right]}{\frac{1}{n}} \cdot 1{,}000,$$

where P_i = period of the i-th cycle (ms) and n = number of periods in the sample.

Put into ordinary language, the numerator is the sum of the absolute value of the differences between successive periods divided by the number of differences measured $(n-1)$. In short, it is the average magnitude of perturbation. The denominator is the sum of the periods, i.e. the mean period. Multiplication by 1,000 only serves to make the resultant ratio larger as a matter of convenience.

Titze [1991] found that the sources of fluctuations in amplitude and frequency of the vocal output are the following: (a) random movement of the mucus in the vocal folds; (b) acoustic and biomechanical coupling between the sources of the vocal tract; (c) instability in the turbulence in the air stream; (d) asymmetry in movement between left and right vocal folds; (e) the neurological input to the laryngeal and respiratory muscles, and (f) non-linearity in the biomechanical oscillators (chaos).

4.4.6
The Measurement of Neural Variability:
Time Latency Jitter and Related Parameters

4.4.6.1
The Interpretation of Standard Deviations

In relation to a semiological application and in line with the above-mentioned studies, we can try to define some criterion allowing us to identify the parameters more closely related to the intrinsic variations in latency time, response duration and its F_0.

We have previously analysed the voice jitter and its measurement modalities. We assume now that also the neural CCP-linked variations can be expressed as jitter. In fact this term is currently used in neurophysiology to indicate the variations in time intervals of spiking of two adjacent muscle fibres. With reference to verbochronometry, the variations could be localized by the degree of synchronization-desynchronization of the activity in channels with PDP.

Secondly, the variations could occur at the level of pairs of coordinated muscles that contribute to modify the shape of the vocal tract. The resulting variations will be expressed in the SD of mean latency times.

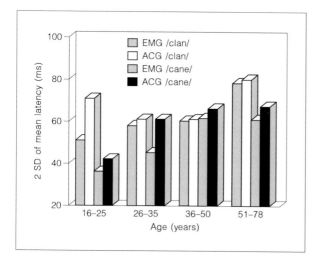

Fig. 43. Mean intra-individual ACG and EMG reaction time variability of immediate verbal reactions to the words /clan/ and /cane/ (first trial, with fore-period = 0) in 34 healthy subjects divided into four age groups.

4.4.6.2
Variability of Acousticogram and Electromyogram Latencies in Immediate Verbal Reactions Measured as Standard Deviations

In the diagram of figure 43, we report the SD for mean values of EMG and ACG latencies of /clan/ and /cane/ in immediate reactions (foreperiod = 0) for normal subjects, divided into four age groups: 16–25 years (8 subjects), 26–35 years (10), 36–50 years (7) and 51–78 years (9).

It can be appreciated how SD is greater for /clan/ in the group of the youngest and of the oldest subjects and how it increases for /cane/ with aging.

4.4.6.3
The Heuristic Value of Standard Deviations in Foreperiod Reactions

In normal subjects, the neural jitter related to the CCP variability factor will be expressed in the SD of mean latency times in delayed reading reactions with very short foreperiods. On the other hand, the neuromotor jitter related to the intermediary pre-executive and executive phases of word utterance will be reflected in the SD of mean latency times in delayed reading reactions with foreperiods >0.4 s.

On the other hand, in line with the proposal taken into consideration in 2.2 – and with particular reference to pathological conditions like schizophrenia – the SD of mean latency times in simple reactions seems the most adequate specific indicator of the neuromotor jitter related to the executive phase of the word utterance.

We must stress again that the intrinsic neural jitters could actually be identified by adopting a neutral task and trying to avoid at the same time all possible contingent interfering factors.

Two further questions, pertaining to two orders of functional biological factors, must be taken into consideration:

(A) Is there a variability in the 12-trial mean values and SD occurring at rather short periods during the life of the subject?

The origin of this variation might be double: (1) an exercise effect; (2) some psychological-functional variations in the subject's personality.

To answer this question about intra-individual variability requires a longitudinal investigation with repeated tests in the course of a convenient period that could be chosen in the range of 1 year. We will deal with this study in 5.3.

(B) How much do the 12-trial mean values and SD change as a function of age, i.e. in the course of maturation and aging?

This study will be carried out with interindividual cross-measurements (see Sections 6 and 7).

5

Multiple-Delayed-Reaction
Verbochronometry

Word Reading as an Intrinsically Complex Task and Foreperiods as Supersensitive Detectors

The substantial differences between verbochronometry and the most usual methodology of reaction times are threefold. The first difference concerns the task to be carried out by the subject. The second difference consists in the foreperiods we can interpose between the presentation of the target and the execution signal, some of the foreperiods being shorter than the time taken by the CCP *(very short foreperiods)* and some exceeding the CCP time. In their turn, some of these *long foreperiods* were chosen with a relatively short duration, others with a longer-lasting duration. The corresponding values were identified by original tentative experiments intending to identify two points: (1) the long foreperiods with short duration or foreperiods between 0.4 and 3 s were used to measure the time during which the ongoing internal flow of impulses reaches an optimal facilitating effect; (2) the longest foreperiods (3–4 and sometimes 10 s) were tested to discover the *temporal* decay of the encoded patterns of signals. These procedures will be analysed in 5.2 and 5.3.

5.1.1
The Task to Be Performed by the Subject

The task requested in our MDRV during the first study period was the utterance of a disyllabic word appearing at random on a PC screen out of a couple of similar words. More recently, we have adopted a threefold task with a syllable, a disyllabic word and a sentence having the first syllable in common. In this way, phonological and grammatical formulator processes were analysed.

The brain processes and the neuromotor executive performances of such tasks are much more complex than those of the usual reactions of pressing a key [Welford, 1980], of moving our foot [Saltzman and Kelso, 1987] or our eyes and hand [Aldridge et al., 1980]. In fact, the task of uttering a word in choice reactions implies a *more differentiated mental* activity with implicit semantic reference. Moreover, the corresponding cerebral activity of CCP, at variance with other actions like oculomotion, gait or pressing a key, is involved in a complex chain of operations: each syllable of the word must be matched with the corresponding cerebral representations of a set of muscles which must be coordinated to provide the correct utterance. Also, the brain must chronologically order the sequence of operations for the successive syllables. To become aware of the complexity of this task, one must underline that it includes a calculation by the brain itself of the cyclic time of excitation and inhibition of the neural structures delivering the invariant commands. Eventually the adaptation processes depend also on the muscular contraction time, on relaxation time and on the retrieval of the neuromuscular coordinated synergy.

Moreover, a circular integration with impulses coming from exteroceptive and proprioceptive receptors has been operating continuously since the starting phase. Information about whichever obstacle altering a kinematic condition (the so-called 'pipe-in-the-mouth phenomenon') will modify, already in the first trial, the specific invariant commands to the motor units. On the other hand, when the articulatory programme is already under execution, afferent external trigeminal stimuli, at least at low intensity, will not interfere with the ongoing coordinating action. On the contrary, a suppression effect is exerted by stimuli of an identical intensity during a more automatic powerful movement like chewing [Pinelli and Ceriani, 1992] (see also 4.4.4).

5.1.2
Implementation Modalities

The mean latency time of the ACG onset corresponds to the total time spent by the conduction and transmission of the impulses from the retina (input) through PDP in associative loops to CCP of the programming system (corresponding to the hidden unit layer of the artificial network) and hence to the motoneuronal system providing the innervation of the muscles (output). The resulting air vibrations are directly recorded as ACG.

We have previously explained how it is possible to measure separately the input, the 'hidden' and the output processes by asking the subject to perform not only immediate, but also delayed reading reactions. In this case, the subject does not pronounce the word immediately after its presentation on the PC, but he does it after a precise interval, exactly when a 'go' signal (a few asterisks) is shown on the PC.

In our present routine methodology the stimulus task is constantly maintained on the PC screen during the whole interval and also with the appearance of a series of asterisks below and over the stimulus task. This modality was chosen in order to avoid the involvement of the short-term memory which, on the contrary, is activated when the stimulus task is removed after a few seconds of presentation. A possible component of a short-term-memory-like process in the attention implied in the readiness answer will be discussed in 5.2.

With the most suitable intervals (very short foreperiods, foreperiods between 0.4 and 3 s and foreperiods lasting 3–10 s), we increase markedly the analytic capacities of the tests in two areas of investigation: (1) separating the measurement of the brain central computational processes from that of the effector processes; (2) evaluating the degree of parallelism (or synchrony) of several operative brain processes, that is the acceptance capacity of the brain for simultaneous multiple functions inherent to the same task.

5.1.3
Long Foreperiods

We found that in normal adult subjects foreperiods from 500 to 1,500 or even 4,000 ms give rise to the best performance with the shortest latency time (of ACG and EMG). A more precise identification of the 'best' foreperiod was obtained in relation to the type of task to be carried out by the subject and particularly the frequency of use of the word stimulus.

A 500-ms foreperiod can work for the most usual words, whereas a 1,500-ms foreperiod was requested for words with low frequency of use. On the other hand, prolongation of the foreperiod to 3,000 ms did not significantly change the latency times (of ACG and EMG), while longer ones (beginning with 4,000 ms) could give rise to slightly longer latency times, even if always below the ACG latency of the immediate responses.

The decrease in latency time with foreperiods longer than the CCP time with respect to that of the immediate reactions (foreperiod = 0) was expressed with the ratio of intermediary processes of ACG latency at $FP_{1.5}$ to ACG latency at FP_0 that was found to be <0.9 in normal subjects. The explanation of the decrease in ACG latency with the 1.5-second foreperiod requires a further analysis of the processes of the earliest brain operations, of the afteractivity and the associated intermediary internal circuits that develop during the foreperiod. In fact, at the moment of the 'go' signal, the subject has already performed perceptive and central computational processes and has created a homogeneous low-threshold neuronal assembly in the sense of Hebb [1949].

In the usual box models, at the intermediary phase, an operative buffer is drawn: with reference to this concept we have already mentioned the hypothesis of the articulatory buffer in Levelt's blueprint of speech formulation. Anyway, in accordance with the critical analysis developed in the previous chapter, it seems more realistic to focus our evaluation of the intermediary processes mainly on the low-threshold neural assembly produced by reverberating CCP cycles. Owing to the different contexts and the functional meaning of the CCP, we used in that case the term 'intrinsic facilitating feedbacks'. The related function – as we mentioned in 2.5 – was analysed further by Hinton et al. [1993] who improved the validity of brain PDP models by introducing into the hidden unit layers a sweep circuit of *clean-up units* (see fig. 17, section 2). Now, trying to perfect the evaluation of the temporal course of these different processes, it seems necessary to consider the chain of events and the final triggers in more detail.

....

Sensorimotor Transformations, Triggering and Retrieval Processes

To follow the analysis of the functional multiple-delayed-reaction processes and of the corresponding brain structures and the operative times, the reader may refer to the figures reported and described in Section 2.

5.2.1
The Chain of Events in Immediate and in 1,500-ms Delayed Reading Reactions

The immediate-response latency time (total t) includes:

$$t = V + eCCP + IL + E, \tag{1}$$

where V is the visual perceptive process, eCCP indicates the early central processes, IL corresponds to internal intermediary processes and E indicates the executive processes including a triggering pre-executive phase.

The latency time of a 1.5-second delayed reading response (ACG latency at $FP_{1.5}$) includes perceptive + executive processes.

In the meantime, in the foreperiod between the visual signs of the word and those of the 'go' signal, a certain number of CCP occurs: they maintain the transformed visuomotor patterns and facilitate the corresponding neural substrate. Thus, it seems opportune to differentiate the internal intermediary processes (IL) from delayed intermediary processes (DL), by the following equations:

$$IL = 1 \text{ invariant-to-variant CCP,} \tag{2}$$

$$DL = nCCP \text{ of foreperiod,} \tag{3}$$

where nCCP = a certain number of central processes occurring during the foreperiod.

The ACG latency at $FP_{1.5}$ can significantly depend on eCCP and IL only if a fundamental condition d1 is respected: perceptive + executive process times are eCCP and IL times. Only under condition d1 is ACG latency at $FP_{1.5}$ shorter than ACG latency at FP_0; this means that the previous nCCP in the foreperiod must have time enough in multiple delayed reactions to occur regularly, letting the programmed visuomotor patterns of impulse activate neural assemblies.

The time taken by the CCP can thus be obtained as the difference between ACG latencies at FP_0 and $FP_{1.5}$, i.e. $(V + eCCP + IL + E) - (V + E) = eCCP + IL$. In this equation we assume that, in multiple delayed reactions, a perceptive process occurs, with an identical value during both immediate and delayed reactions: in the delayed reaction it starts just when the subject perceives the 'go' signal (which is represented by the asterisks appearing above and below the word).

The value eCCP + IL, according to equations 1–3, corresponds to nCCP. This inference is valid as long as the condition d1 is respected.

5.2.2
The Chain of Structures Implied in the Delayed Reactions and Related 'Active Memories'

The neural structures underlying the previously described events have recently been well described by Fuster [1993].

In the posterior cortex, representations of perceptual memory are probably organized hierarchically, much as perceptual processing. The simplest unimodal sensory memories would be represented at the earliest processing levels, in primary sensory and higher-order sensory areas, while the most complex multisensory memories would reside in the networks of the higher associative cortex of temporoparietal regions.

Motor representation in frontal areas appears to be organized symmetrically to that of perceptual presentation in posterior areas, as if one were the mirror image of the other. Thus, whereas the prefrontal cortex represents broad schemes of sequential temporally organized movement (area 1), the premotor and motor cortices represent more specific movements that are discrete in terms of somatotopy and trajectory. In spoken language, the syntax, the ideas, logical statements and perhaps even sentences would be represented in the prefrontal cortex, whereas the words (morphemes and phonemes) would be represented in the premotor and motor cortices. (Broca's area, with its articulatory function, is located like the premotor cortex at an intermediate stage between the prefrontal and oropharyngeal motor cortices.) Implicit in this hypothetical arrangement is the notion that the processing of action flows from prefrontal to motor areas, from the general to the specific. Also implicit is the notion that, in the organization of temporally extended behaviour or of language, the cognitive function that bridges percepts and movements across time should be most evident and necessary in the prefrontal cortex, where the global scheme of action is presented and monitored during execution (see second part of Section 6). So, the short-term memory and motor set functions of the prefrontal cortex seem 'to lay the bridge from perception to action over time' [Fuster, 1993], closing at its highest level the cycle of perception and action. There is consistent neurophysiological evidence for these assumptions.

Although most of the cortical processing of movement probably runs through parallel streams, again in analogy with perceptual processing, and involves subcortical nuclei, successive populations of neurons are recruited down the frontal hierarchy before a given motor act is generated (areas 1, 18, 19). In the *delay tasks,* where a stimulus precedes the response by seconds or minutes, cells are first activated in the prefrontal cortex (areas 9, 46), then in the premotor cortex and finally the motor cortex.

From this order of cellular engagement, it has been suggested, that prefrontal neurons specialize in the memory of sensory and temporal information, whereas premotor and motor neurons specialize in planning responses or so-called 'set' processes (area 18).

As already mentioned, however, all three major frontal stages of the motor hierarchy appear to be involved in active memory and set. What differs in these stages is the temporal range of these two cognitive functions. They span the longest time in the prefrontal cortex where global schemes of behaviour are represented and where, during enactment, perceptions and movements are integrated over the longest periods. Memory and set span the shortest time in the motor cortex, where the 'microstructuring' [Brown, 1987] of movement takes place.

In the context of motor processing, the active aspect of memory needs to be emphasized. During operation of the perception-action cycle, Fuster [1993] assumes that the neuronal substrate of sensory and motor memories must be temporarily in the active state, as single-unit studies strongly indicate. The substrate may coincide to a large extent with that of long-term memory. The neurons of a cortical long-term storage network, to which frontal neurons belong in as much as the network represents movement and its perceptual antecedents, are induced to fire above the resting rate for as long as memory needs to be retained to implement current behaviour. (The term 'active memory' is preferable to that of 'working memory', because working memory may imply a separate neural substrate and memory system, whereas active memory simply implies, more appropriately, a different state of the very same substrate that stores permanent memory.)

Set also implies a kind of active memory: the 'memory' of forthcoming responses or movements in preparation. It has been called 'memory of the future' [Ingvar, 1985]. Thus short-term memory and motor set would represent two mutually complementary functions of the prefrontal cortex.

5.2.3
The Decoding-Triggering Processes

A further point to be considered in the evaluation of the results that can be obtained by our methodology is the inclusion of a decoding-triggering process occurring in the 1.5-second delayed reading reaction. However, a correct neurophysiological analysis of the events corresponding to this decoding-triggering process demonstrates that it requires such a very short period of time that it could be disregarded with reference to the difference ACG latency at FP_0 – ACG latency at $FP_{1.5}$. One must keep in mind that a retrieval time is implied in the triggering process, but it may be considered equivalent to the retrieval process included in the intermediary processes.

5.2.4
Roelofs's Derivation of the Expected Retrieval Latency

On the basis of a series of experimental researches carried out with the methodology of *stimulus onset asynchrony* [Levelt, 1993], Roelofs [1992] presented a mathematical formula for the derivation of the expected retrieval latency in speaking. The symbols used are those of the proportional calculation [Hofstadter, 1991]:

Let T denote time, let s be the sth time ($s = 1, 2, \ldots$) and Δt the duration of a time step (ms).

Definitions:

$f(s) = p$ (selection at s) and

$h(s) = p$ [selection at s | $\neg \exists u : (u < s \wedge$ selection at u)],

respectively, the probability mass function and the hazard rate function.

Derivation of $f(s)$ from $h(s)$:

$$h(s) = p \text{ [selection at s} \mid \neg \exists u : (u < s \land \text{selection at } u)]$$

$$= \frac{p \text{ [(selection at s)} \land (\neg \exists u : [u < s \text{ selection at } u])]}{p \text{ [} \neg \exists u : (u < s \land \text{selection at } u)]}$$

$$= \frac{p \text{ (selection at s)}}{p \text{ [} \neg \exists u : (u < s \land \text{selection at } u)]}$$

$$= f(s) \Big/ \prod_{j=0}^{s-1} [1 - h(j)]$$

$$\Rightarrow f(s) = h(s) \prod_{j=0}^{s-1} [1 - h(j)],$$

where $h(0) = 0$.

For the expectation of T holds:

$$E(T) = \sum_{s=1}^{\infty} f(s) \, s \Delta t$$

$$= \sum_{s=1}^{\infty} h(s) \left\{ \prod_{j=0}^{s-1} [1 - h(j)] \right\} s \Delta t.$$

The propositional definition of the alternative pathways of the different neural processes from the mental representation to the utterance of the corresponding words was formulated with reference to the spreading-activation connection model of Dell and Juliano [1991]. It represents a comprehensive point of reference for the experimental clinical research of the neural processes involved in sentence formulation and the related occurrence of errors, the time latency of the different phases and the duration of the sequence requested by the task.

Measuring Reverberating Circuits

> In the brain, we assume that there is an iterative process, and we simulate this by dividing time into many small steps and updating the activation of each unit once in each time step, based on the activations of other units at the previous step. In the case of networks with symmetrical connectivity, this causes them to settle, after a pattern is presented, into a stable condition or *attractor*, in which the relevant patterns are active in all parts of the networks.
>
> [McClelland, 1994]

5.3.1
From the Conceptualizer to the Formulators

In a preliminary design of the CCP or reverberating circuits, we will refer to spontaneous speech. The analogous mechanism in word reading reactions will be considered in Section 6.

The translation of the impulse pattern from the mental representation ('mentese' according to Pinker [1995]) in the 'conceptualizer' [Levelt, 1989] to the grammatical and phonological representations in the formulators corresponds to a flow of impulses that is homologous to a 'mental late activity': the nature of this activity has previously been defined with regard to the delayed reactions, as intermediary processes. This remains true however fast the translation from the conceptualizer to the formulators may be. On the other hand, some differences may occur in the course rate and in the amplitude of the neural events characterizing spontaneous speech and delayed reactions, respectively.

The activation of the formulators will correspond to a decoding-triggering process of the facilitated neural assembly in word reading reactions.

5.3.2
The Internal Circuits

All things considered, the dynamic internal circuit theory of the mental activity, proposed by Pinelli [1970–1971] and McKay [1987] and recently developed in a model by Rosenfeld [1993], appears to be a reliable landmark also for the interpretation of the decoding-triggering process. A stream of impulses runs in internal programming circuits of corticogangliobasal loops. This internal circuit (corresponding to a latent mental activity) can be connected to the executive output by one of the following systems, partly decisional and partly automatic: (1) the conceptualizer [Levelt, 1989]; (2) an external more or less conditioned stimulus acting on the hebbian assembly; (3) an internal impulse of emotional nature. These three systems, related respectively to the frontotemporal-parietal cortex, the corticosubcortical circuits and the limbic-frontobasal circuits, provide what we might call in psychological terms a voluntary decisional act, short-circuit automatic behaviour or emotional reaction.

Different situations can occur when one system prevails or when, on the contrary, all systems contribute to different degrees to trigger the final executive process. At the same time, the ascending reticular system provides interacting impulses of attentional nature.

5.3.3
The Circuits for Low-Threshold Neural Assemblies Reverberating from 1 to 6 Times

On the grounds of the previously defined patterns, we can look more closely at the events occurring in the intermediary foreperiod of verbal reactions (Section 2, fig. 13–15).

As we mentioned, the minimal ACG latency response was obtained with foreperiod values of 500–1,500 ms. This last value seems the optimal one for delayed reading reactions of unusual words: in this interval the facilitation process develops its full activity. To embark on the interpretation of the underlying brain activities requires the analysis of what occurs in this interval in order to formulate a more correct general model of the facilitation process.

From the moment of the word stimulus presentation on the screen of the PC monitor to the appearance of the 'go' signal around it, CCP are activated with a latent mental activity (unconscious thinking) going on. An internal stream of impulses is conducted and transmitted in the central computational systems co-activated for the word control. These flows of impulses lower the synaptic threshold of the related hebbian assemblies and make them ready to react. In artificial neural networks, this process is named 'lowering of weight' or synaptic threshold. This facilitation involves homogeneously a large number of neurons that become integrated in an assembly answering Hebb's [1949] criteria: thus, we call it a 'lowered-threshold neural assembly'. An equivalent, even if maybe less precise term, used by some authors and by us in the course of this book, is 'facilitated neural assembly'.

In order to effect this facilitation, the flow of impulses has to pass through the neural assembly a certain number of times. The circuits reverberate during a different period of time, according to the more or less available representations. After a low-threshold neural assembly has been obtained, when the 'go' signal has been perceived by the subject, his programming internal circuit triggers the discharges of the assembly that will be conducted and transmitted to the executive systems.

According to our experimental data, for the most usual words a value of 500 ms seems to be a sufficient period of reverberating circuits to effect the facilitatory processes of neural assemblies. In contrast, raising the threshold for less usual words may require foreperiods as long as 1,500 ms. This finding allows us to find out how the number of recurring internal intrinsic facilitating feedbacks can be calculated.

In the previous chapter we have given an idea of the time taken by a single CCP process. Now we will identify the successive stages of activity. We will start our calculations with those occurring during a period as long as 1,500 ms: (a) the subject has perceived the stimulus word on the PC: this event requires about 100 ms, taking into consideration the modality of the PDP already mentioned; (b) he has also performed the passage from the visual areas to Broca's centre, taking a further 30 ms; (c) CCP implies a cortical-gangliobasal-cerebellar loop requiring about 100 ms; (d) the phonological operation is accomplished by the formulator in about 30 ms; (e) the further computation of the temporal order of succession of discharges for the word might last about 30 ms.

Thus we have an idea of the *cumulative time* of the operation involved in the CCP: $100 + 30 + 100 + 30 + 30 = 290$ ms.

Then the time during which the reverberating intrinsic feedbacks are running would be $1{,}500 - 290 = 1{,}210$ ms. A single CCP recurring in the complete loop of the phases previously named (c, d, e) comprises 160 ms, and hence the number of times of recurrent CCP cycles would be $1{,}210 : 160 = 7.5$. This means, in line with Hinton's model [Hinton et al., 1993], that a 7 times reverberating circuit (or internal flows of impulses, or internal feedbacks) is the optimal condition to accomplish the process of hebbian facilitation of low-threshold neural assemblies in unusual tasks and to avoid all possible later decays as those appearing with a longer foreperiod (>400 ms). These decays might be due to intrinsic properties or some negative interfering effects: in psychological terms one could speak of fading or inhibited attention.

The next and final stage is the execution of the reaction to utter the word, after having perceived the 'go' signal. Triggering the 'prefacilitated' low-threshold neural assembly can be compared to an Exner-Cattell prepared reflex [Pinelli, 1964]. Without the 'go' perceptive time and the executive time, what remains is the time taken for the transmission from the occipital internal circuit to Broca's area. This transmission time from occipital lobe to Broca's area might last about 15 ms. Broca's area will in turn produce the final triggering discharges.

Intra-Individual Variations of Verbochronometric Parameters

In a quantitative evaluation of brain functionality with MDRV, a fundamental question addresses the degree of constancy of the resulting values in a single subject. To answer this question, we must find out how much a trial mean value and SD can vary when we repeat the same examination after a determined period of time. In this way, we can check if, and within which limits, MDRV allows us to identify a functional marker of brain functions in one individual subject.

In this chapter, we will study the possible variations in MDRV results obtained from one individual subject submitted to several identical investigations in the course of 1 year.

On the other hand, the static factors, of both genetic and epigenetic origin, responsible for *interindividual* differences will be treated in 6.1.

Eventually, *intra-individual* variations during life, corresponding to the biological cycle of maturation and aging, will be treated later on, in 6.4 and 8.1.

5.4.1
Repetition of the Same Series of Reactions at 1- to 12-Month Intervals

To compare the results of the series of reading reactions in one single individual, at a first basal examination and after determined periods of time, is of great interest, in line with various questions [Georgopoulos et al., 1981].

A comparison between basal and later results allows us to measure the range of the reliability of mean and related SD values that should characterize the subject as far as brain functions in speech production are concerned.

Still more important is the need to know the individual range of spontaneous variability of ACG latency in follow-up studies aiming to evaluate the course of the disease, the effects of the treatment or more generally the effects of drugs or neurotoxic substances on that particular subject.

At the interface between applied neurophysiology and cognitive psychology, the study of the effect of repetitions of multiple delayed reactions might yield new cues for the nature of what appears as a spontaneous normal variability. An acceleration of neural processes and particularly a diminution of SD could occur after preliminary exercises, and before a marked facilitation of hebbian neural assemblies (leading to learning effects) or changes in strategies of reaction performance take place.

We will limit the study of the intra-individual variability of a 12-trial mean value and SD to a 2–3 times repeated series of reactions at a 1- to 12-month interval.

Real processes of learning may occur with a higher number of repetitions, a topic that we will treat later on (see 8.3).

Apart from facilitatory prelearning factors, other effects on the 12-trial mean value and SD in 2–3 repetitions could be produced, with opposite signs, by adverse contingent conditions, like stressing factors and migrainous disturbances.

Table 9. Repeated investigations of /mare/ and /muro/ reactions (ms): basal (0) and successive-month intervals

No.	Case	Sex	Age years	At month	ACG latency at FP_0				ACG latency at $FP_{0.1}$				ACG latency at $FP_{1.5}$			
					mean	%	SD	%	mean	%	SD	%	mean	%	SD	%
1	O.S.	F	27	0	437		56		471		64		354		27	
				1	414	−5	48	−14	395	−16	38	−40	305	−13	30	+10
2	D.A.	M	32	0	381		64		374		52		291		30	
				7	346	−9	31	−51	341	−8	25	−51	260	−10	18	−40
3	C.A.	F	26	0	354		38		–		–		283		27	
				12	361	+2	29	−23	–		–		289	+1	22	−18
4	P.I., migraine	M	39	0	351		43		334		45		205		5	
				12	281	−20	27	−38	341	+2	36	−15	192	−5	5	0
5	I.M., migraine	M	42	0	360		26		369		35		269		20	
				2	401	+11	71	+173	402	+8	49	+29	329	+18	40	+50
6	R.C., migraine	M	36	0	362		55		329		17		326		19	
					(356)		(73)		(327)		(17)		(335)	(29)		
				11	335	−7	35	−36	355	+7	20	+20				
					(332)	(−8)	(50)	(−31)	(302)	+7	(−28)	(+40)				
				14	302	−16	27	−50	278	−12	32	+90	258	−23	36	+8
													FP_3			
7	F.E.[1] epilepsy	M	33	0	681		87						702		62	
				3	603	−11	85	−3					576	−18	108	+45
									$FP_{1.5}$				FP_4			
8	M.L., spastic dysphonia	F	60	0	1,372		120		1,038		92		949		64	
				1	961	−67	78	−30	840	−19	52	−42	904	−10	18	−72

Figures in parentheses indicate ACG durations.
[1] See figure 44.

5.4.2
Intra-Individual Variations in Normals and Patients with Migrainous, Epileptic and Spastic Dysphonia

The results of two series of /mare/ and /muro/ reactions carried out in different periods by the same subject are reported in table 9 and figure 44.

The results pertain to 3 normal subjects, 3 patients with migraine (ophthalmic type), 1 epileptic (F.E.), who was under treatment with 0.8 g/day Tegretol, free of fits in the whole period of 3 months, and 1 patient with spastic dysphonia, investigated with MDRV 1 month after local treatment with botulinum toxin.

The 3 normal subjects had a similar level of education (middle school), IQ values (102–109), with normal findings at the anamnestic and clinical investigations. Cases 4, 5 and 6 were affected by migraine (ophthalmic type); in case 6, the number of migrainous attacks was about 2 per week; in patients 4 and 5 it was about 1 attack per month. The main results of MDRV worthy to be mentioned are the following:

(1) In the interval between in the two investigations, the first 3 subjects showed changes in ACG latency at FP_0, from +2 to −9% without a correlation with the time elapsed between the two investigations (1–12 months). The changes in SD were more ir-

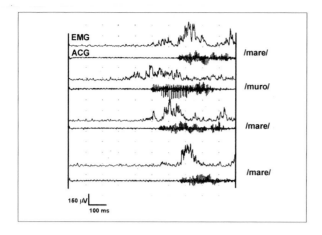

Fig. 44. Immediate reactions to /mare/ and /muro/. A retest. Subject F.E., male, 33 years old, affected by epilepsy (No. 7 in table 9).

regular, with higher dispersion: from –12 to –51% without correlation with the duration of the interval between the two investigations.

The changes were also evident in the delayed reactions and particularly at $FP_{1.5}$ (+1 to –13%) with rather large changes in SD (+10 to –40%). One can differentiate between two groups: (a) the normal subject C.A. (No. 3, interval 12 months) does not show any significant change, i.e. the mean ACG latency change is +2% at FP_0 and +1% at $FP_{1.5}$ with SD changes of –23 and –18%; (b) the normal subjects O.S. (No. 1, interval 1 month) and D.A. (No. 2, interval 7 months) show rather moderate decreases at FP_0 (–5%; –9%) and a little more marked ones at $FP_{1.5}$ (–13%; –10%); decreases in SD reach values of –40% to –50%.

(2) In the cases with migraine, the changes in ACG latency at FP_0 were more marked. In case 4, the decrease in mean value was –20% and in SD –38%. In contrast, case 5 showed a moderate increase in mean value (+11%) with an exceptionally high increase in SD (+173%). Case 6 was basically characterized by a relatively high intermediary process ratio (0.9), a point that will be discussed in Section 9. This case was 3 times investigated with MDRV and showed a progressive decrease in both mean values and SD. On the other hand, the intermediary process ratio remained practically unchanged (from 0.9 it decreased to 0.85). This last result is at variance with the increase in this ratio found in normals, in >4 repetitions of the same task, that in fact was due to a significant decrease in ACG latency at FP_0, without a correspondent decrease in ACG latency at $FP_{\geq 0.4}$. As we will discuss later (in 8.3), these changes reflect a learning effect.

On the grounds of these findings, the migrainous patients can also be separated into two groups: (a) 2 migrainous subjects, R.C. (No. 6, intervals 11 and 14 months) and P.I. (No. 4, interval 12 months), show rather marked decreases at FP_0 (–16% at the third examination with respect to the first and –20%, respectively); (b) 1 migrainous subject, I.M. (No. 5, interval 2 months), shows a moderate increase at the immediate (FP_0) and delayed reactions ($FP_{0.1}$, $FP_{1.5}$).

The patient with epilepsy (frontal bilateral foci), F.E. (No. 7, interval 3 months), had a rather high ACG latency at both immediate and delayed reactions (FP_3); the decrease at the second examination was rather moderate.

Patient M.L. (No. 8, interval 1 month) with spastic dysphonia *was treated with local injections of botulinum toxin* and showed a very marked decrease in ACG latency at FP_0 (see 9.2.1).

Increasing the Types of Stimuli within the Bounds of Reaction Ability and Reliability of Diagnostic Data

....

Picture Naming and Word Reading: Relevance of the Tasks and Interindividual Variations

> Verbochronometry with delayed reactions competes with EEG of speech-related events, spectrographic functional MRI and PET to differentiate functional changes in sensorimotor processes, active short-term memory and working memory. Interindividual variations may arise from both genetic and acquired factors.

6.1.1
Picture Naming Tests Occupy a Consistent Place in Verbochronometry in Association with Word Reading Reactions

There are two main reasons to include picture naming reactions in our methodology. The first arose when we started examining children at preschool age. The second reason emerged during the meeting of the World Federation Group of Organization and Delivery of Neurological Services in New Delhi (1994), when we wanted to extend the verbochronometric investigations also to illiterate people.

Picture naming tests with multiple alternatives were applied in association with word naming (reading) tests by the Nijmegen team of speech scientists: they called them the 'double naming tests'.

6.1.1.1
The Double Naming Tasks (Nijmegen Test)

6.1.1.1.1
Picture Naming

In the picture naming task at the Nijmegen laboratory, an intertrial interval of 1,500 ms was used after which a 1,000-Hz tone of 100 ms signalled to the subject the appearance of an arrow on the screen pointing to one of four possible pictures on a plastic frame. The subject had to name the picture as soon as the arrow appeared.

Sixteen different pictures of words with primary stress on the first syllable were used. They were grouped to 4 series: (1) monosyllabic; (2) disyllabic simple; (3) disyllabic complex; (4) trisyllabic.

Each block consisted of 12 repetitions. Block sequence and position on the picture frame were randomized in a balanced incomplete Latin square per subject. All words were classified as being of low frequency and belonged to the syntactic category of nouns. Each block was preceded by a learning session in which the subject had to learn the 4 combinations of pictures and words by heart, until he could name all 4 pictures without hesitation or errors. In general, each learning session lasted less than 1 min.

All subjects were instructed to focus on the middle of the screen before and after the arrow appeared.

The series of words were Dutch. It would be impossible to find the equivalents in the Italian language, but we guess that a test could be proposed with northern Italian dialects. A possible example is given:

(1) pont (ponte), occ' (occhio), nas (naso), pä (piede);
(2) canton (cantone), capel (cappello), casel (casello), soldat (soldato);
(3) ombrel (ombrello), baston (bastone), teston (testone), bestion (bestione);
(4) campanar (campanaro), frumenton (frumentone), bottiglion (bottiglione), bastiment (basti-mento).

6.1.1.1.2

Word Naming

The word naming task had an intertrial interval of 200 ms. A 1,000-Hz tone of 100 ms was followed by the appearance of a target word (out of a set of 32 possible target words) on the screen. The subject had to name the word as soon as it appeared on the screen. All 32 words were repeated 3 times and presented in a random order in two blocks of 48 trials each. They were balanced with the words in the picture naming task with respect to word type, word frequency, initial phoneme and number of sounds.

Preliminary learning trials were performed, like those of picture naming.

For both tasks, the response period lasted 1,000 ms after which the stimulus disappeared, followed by a silent period of 1,500 (pictures naming) or 2,000 ms (word naming).

6.1.1.1.3

Results

The mean values of *word duration* were similar in picture naming and word naming: series 1 = 435 ms; 2 = 640 ms; 3 = 740 ms; 4 = 670 ms. The SD were higher for picture naming (70–100 ms). In word naming *speech reaction time* (ACG latency) increases from 1-syllable words (550 ms) to 2-syllable words (565 ms) and to 3-syllable words (580 ms). In contrast, in picture naming, ACG latency for 3 syllables decreases with respect to 2 and even to 1 syllable: series 1 = 725 ms; 2 = 750 ms; 3 = 710 ms. This represents the so-called *inverse length effect.*

6.1.1.2

A Two-Alternative Picture Naming Test (Veruno Test)

Taking into account the need for verbochronometric tests to be applied to children at preschool age and to illiterate people, we devised tests simpler than those of the Nijmegen researchers. The leading idea was to present only 2 pictures of very familiar subjects, recurring 12 times each, in a random course. A detailed description of this test will be reported in 8.4 when dealing with the study of preschool age children.

6.1.2
The Impact of the Task on the Reading Reaction Parameters

6.1.2.1
A Preliminary Control: Jaw Movements in Speaking and Chewing

Reading reactions to /mare/ and /muro/ were compared with choice reactions where the subject was asked to open or close his jaw in response to a stimulus to open or close. The rationale of the initial project was based on the consideration that opening and closing the jaw was a common performance in both kinds of reactions, whilst verbal related processes were a specific component in the reactions to /mare/ and /muro/. If other conditions were the same in the two kinds of reactions, one could hypothetically calculate the time of the verbal operating processes from the difference between EMG latencies in verbal reactions and in chewing reactions. In both groups of experiments we recorded the EMG from the temporal and the digastric muscles.

However, the results of these experiments showed that other relevant factors differentiate the *artificially* isolated elementary jaw movements from the articulatory jaw movements during speech. In fact, we found that EMG latency is longer in the simple opening and closing of the jaw than in the analogous automatic movement of speaking. The most likely explanation of this finding is that genetic endowment and, even more, the long educational training of speaking created well-organized neuronal hebbian assemblies at a low triggering threshold, which do not exist for isolated non-purposeful movements. In fact, the jaw movement requested in our non-verbal reactions were outside the natural performances of mastication.

6.1.3
Immediate Verbal Choice Reactions: Latencies of Electromyogram and Acousticogram

6.1.3.1
The Activation Order of the Different Neuromuscular Executors for a Single Word

The activation order of the different muscles in the subglottal, glottal and supraglottal sectors of the vocal tract might vary according to the multitrajectory degree of freedom. Greater changes have been observed under different starting conditions of the executors [Georgopoulos et al., 1981].

The order of activation was found to undergo several types of changes in abnormal conditions like stuttering. More consistent impairments of coordination were found not only in cerebellar diseases but also in cases of phonetic disintegration of cortical origin [Schönle et al., 1992; Schönle and Grone, 1992].

6.1.3.2

Latency Time of the Onset of the Electromyogram

6.1.3.2.1

A Preliminary Distinction

Our first concern was to check if the EMG recorded from the orbicularis oris muscle had something to do with an alarm reaction. This possibility was in fact ruled out since it never correlated with the occurrence of generalized signs of alertness like neck muscular activity [Pinelli and Ceriani, 1992]. Moreover, the values of EMG latency time displayed rather specific changes in relation with the different words. The mean EMG latency was found indeed to correspond to the preparatory phase of the verbal reaction.

6.1.3.2.2

The Preparatory Electromyogram

On the grounds of previous analyses (e.g. Section 3) we consider the first part or 'dome' of the EMG to represent the early tonic short innervation which modulates the basal tension of the muscles required for the utterance of the word stimulus. This innervation corresponds to the first phase of the CCP activity in the brain and we have analysed in previous chapters how it provides the tuning regulation of the stiffness, an operation differing from the executive successive processes in being less modulated in its development. In the further course of the text, we will indicate the latency time of the EMG onset as EMG latency.

6.1.3.2.3

The Executive Articulatory Phase of the Electromyogram

We analysed previously how the second 'dome' or spindle of the EMG might be considered to reflect the finer and more syllable-specific innervation of the executive articulatory phase. (A more neurophysiologically oriented analysis will be made in 7.3.2.) This innervation will produce the muscle contractions causing the changes in shape of the vocal tract required for the utterance of the first letter in the word target. The time taken by the CCP in the brain to generate this executive contraction after the preparatory phase could be denominated the shaping time, and it can be measured as the difference between the latency time of the ACG onset and the EMG latency. Of course, since the times of occurrence of motor unit electrical discharges (EMG) and muscle contraction (equivalent to the ACG) are different, we must subtract from EMG latency – ACG latency a delay of 60 ms, corresponding to the interval between the electrical impulse and the muscle contraction.

Preliminary investigations showed that the shaping time undergoes different changes in pathological conditions like spasticity, rigidity and ataxia.

6.1.3.3

Total Latency Time of the Acousticogram

The mean ACG latency time in immediate responses, calculated from 12 successive trials, can be significantly affected by numerous factors that will be listed below.

6.1.3.3.1
Frequency of Use of the Word

Words with a high frequency of use are taken out from the encyclopaedic buffer [Levelt, 1989] during verbal reactions with a shorter time than that required for more rarely used words. Differences as great as 25 ms were found between the two classes of words.

6.1.3.3.2
Length of the Utterance

With reference to the effects of the length of utterance one can state that it proportionally increases ACG latency, but there are numerous different factors that are worth considering.

6.1.3.3.3
The Syllable Effect in the Word

The length of the word to be pronounced increases the ACG latency in the order of 10 ms for each syllable [Sternberg et al., 1978]. It has recently been found that this rule is not completely respected when the word is pronounced within long sentences.

6.1.3.3.4
The Accenting Effect

When one reads to words with an equal number of letters and equal frequency of use, the word with the accent on the last syllable shows a 15-ms increase in ACG latency. This prosodic mechanism seems to imply a specialized CCP.

6.1.4
Phonological, Semantic and Linguistic Factors: Different Tasks and Their Effects on Reaction Times

6.1.4.1
Artificial Word Stimuli without Meaning

Verbal reactions to artificial word stimuli or pseudo-words were thought to bypass the semantic analyser, a stage that should be included in verbal reactions to natural meaningful words with a similar phonological conformation. A comparison of the results of these two different kinds of reactions should allow us to detect the operative time taken by the semantic analyser.

However, this hypothesis underwent a radical revision in the course of our research.

In fact, to comprehend the meaning of a word is not compulsory in the experiment of reading repetitively a single word even if it is presented at random as it occurs in our tests of verbal reactions. It is more correct to assume that the reader performs his task automatically. In fact, the calculations we developed from the whole series of processes of speech control in verbal reactions do not include a semantic stage.

The greatest difference between words and non-words in relation to the production of their utterance is represented by a zero value for the frequency of use of the latter. This difference would produce an increase in ACG latency at variance with the saving of time expected by the absence of a semantic phase. A trend to an indirect use frequency > 0 could be due to a possible association between the non-word and a used natural word according to the research on prototypes we previously reported. The interpretation of all these factors makes the experiments of comparison between word and non-word reactions appear to ambiguous for the identification of a semantic stage.

6.1.4.2
A Way to Assess the Semantic Stage

A task for verbal reactions implying the activation of the semantic analyser could be found in some denomination trials or in the presentation of incomplete phrases where one word was omitted; the subject was then asked to pronounce the missing word.

The search for a comparative task, similar in visual perception and reading but not implying a semantic stage, should include a suitable phase of preliminary learning.

6.1.4.3
Concrete versus Abstract Words

There is neuropsychological evidence that the production of concrete words like /mare/ and /muro/ is processed mainly in the non-dominant hemisphere, whilst the abstract words like /virtù/ and /vizio/ or /male/ and /mito/ are processed in the dominant one (see also 4.4.2.1). Thus, it becomes possible to evaluate whether a CCP impairment prevails or is confined in only one hemisphere by comparing verbal reactions with these two different pairs of word stimuli, i.e. concrete and abstract.

A relevant factor that must be taken into consideration is the emotional meaning linked particularly to abstract words, like for example 'freedom'. On the other hand, sexual emotion is obvious for pornographic words.

As it will be discussed later in Section 8, we found, with this methodology, that crossing interhemispheric effects of facilitating and hindering nature can occur. An example of the results with /mare/ and /muro/ and with /male/ and /mito/ is given in figure 45.

6.1.4.4
Length Effect and Inverse Length Effect

Van Lieshout et al. [1991] carried out several studies on the effects of word length on ACG latency. Usually word size is discussed as a linguistic variable [Peters et al., 1991], but within the area of motor control of speech a different perspective is used. Crucial to such an approach is the concept of a *motor plan* by which the speech articulators are controlled [Klapp et al., 1973; Rosenbaum et al., 1987; Sternberg et al., 1978]. This motor plan is an 'abstract code or structure that, when executed, results in movement' [Schmidt, 1988, p. 266].

Kelso et al. [1983] criticized this view of motor programming and proposed a 'dynamic pattern' perspective on control and coordination of movement.

A basic notion, supported by some findings, concerns the *advance response preparation* [Keele, 1982; Schmidt, 1988]. For speech, it was found that by increasing the size of a word in its number of syllables, normal-speaking subjects showed longer ACG latencies [Klapp et al., 1973; Klapp, 1974; Klapp and Wyatt, 1976].

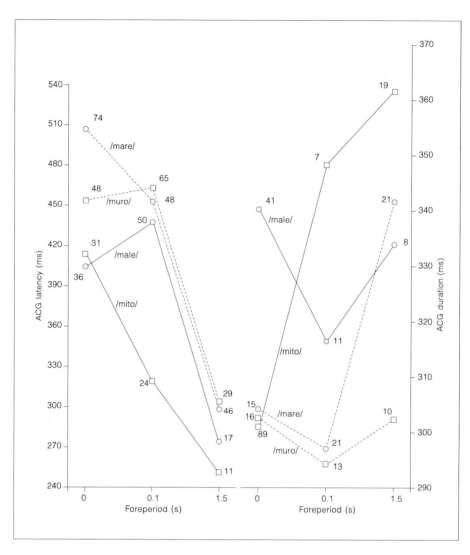

Fig. 45. ACG latencies and durations of /mare/ (--○--), /muro/ (--□--), /male/ (—○—) and /mito/ (—□—). Subject A.F., male, 41 years old. Figures near symbols indicate SD.

In our experiments [Pinelli and Ceriani, 1992], as reported in table 1 (see 3.2.2), the increase in ACG latency of /camel/ with respect to /clock/ was present in 3,000-ms foreperiod reactions with a value of 15 ms, with an equal ACG duration. Since in a 3,000-ms foreperiod-reaction the preparation has already been performed, one would rather stress the role of the dynamic pattern. Anyway it was argued that the syllable is the basic unit of motor control of speech: thus, in adding syllables, the number of motor plan units would increase and therefore subjects would need more time to prepare the total motor programme.

The assumption that syllables form the basic unit of the speech motor plan was questioned by Sternberg et al. [1978]. They showed that the effect of word size (in number of syllables) on the total speech reaction time was added to the effect of increasing the number of words or stress groups (a segment of speech associated with a primary stress) within an utterance. In view of further original findings, Sternberg et al. [1978] proposed the four-stage model for motor control of speech.

In the first or *motor-programming* stage, a motor or phonetic plan, as Levelt [1989] called it, is assembled and incorporated in a motor memory buffer. In the second or *retrieval* stage, the motor plan is retrieved from the memory buffer. In the third or *unpacking* stage, each unit is unpacked or fractionized into smaller parts or subunits (syllables, articulatory gestures, sounds) which are transferred to the fourth or *neuromotor command* stage in which each subunit results in neuromotor system actions and the execution of the intended movements.

Within the third stage, the processing time will be influenced by the size of the motor plan unit, as determined by the number of syllables of a word or stress group [Sternberg et al., 1978; Levelt, 1989].

According to Sternberg et al. [1978], what is exactly specified within a motor plan is not considered to be critical to the model. To understand specific motor production factors for speech at the level of motor execution would require an incursion in the correlated neurophysiological processes.

The different phases are considered to be independent from each other, and therefore the total time needed to prepare a response is the sum of each time interval resulting from the separate phases. Motor execution times must also be added when computing the total ACG latency.

6.1.4.5
Higher-Level Linguistic Processing

Peters et al. [1989] assumed that higher-level linguistic processing is going on in parallel with lower-level motor programming of speech and can interfere with it. They carried out some experiments allowing to investigate the effect of varying the size of a word (number of syllables or number of sounds) as well as the effect of linguistic complexity on the time interval between stimulus presentation and speech onset (ACG latency). Two criteria were therefore adopted.

(1) In varying the number of sounds without changing the number of syllables in a word, one should be able to differentiate the effects of within-word variations in terms of number of syllables (the manipulation of word size) and in number of sounds and articulatory effort (the manipulation of sound cluster or word complexity): longer ACG latencies for words with more sounds but the same number of syllables would suggest either a smaller subunit in motor control of speech than the syllable or that the phonological structure of sound clusters have to be considered in preparing a word response, as we suggested by Yaniv et al. [1990].

(2) To estimate the effects of linguistic complexity on ACG latency, the authors used two different naming tasks, i.e. a picture naming task and a word naming (reading) task. In picture naming, due to a different order by which semantic and phonological codes are accessed, more extensive linguistic processing is needed than in word naming [Kroll and Smith, 1989; Smith and Maggie, 1986].

Furthermore, as Klapp et al. [1973] suggested, in using picture naming tasks, possible effects of implicit speech and reading differences that can be present in word naming tasks are circumvented.

6.1.4.6
Synopsis of Word Reading and Picture Naming Reactions

The increase in ACG latency for 2-syllable words in comparison to 1-syllable words is well established [Klapp et al., 1973]. It was also confirmed in our experiment for the same increase of 15 ms (table 1, 3.2.2).

The decrease in 3-syllable words in the picture naming task, as opposed to the word naming task, is more difficult to be understood, as two different aspects are involved: first, the difference of the naming task in ACG latency for 3-syllable words and, second, the decrease in ACG latency itself.

Concerning the first aspect, it is important to realize that in a choice reaction of a word naming task differences of ACG latencies might not simply reflect differences in response preparation but also differences in other processes. Possible disturbing influences in this respect may arise from implicit variations of speech and reading time [Klapp et al., 1973]. Therefore, differences in word size as responsible for differences in ACG latency of word naming tasks must be considered with much caution, unless sufficient control conditions can be supplied with respect to the factors just mentioned. In using picture naming tasks, this problem may be circumvented: effects of word size in picture naming seem to be more reliable with respect to response preparation [Klapp et al., 1973].

Taking into account these factors, van Lieshout et al. [1991] tried to explain the *inverse length effect* found with 3-syllable words in the picture naming task. In fact, a possible answer to this question is implicit in a study carried out by Rosenbaum [1987]. With rapid finger responses, he found that the latency (comparable to ACG latency), of the first response in a choice reaction time task *decreased as the length of the required sequence increased.* In order to explain these findings he introduced the notion of 'scheduling strategies'. These strategies are based on the principle that during the execution of a series of responses, later responses can be edited (= prepared) in such a way that 'means and variances of interresponse times can be minimized' [Rosenbaum, 1987, p. 176]. In plain words, if more responses can fill the time interval needed to prepare any following responses, the execution of the first response can start earlier. Similar suggestions in terms of interresponse programming were made in earlier research by Klapp and Wyatt [1976].

A more recent study by Kornbrot [1989] revealed that the effect of the number of units prepared within a single motor plan depends on how the subjects can organize the motor task they have to perform. So, the same number of syllables per word can have different effects on ACG latency according to the way individual syllables can be grouped together at a higher organizational level, e.g. with respect to place or manner of articulation. The number of nodes at the high level determines the reaction time [Kornbrot, 1989].

In other words, the size of the motor plan unit may vary according to the specific motor task, and it might be difficult to compare two tasks if there are differences in the way subjects have organized speech motor control processes for both tasks. The fact that in the picture naming task a 4-choice reaction time paradigm was used, whereas the word naming task used a more complex one, could have induced subjects to use different (even unknown) motor control strategies for each naming tasks, which might explain the differences in ACG latency for 3-syllable words.

6.1.5
Interindividual Variations: Psychomotor Traits, Level of Education and Strategy of Performance

In order to obtain reliable mean values of the MDRV variables, we should refer to homogeneous groups of subjects taking into account also constitutional psychomotor traits and the degree of education.

A detailed analysis of these factors will be carried out later, in 7.1.

Interindividual differences may even be at variance with Sternberg's law [1966, 1969] of correlation between reaction time and length of the word; systematic investigations by Japanese authors showed 15–25% exceptions to this rule. Several factors may explain the exceptions: not only genetic endowment but also different psychological attitudes and acquired psychomotor abilities may influence the threshold and availability of the representations in the brain, with positive or negative effects [Collins and Quillian, 1969; Cohen and Faulkner, 1983].

The Grammatical Tasks

6.2.1
Edelman's Principle: Enunciation of a Sentence Overcomes Phonological Formulation of a Word or Syllable

The law of direct proportionality between length of utterance and reaction time maintains its value only when *restricted to the field of executive processes.*

In contrast, the linguistic domain prevails over a factor merely dependent on phonetics. We proved the validity of this statement with a threefold task, including both phonetic and grammatical performances.

Normal adults who read aloud a series of 3 word stimuli with different lengths, as /ma/, /mare/ and /mare è bello/ – each item presented at random – in each series of 10–12 reactions may show equal or even longer ACG and EMG latencies with /ma/ than with /mare è bello/. The results are given in figures 46–49, for 4 normal subjects of different ages.

With immediate reactions, ACG latency for sentences is the shortest in subject R.C. (fig. 47), shorter than for the monosyllable in subject D. (fig. 48) and for the disyllable in subject L.V. (fig. 49); in M.G. (fig. 46), ACG latencies are practically equal for all three tasks. The values of EMG latency show a similar trend and are never the longest for sentences.

With 100-ms foreperiod reactions, an increase in all ACG latencies is observed in cases M.G., L.V. and, at a lower rate, in D.: it is longer for monosyllables or for disyllables but never for sentences.

With the 1.5-second foreperiod, ACG and EMG latencies are the shortest for sentences. In cases M.G. and D., ACG latencies for sentences are intermediary, whereas in case R.C. a positive correlation for both ACG and EMG latencies with the length of the task was found.

In figure 50, ACG and EMG latencies of 1.5-second foreperiod reactions are compared for a young man and an old normal subject: the courses of ACG latencies are represented in figure 51. R.C. was one of the rare cases who, in 1.5-second foreperiod reactions, showed an increasing ACG latency from the monosyllable to the disyllable and sentence. This peculiar behaviour will be discussed in 6.4.

The finding of a significant decrease, or no change, of ACG latency with sentences with respect to mono- and disyllables is a proof of a lower threshold of the grammatical representation with respect to that of the simple syllable or the disyllabic word. This is the same as saying that the speech unit seems to correspond, under certain conditions of reading, to a sentence rather than to a syllable or a word.

In these experiments, we are dealing with a sentence conceived as a rather undetermined representation that is supposed to take place in the tertiary cortical area; the analysis given by Plato of the *idea* in comparison to an *aesthesic image* (localized in primary cortical areas) might yet help to understand this stage of brain processes.

In fact, the above-mentioned findings prove that the law of a positive correlation between ACG latency and length of utterance is valid only in the domain of the *phono-*

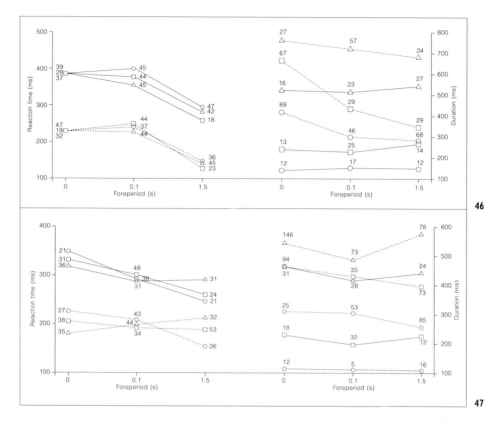

46

47

Fig. 46, 47. Reaction times and durations of 3 word stimuli presented to normal adults. —— = ACG values; ------ = EMG values; ○ = /ma/; □ = /mare/; △ = /mare è bello/. Figures near symbols indicate SD. **46** Subject M.G., female, 21 years old. **47** Subject R.C., male, 36 years old.

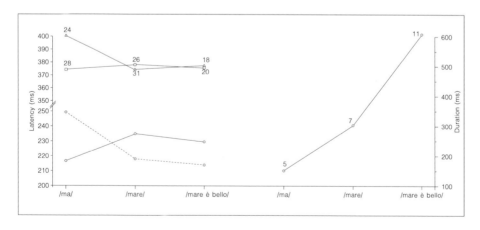

Fig. 48. ACG and EMG (reported only for $FP_{1.5}$) latencies and ACG duration at different foreperiods. —— = ACG; ------ = EMG; △ = FP_0; □ = $FP_{0.1}$; ○ = $FP_{1.5}$; figures near symbols indicate SD. Subject D., 32 years old.

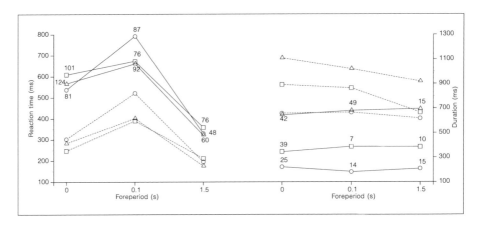

Fig. 49. Reaction times and durations of subject L.V., female, 67 years old. For explanations, see figure 46.

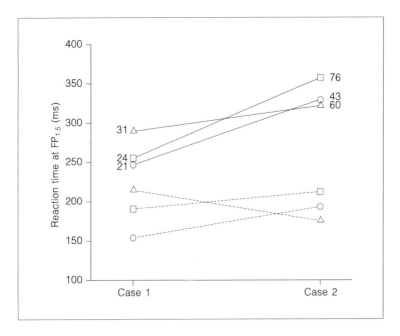

Fig. 50. Reaction times at FP$_{1.5}$ of a young (case 1, R.C., 36 years old) and an old normal subject (case 2, L.V., 67 years old). —— = ACG; ------ = EMG; ○ = /ma/; □ = /mare/; △ = /mare è bello/. For individual case data, see figures 47 and 49.

logical formulator. Sometimes it becomes even valid for grammatical tasks in delayed reactions with long preparatory intervals.

In the domain of the *grammatical* formulator, ACG latency is shorter than in the domain of the phonological formulator; thus, when we compare the ACG latencies of the two performances, since a sentence is longer than a simple syllable and short word, we ob-

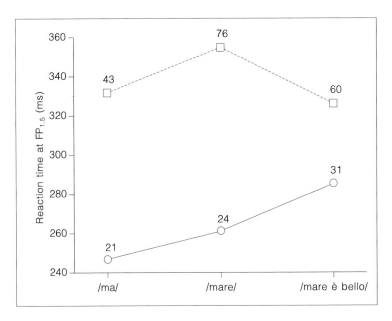

Fig. 51. ACG latencies obtained from a young (○, R.C., 36 years old) and an old normal subject (□, L.V., 67 years old) for triple-stimulus reactions.

tain the paradoxical finding of independence or inversion of the law relating ACG latency to length of utterance.

Edelman's principle [1992] might therefore be applied to the interpretation of the *priority of the enunciation with respect to the phonological organization:* the more automatic speech unit is represented by the sentence. Then one could hypothesize that a subject, requested to read a syllable or a simple word, would extract them from a related sentence, that is an actual semantic representation connected to the area of conceptualization. This extraction could in fact imply a suppression process in the sense of Edelman's theory. As it is reported in figures 47 and 50, the better trained subject R.C. who was able to reach a lower ACG latency for mono- and disyllables, with a 1.5-second reaction, might probably extract the phonological unit (that we should more correctly name subunit) from the sentence. In this case, we should hypothesize that in the interval of 1.5 s from the task presentation to the 'go' signal, in the brain not principally a low-threshold neural assembly facilitation but rather a rehearsal of the representations related to the subunit occurs.

A further confirmation of this interpretation was found with a different threefold series of reactions, in which the subject was asked to read non-words with a number of syllables equivalent to the previous /ma/, /mare/ and /mare è bello/. The actual tasks were /me/, /mece/ and /mece a bille/. The task was carried out by the subject with immediate and the usual delayed reading reactions. The findings were at variance with those obtained with /mare è bello/ and correspond to the law of increase in ACG latency with the longer utterance /mece a bille/, as it occurs in the phonological domain without semantic implication. The only Italian-speaking subject, expert in Danish, who did not show any significant increase in ACG latency with the pseudo-sentence, asserted that he mentally associated the non-words with a phonetically similar sentence: he interpreted the sentence /mece a bille/ as 'la merce è conveniente' (the goods are cheap, i.e. *billig* in Danish).

6.2.2
Extracting the Phonological Subunit from the Grammatical Unit

Peters et al. [1989] investigated immediate and delayed reading reactions of a 1-syllable word, a polysyllabic word and a sentence under two conditions of time pressure (high and low). They found that ACG and EMG latencies are longer at high pressure in immediate reactions than in delayed reactions and that they proportionally increase from the monosyllabic to polysyllabic word to the sentence. In adult stutterers, the values are increased, but with a statistically greater increase in the sentence task. The heuristic principle that the authors infer from their experiments is that an abnormal increase in latency times, appearing significantly greater for the longest utterances, can be considered as a indication of difficulties in motor programming of speech behaviour.

In the light of our results (fig. 40–50) this statement must be revisited with a better definition of the conditions requested for the accomplishment of the trials and the principles of their interpretation.

In fact, the *sentence* rather than the word or the syllable seems to correspond to neural assemblies that in normal adults are more facilitated, i.e. to low-threshold neural assemblies that can be more easily and more automatically activated in a first-hand trial during the CCP. On the contrary, there is no doubt that the final executive articulation will require an operative time directly proportional to the length of utterance.

Thus, reading a sentence in a delayed reaction with a foreperiod >0.5 s allows a preliminary decoding of the phonological units, and the three different tasks can then be carried out as phonetic performances of increasing length.

If we wanted to develop a methodology able to calculate the CCP latency of the *best* low-threshold neural assemblies, one should adopt as task *two sentences* presented at random, like /il mare è bello/ ('the sea is beautiful') and /il mare è mosso/ ('the sea is churned up'). The immediate reading reaction will include only the computation and timing of the easily available low-threshold neural assembly. The difference of ACG latency at FP_0 – ACG latency at $FP_{1.5}$ will be equal to the CCP latency.

Moreover, the results reported in figure 49 show that the production of the syllable utterance is markedly slowed in 0.1-second delayed reading reactions. In fact, the corresponding central computation requires a supplementary time to extract the phonological unit from the sentence.

It ensues that, when the PDP are not quite efficient, as in old subjects (fig. 49), the increase in ACG latency will be greater for the syllable than for the sentence. In our methodology, this means that to detect a subclinical early deterioration of PDP would be easier with a task like /m/, /mu/ than with words and sentences. Of course this will be true for an aspecific deterioration; in contrast, a specific impairment of particular linguistic performances might preferentially affect different corresponding tasks.

Besides the slowing down of reaction times, the occurrence of errors in responses or the total failure of some responses represent signs of severer disorders in brain functions. Errors and pauses can also be found in normal conditions, and their analysis represented a hard but also intriguing task for the earliest researchers in speech science.

....

Errors and Pauses

6.3.1
Errors in Brain Processes Occur as in Artificial Neural Networks

During the development of the internal programming circuits in the brain, two orders at least of *internal feedbacks* co-operate to assure the conformity between the instructions given by the preprogramming CCP and the last-order invariants produced by the formulators (or convertors), i.e. the intermediary neural processes in Levelt's blueprint [1989]. In fact, owing to the stochastic, trial-and-error functioning of the brain (see Section 4), the *occurrence of errors* is a normal event in analogy with what occurs in artificial neural networks and the analogue computer [Banks, 1991]. In the human brain, as in artificial networks and analogue computers, several systems of correction are operating in series.

An ultimate *overt feedback* operates from the final product, (i.e. the word pronounced), and it is produced by acoustic impulses. In the previous stages, the corrections imply only some *pause*, while in the last it becomes impossible to avoid misutterance and the subject can only correct the occasional overt error.

6.3.2
A Classification of Pauses

The adjustment of ongoing operations, taking place before the word stimulus has been pronounced, was in fact proved by the identification of pauses occurring in the course of speech. The identification of such pauses, independent of intentional prosodic or occasional contingent pauses, was performed by pioneers of the scientific objective approach to the study of speech production [Baars et al., 1979].

These pauses could be named *adjusting pauses* and represents a clear demonstration of the trial-and-error way of functioning of the CCP, corresponding strictly to analogous computers. These in fact differ from digital computers in being capable of autoprogramming and learning but making some occasional slips and errors.

The other order of *functional pauses* should be defined, according to the corresponding physiogenesis, as intentional, prosodic or contingent pauses.

6.3.3
The Acoustic Feedback

Experiments carried out with acoustic masking proved that under conditions of acoustic deprivation the accuracy of the word utterance is decreased and the preparatory innervation undergoes broader variations associated with marked changes in the degree of motor unit recruitment. On the contrary, the ACG latency time is only slightly increased [Pinelli and Ceriani, 1992].

6.3.4
Effects of Pre-Existing or Interfering Stimuli on the Control of Speech

Speech production requires not only facilitated neural assemblies able to activate the executors but also ongoing information about the actual conditions of the executors to reach the CCP that ensure the flow of programming impulses. If an obstacle (like a pipe in the mouth) reduces the range of organ (mandibular) mobility, the motor programme will be properly modified thanks to the contribution of the exteroceptive and proprioceptive afferent impulses.

Thus, the requested ratio of innervation will be realized from the first trial by the subject who transmits a greater load to synergistic muscles. On the other hand – as we have already reported in 4.4, fig. 39–42 and table 8 – the effect of external stimuli occurring when the programming commands have already been delivered is quite restricted during speaking [Pinelli and Ceriani, 1992]. At variance with the inhibition exerted by external trigeminal stimuli on ongoing masticatory activity, it was found that the descending commands for speaking stimuli prevailed (see Section 4). Therefore the utterance of the word remains nearly unmodified in spite of interfering simultaneous external stimuli.

···

Interindividual Variations: Maturation and Aging Effects

6.4.1
Aging, Maturation and Latency of the Acousticogram

MDRV proves to be a privileged means of investigation of age-dependent changes in CCP, responsible for a slowing down, prevalent in immediate verbal reaction times.

6.4.2
Verbochronometric Values in Homogeneous Groups of Subjects

Until now our investigations have been focused on rather homogeneous groups of healthy subjects as far as education, language and character are concerned. All people were Italians with a middle degree of school education. Hypomanic or extremely phlegmatic persons were excluded.

However, an individual trait that was not taken into consideration from the outset is a psychomotor variable linked to a constitutional speed of action. It will be analysed in 8.1, under the name of *kinetic factor*. (In the following discussion we prescind, for the moment, from this factor.)

The SD of the mean values reflects the stochastic functioning we analysed in the preceding chapters. In fact, no effects of learning or fatigue were observed during the series of 12 trials that were always carried out after a preliminary training.

The occurrence of interindividual differences in mean values among homogeneous groups of the same language, middle education and character traits speaks in favour of individual 'styles of speaking' with a more or less automatic reading ability on individual velocity of performance and accuracy of utterance.

6.4.3
Mean Values of Acousticogram Latencies in Immediate Verbal Reactions of Children (4–12 Years Old)

As usual in adults, the research was performed with the written word pair /mare/ and /muro/ shown on a PC screen to school age children (6 and 12 years old). On the other hand, to preschool age children (4 years), some geometric pictures, schematically representing the image of a male and a female, were shown as stimuli on the PC screen, and the child was asked to react immediately and with a 1.5-second delay with the utterance 'father' (*padre* in Italian) or 'mother' (*madre* in Italian).

The results of these two orders of verbal reactions are reported in figures 52, 53a–d and 54 and table 10. More detailed data, with a comprehensive evaluation, will be reported in 8.4.

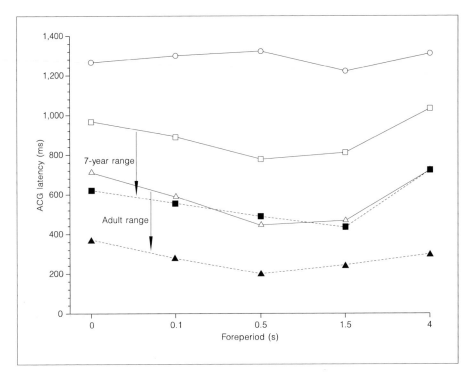

Fig. 52. ACG latencies of /muro/ paired with /mare/ presented to children and adults. ○ = T.L., 6 years old (non-hierarchical planning phase of psychomotility); □ = C.P., 7 years old; ■ = S.M., 7 years old; △ = F.L., 33 years old; ▲ = F.A., 23 years old.

6.4.4
Mean Values of Acousticogram Latency in Immediate Verbal Reactions of Young (16–25 Years Old) and Middle-Aged Subjects

We must now turn back to the results of the research carried out in 1992 with the word pair /clan/ and /cane/ as reported in table 2 (see 3.2.3.1). Additionally in figure 43 (see 4.4.6.2), the mean intra-individual variations have been reported (expressed on the ordinate as 2 SD). We will now analyse the two groups of subjects aged 16–25 and 26–35 years among the four groups subdivided in this first study, with 8, 10, 7 and 9 subjects, respectively.

The results obtained with the word pair /mare/ and /muro/ in the research carried out in 1993 are reported in figure 55, collecting the data of 12 normal subjects aged

Fig. 53. Responses of subject T.L., male, 6 years old, to /muro/ at FP_0 (**a,** 15th reaction), $FP_{0.1}$ (**b,** 11th reaction) and $FP_{0.5}$ (**c,** 1st reaction) as well as to /mare/ at $FP_{1.5}$ (**d,** 13th reaction). Figures on the right, from top to bottom, indicate latency time (ms) of the onset of the responses, latency time (ms) of the end of the responses and duration (ms) of the responses. Duration of the EGG includes the glottogram and final motor artefacts. EGG = Electroglottogram; EMG1 = orbicularis oris muscle; EMG2 = digastric muscle.

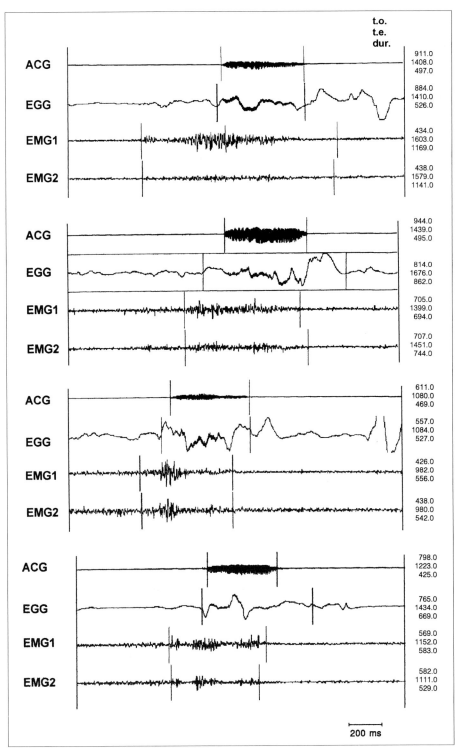

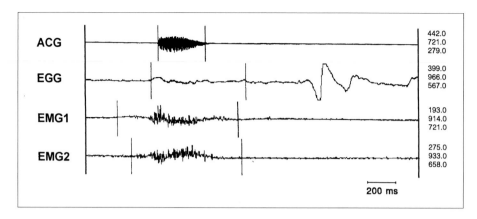

Fig. 54. Responses of subject S.M., male, 7 years old, IQ 107, 2nd class school, to /mare/ at $FP_{1.5}$. For explanations, see figure 53.

Table 10. S.M., male, 7 years old – EMG and ACG reaction times to /mare/ and /muro/

	Foreperiod				
	0	0.1 s	0.5 s	1.5 s	4 s
ACG latency, ms					
/muro/	580.5 ± 91.1	549 ± 170	455.8 ± 89.3	450.2 ± 62.3	715 ± 98.1
	(391 – 690)	(369 – 707)	(378 – 591)	(370 – 527)	(600 – 857)
/mare/	627 ± 63.9	553.3 ± 158.8	451.5 ± 34.6	443.3 ± 24.5	715.5 ± 55
	(529 – 713)	(425 – 731)	(413 – 496)	(415 – 458)	(636 – 789)
EMG latency, ms					
/muro/					
Orbicularis oris	380.5 ± 86.3	273.6 ± 78.5	279.2 ± 11.9	264 ± 42.7	492.2 ± 128.6
	(192 – 497)	(184 – 330)	(155 – 460)	(204 – 315)	(355 – 672)
Digastric	385.1 ± 69.7	309.6 ± 70.8	307 ± 111.1	232.4 ± 39.6	518.6 ± 120.1
	(251 – 473)	(229 – 362)	(207 – 491)	(188 – 279)	(387 – 695)
/mare/					
Orbicularis oris	455.4 ± 64.2	364.3 ± 115.5	287.5 ± 68.9	273.3 ± 78.9	492.7 ± 35.1
	(377 – 580)	(250 – 481)	(209 – 372)	(208 – 361)	(455 – 543)
Digastric	417.1 ± 66	331 ± 133.4	306.5 ± 64	298 ± 69.3	538.5 ± 46.1
	(287 – 524)	(250 – 485)	(222 – 369)	(233 – 371)	(490 – 595)
ACG duration, ms					
/muro/	380.2 ± 53.7	287.7 ± 13.3	281.8 ± 27.6	284.2 ± 17.5	275.8 ± 39.7
	(278 – 480)	(273 – 299)	(233 – 301)	(265 – 312)	(218 – 325)
/mare/	360.4 ± 29	280.3 ± 48	261.7 ± 64.4	264 ± 24.8	273.5 ± 26.1
	(321 – 403)	(225 – 310)	(194 – 346)	(245 – 292)	(247 – 313)

Results are means ± SD, with ranges in parentheses.

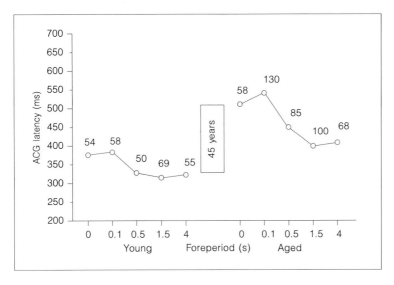

Fig. 55. ACG latencies of /mare/ and /muro/ obtained from young (18–44 years old, n = 12) and aged subjects (45–81 years old, n = 12). Figures near symboles indicate SD.

18–44 years and 12 aged 45–81 years. Figure 56 shows the results of an enlarged population of normal subjects: 6 subjects 46–60 years old and 6 aged 61–81 years were added in this study, subdividing the total population into three age groups. In figure 57, the corresponding values of ACG duration are given.

It can be seen from the tables that the ACG latency of /mare/ and /muro/ (fig. 55, 56) is shorter than that of /clan/ and /cane/ (fig. 2): for the latter word pair the cumulative mean value is 461 ± 51 ms, whilst for the former it is 376 ± 51 ms. The longer ACG latency for /clan/ and /cane/ might be related to the more complex change in vocal tract shape required to produce the consonant /c/ in comparison with /m/. In fact, this phonological element can be produced with an oromandibular action, whilst the /c/ element implies a strong and long-lasting coordinated action of the dorsal back upper part of the tongue in contact with the palate. The rare use frequency of /clan/ can also play a role in the longer ACG latency.

The phonological difference between /clan/ and /cane/ is greater than between /mare/ and /muro/: the subject uses a common characteristic neural pattern for the first letter of the syllables /ma/ and /mu/ whilst the passage from the /cl/ to /c/ articulation for /clan/ and /ca/ implies different characteristic neural patterns. Hence, the subject under trial needs a longer motor control preparation for /clan/ and /cane/ than for /mare/ and /muro/. Eventually, the lower use frequency of /clan/ can also influence the longer ACG latency.

A further observation concerns the shorter EMG latency in the 25- to 35-year-old subjects than in the youngest in relation to the /c/ phoneme. This difference could be attributed to a better automatic shaping of the corresponding vocal tract in mature subjects. A role of the degree of accuracy should also be investigated.

On the other hand, the role played by the programming and executive neural processes might be better analysed taking also into account the results of the delayed reading reactions.

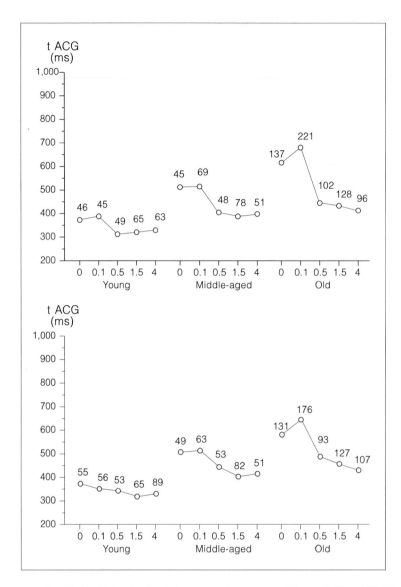

Fig. 56. ACG latencies (t) of three normal age groups (18–44, 45–59 and 60–80 years old) in response to /mare/ (**a**) and /muro/ (**b**) with different foreperiods. Figures near symbols indicate SD.

6.4.5
Mean Values of Acousticogram Latency of Immediate Verbal Reactions in Old People

The verbal reactions with both word pairs /mare/ and /muro/ and /clan/ and /cane/ were analysed in the two older groups of normal subjects. One represented the presenile period; it included 11 subjects, 44–59 years old, who performed the /mare/ and /muro/ test,

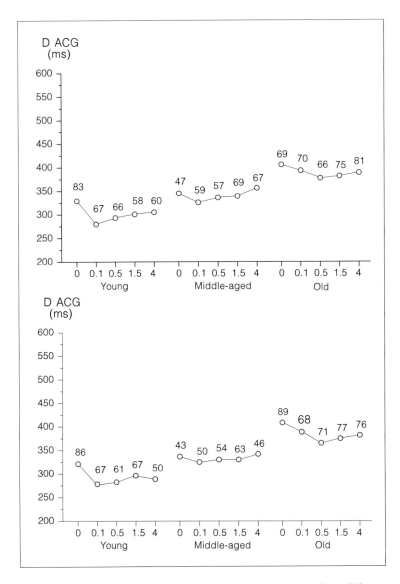

Fig. 57. ACG durations (D) of the same three age groups as in figure 56 in response to /mare/ (**a**) and /muro/ (**b**).

and 7 subjects aged 36–60 years, who performed the /clan/ and /cane/ test. The second group represented the senile period; it included 5 subjects, 60–80 years old, who performed the /mare/ and /muro/ test, and 9 subjects, aged 61–78 years, who performed the /clan/ and /cane/ test (table 2).

A change shown in all these trials is an increase in ACG latency in all groups of old subjects and all word stimuli in comparison with the group of young subjects. In fact, the change for /clan/ and /cane/ is from 463 ± 51 to 540 ± 52 ms and for /mare/ and /muro/

from 376 ± 51 to 496 ± 69 ms for subjects of the presenile period, and to 569 ± 53 and 619 ± 169 ms, respectively for those of the senile period.

It is quite evident that the changes are much greater for /mare/ and /muro/ than for /clan/ and /cane/. This divergence reaches such a high level that – in spite of the higher ACG latencies of /clan/ and /cane/ in the young subjects – the ACG latency values of /mare/ and /muro/ become equal to those of /clan/ and /cane/ in the presenile age and even higher in the senile period. Eventually, it must be stressed that in the case of /clan/ and /cane/ reactions, the change is very marked between the mature and the presenile periods and barely significant between the presenile and the senile ones.

A tentative explanation of this divergence and reversion might be given according to the executive constraints of the two different consonants /c/ and /m/. One could argue that in old age the oromandibular myo-articular elements deteriorate more than the tongue and palate. If this were really the case, the investigation with foreperiod reactions should reveal relatively higher ACG latencies for /mare/ and /muro/ than for /clan/ and /cane/. As we will report later on, this result was confirmed by our experiments.

The recourse to long foreperiod reactions should also provide the necessary data to analyse at which stage of brain operations the increase in total time for the production of ACG takes place in old patients.

6.4.6
Duration of the Acousticogram

6.4.6.1
A Premise on the Central Timing and Diadochokinesis: Functional Substrates

The parameter ACG duration is regulated by two main processes: central timing and diadochokinesis.

In fact, central timing is included in the CCP of the motor programme, whilst diadochokinesis is guided by the executive phase where servo-mechanisms and the descending motor discharges provide the correct temporal pattern of coordinated myokinetic activities required for the pronunciation of the word syllables.

The central timing processes develop in many cerebral areas. The frontal cortex represents a *prognostic* computer, as much as it determines the precise time intervals which pace the delivery of each pattern of discharges for the single phoneme in succession. However, this computation is not carried out isolately by the frontal cortex: it needs the contribution of the cerebellum in a loop that includes the supplementary motor area and the basal ganglia with the thalamic afferent pathway to the cortex.

The internal timing circuit acts inside a huge population of neurons and synapses and exerts modulatory effects in relation to a series of variables that we will further analyse in the following chapters.

At the end of the central timing processes emerges the right, alternative and cyclic succession of movements between agonist and antagonist muscles that the neurologist, beginning with Holmes [1922], termed diadochokinesis. Its final regulation depends on the spinal and supraspinal coordination of the stretch reflexes and reciprocal innervation, starting from the neuromotor spindles and tendinous Golgi receptors and implying the tuning mechanisms with $\gamma 1$ and $\gamma 2$ neurons. In its turn, this great loop converges on the cerebellar system.

Duration of the Acousticogram at Different Ages

ACG duration was measured in three age groups of subjects (18–44, 45–59 and 60–80 years) who were investigated with verbal reactions to /mare/ and /muro/ (fig. 57). As it is shown in table 7, we found that, in the third group of the oldest subjects, ACG duration is significantly increased: from 323 ± 76 and 339 ± 77 ms of the first two groups, it rises to 446 ± 85 ms in the third group.

It becomes therefore important to determine in which phase of the neural chain of speech control, central time or diadochokinesis, the increase in ACG duration occurs. The use of delayed reactions has provided enlightening data, but the whole problem of slowing down in CCP deserves a more detailed discussion.

6.4.7
A View on the Manifold Causes of Slowing Down in Central Cerebral Processes

6.4.7.1
How Information Loss and Modular Impairments Are Related to Changes in Parallel Diffuse Processes and Algorithmic Processes

Taking into account the intrinsic variability of the CCP (the central neural jitter), as we previously mentioned (Section 4), a first source can be searched in the degree of synchrony among the parallel channels of the hidden units. Whichever kind of desynchronization should occur, it would increase the resulting operative time; the normal performance could be preserved only if the slow-down in verbal processing did not transgress the limit of the tachyphemic law [Lieberman, 1989]. A normal behaviour is in fact ensured by a safety factor that avoids any information loss [Myerson et al., 1990].

A low limit of velocity must also be maintained at the level of the executive systems.

A third condition to allow a normal flow of information in the neural chain of speech concerns the limit of matching at the interface between the CCP and the executor processes. Two differently located slowing alterations can occur and might produce a condition of heterochronism.

6.4.7.2
Heterochronism

Under condition 1, a decrease in CCP speed exceeds a certain value, while that of the executor processes remains in the normal range. Under condition 2, the CCP speed remains normal, while that of the executor processes is abnormally decreased.

Under both these conditions of misalignment, we would be confronted with a situation of heterochronism between CCP and executor processes. However, a negative effect on the global function would be relevant only under condition 2. A disproportionate heterochronism at the corresponding interface, greater than the safety factor, would in fact produce *overloading effects,* when the slowing down affects the executor processes.

Consequently, a backwards slowing down in the associative systems would occur, independently of their intrinsic functional state. The global performance would be impaired with a decrease in the signal-to-noise ratio.

6.4.7.3
Desynchronization in Parallel Diffuse Processes

In paraphysiological conditions like brain aging and, even more markedly, in pathological conditions, the degree in synchrony in PDP can diminish. The resulting abnormal asynchrony might produce a series of deleterious effects in brain functions. These are represented by increased operative times disconnecting normally integrated functions. It can be argued that different kinds of impairments and disorders might ensue at the behavioural level, ranging from inattention to paralytic deficits.

6.4.7.4
Intermediary Disconnectedness

Disconnecting the internal programming circuits at some points could be the origin of many psychomotor disorders. A disconnected point could open artificial internal outputs, a sort of holes in the internal circuits. Abnormal hyperkinetic movements could thus be produced. As far as speech control is concerned, as a consequence of this kind of abnormal holes, speech will be impaired with prolonged pauses, iterations, slips and some kinds of dysfluencies and dysphasic alterations.

Marked repercussions can also occur with alterations of input and final output layers.

In these conditions the modular sequence is not only impaired in itself, but it will also retrogradely affect the function of the *hidden layers*. For a correct interpretation of the data offered by MDRV, it thus becomes essential to identify exactly the distal failures in a preliminary evaluation. This task requires additional neurophysiological investigations usually applied in diagnostic neurology.

6.4.7.5
Associated Investigations: Magnetic Resonance Imaging of the Brain and Motor- and Sensory-Evoked Potentials

Myerson et al. [1990] stressed the importance of determining the possible occurrence of modular slowing down since it can be one of the causes of information loss. A slow-down of conduction velocity along single neural systems can be detected by means of brain MRI that can show demyelination areas. A complementary aid is offered by recording evoked potentials allowing us to measure the increase in latency times at the level of primary, secondary and tertiary stations at both input and output layers. An increase in latency time can depend on a loss of function of the largest fibres or by demyelination. Both events must be evaluated for the interpretation of the results of changes detected with MDRV.

6.4.7.6
Resulting Applications

In fact, all these investigations and analyses are worth being done in view of the precious information they will provide, not only in the field of normal psychophysiology and applied neuropsychiatric diagnosis but also for a better planning of rehabilitative treatment of patients with neurological disorders. The obtained data concern both general principles and the longitudinal assessment of the single case.

A corollary of the concept of heterochronism is that, within certain limits, the global function could be restored by acting on the speed of the normal systems in the chain of speech control. In a condition of heterochronism defined as type 2 in 6.4.7.2, we should try to slow down the CCP, a task that could be accomplished by teaching the subject to perform at a slower rate than he was accustomed to.

In conditions of heterochronism of type 1, no such relevant problems would occur. Anyway, a complementary training might be recommended aiming to provide a good amount of motor unit recruitment in the executive systems that would be otherwise exposed to the negative effects of hypo-activity.

···

Zooming in the Processes of Delayed Reactions

6.5.1
A Trick: Increasing the Sensitivity and Heuristic Value of Verbal Chronometry

In Sections 3 and 4, we have outlined the theoretical arguments justifying the implementation of foreperiod reactions and their methodological achievement.

In routine investigations, delayed verbal reactions with very short foreperiods appeared to represent indeed a very useful tool to detect impairments in PDP functioning during brain control of speaking.

On the other hand, delayed reactions with longer foreperiods allowed us to detect impairments in intermediary processes.

6.5.2
Reactions with Very Short Foreperiods

The investigation of early PDP functioning was done with the introduction of a very short foreperiod in verbal reactions, i.e. shorter than the time taken by the CCP to develop its course. The leading heuristic principle is that a 'go' signal – appearing when the cerebral operation, started at the presentation of the word stimulus, is still in progress – can be accepted by the brain only if the PDP multichannel internal architecture is large enough to let the ongoing processes continue without being disrupted by the new interfering stimuli. If these conditions of acceptance did not occur, the very short delay in reaction onset would induce a significant increase in the temporal variables of the responses.

The short-period delayed reactions were in fact found to yield additional information on the consequences of brain CCP alterations. They will be analysed in a further chapter after having discussed the full functional meaning of the delayed reactions, of whichever length, in comparison to the immediate verbal reactions.

6.5.3
Delayed Reactions with Long Foreperiods

6.5.3.1
A Neurophysiological Premise

A needful investigation in the brain CCP of word utterance is related to the reverberating internal feedbacks corresponding to the intermediary processes. As we have previously discussed in Section 5, the intermediary processes correspond to brain operations developing between programming and executive processes and are named in the scientific literature with different terms like 'working memory', 'assemblage in the buffer' and 'retrieval'.

We have also considered the use of delayed reactions as good means to investigate these intermediary processes. In fact, they develop after the initial programming CCP and the organization of the ultimate invariants.

From a more general point of view, we must also stress that, in the course of *learning*, analogous reverberating internal circuit processes (CCP) produce facilitating influences on the threshold of hebbian neural assemblies.

6.5.3.2
Creating a Hebbian Assembly at a Low Threshold

The excitability level of a neural hebbian assembly depends on the history of a long series of activations with reverberating discharges able to eventually induce neuroplastic changes. Such a reiterative planned homogeneous activation makes the assembly easily available for a final triggered excitation. These epigenetic factors influence the number of internal feedbacks required for the working memory and for the assemblage and retrieval from the buffer.

6.5.3.3
Some Neurophysiological Parameters Related to Differences in Latency of the Acousticogram: The Working Time Requested for Activation of the Assembly

In 5.2, we reported Roelof's [1992] formula of the executor activation times that was empirically elaborated in great details on the grounds of linguistic research. We will now try a neurophysiological approach.

Understanding the nature and identifying the parameters of the activation pattern in the final triggering circuit would require a complex analysis of the most recent neurophysiological, biophysical and biochemical work on the molecular biological mechanisms of short-term memory [Woody, 1982]. Since this task is beyond the aim of our study, I will refer only to some basic elementary principles of 'passive neurophysiology' [Bernstein, 1912] connected to the measurement of some parameters of neuromuscular and reflex excitability in clinical neurophysiology [Pinelli, 1952; Pinelli and Valle, 1960].

A second step of a more complete neurophysiological analysis will be presented in 7.3, dealing with the neural representations activated in reading reactions and with the processes that develop in parallel and sequential series.

The schema of the intensity-duration curve valid for the nerve excitation was extended also to the central nervous system where the polysynaptic organization requires the use of iterative stimuli [Pinelli and Valle, 1960]. Under these conditions, a certain amount of neural impulses is needed to excite the corresponding neural assembly: a defined number of impulses at a determined internal frequency, corresponding to the minimal energy, activates the neuronal assembly. This volley of iterative discharges corresponds to the parameter working time ('temps utile') with reference to the decoding process of the first layer or entry in the hebbian assembly.

To find some reliable cue for the absolute value of these parameters is rather problematic in our experiments. Nevertheless we might succeed in calculating relative values. In fact this is the case when we measure the differences in working time (given by the ACG latency) for tasks of different complexity like that of uttering a word of low frequency of use in comparison with one of high frequency of use.

6.5.4
The Restorative Processes in Cyclic Sequential Activities

While threshold facilitation and working time are implied in the early process related to ACG onset, the further sequence of innervation allowing the word utterance in its total duration depends on a correct development of the underlying physiological processes.

We have previously analysed the central timing processes at the CCP level and the diadochokinetic movements in the final execution. Now we address the elementary physicochemical support of the chain of neuromotor events. This is represented by the repetition of cycles of membrane depolarization and repolarization, neurotransmitter ejection and re-uptake at the level of the single neurons and synapses in the programming and executive assemblies of the brain and distal neuromotor systems.

Successive processes of excitation and inhibition develop in response to CCP, internal iterative feedbacks and adjusting executive processes. Eventually the descending patterns of impulses activate the articulatory executors. The whole series of cycles must be accomplished within the strict limits of time defined by the tachyphemic law [Lieberman, 1991; Pinelli and Ceriani, 1992].

Knowledge of these levels of processes is needed particularly when we evaluate changes assessed by the verbochronometric investigations in paraphysiological or frankly pathological cases. One deals with a difficult, complex diagnostic task that requires always a high degree of caution and criticism. One must take into consideration all levels of possible failure: multiple correlations must be made taking into account the results of all other clinical and laboratory examinations.

6.5.5
Results with Long Foreperiods between 0.4 and 4 s

We defined the duration of the foreperiods in relation to the total duration of the whole series of CCP requested to calculate and execute the verbal reaction (6.4). This time corresponds to about 500 ms: long and short foreperiods were defined with reference to this value of 500 ms.

Moreover, long foreperiods were subdivided into long (0.4–4 s) and very long (4–10 s) in relation to the findings of the greatest decrease in ACG latency observed with respect to the immediate responses and a relatively smaller decrease due to effects of temporal delay. In fact, the meaning of this shortening in ACG latency is related to the threshold of the hebbian assembly and the efficiency of the prefrontal system producing the intermediary processes and related intermediary processes, as discussed in the next chapter.

On the other hand, with the longest foreperiod, ACG latency progressively increases with a return to, or even surpassing, the immediate reaction values. This relative slowing down might yield some cues for the decay of the assembly's response with a parallel increase in the entry threshold.

6.5.5.1

A Key for the Evaluation

As previously reported, the total time required by the brain processes of word reading and utterance is expressed by the ACG latency of the immediate reaction. The corresponding value in normal adults with our word stimuli is about 500 ms, but it can vary with the same word pair between 350 and 600 ms in relation to age.

The shortening of ACG latency in delayed reactions with foreperiods between 0.4 and 4 s which occurs in normal and in most pathological conditions, can be explained by the fact that the perception of the target word and the CCP for the motor programme have already taken place during the interval between the word presentation and the 'go' signal.

With regard to a methodological exploitation of this result, I recall the discussion in this chapter of the heuristic importance of the ratio ACG latency at $FP_{1.5}$/ACG latency at FP_0 (ratio of intermediary processes) in relation to the evaluation of the internal circuit activity developing in delayed reactions.

6.5.5.2

Summary of the Previous Assumptions as a Premise for Chapter 6.6

(1) ACG latency at FP_x = executive time, x being the foreperiod time allowing the shortest ACG latency – in a range from 500 to 1,500 ms – depending on the degree of word frequency; 'executive' indicates the executive processes from the facilitated neural assembly triggering (factor b) to upper and lower motoneuron transmission and conduction, and to muscular contractions.

(2) ACG latency at FP_0 – ACG latency at FP_x = central time. With 'central' we indicate the functional situation of programming and pre-executive processes, being aware that central time may depend on secondary effects (see Section 9).

The precise identification of the pre-executive processes occurring in the x foreperiod represents a challenging task. They may be included in the term 'intermediary processes', but their definition must first of all start from the fact that x delayed reactions imply more than one CCP. They in fact accomplish the rehearsal and 'attentional' processes of the central execution [Baddeley, 1992] occurring in immediate reactions.

In the x foreperiod, a series of pre-executive processes occur until the onset of the triggering activity. In fact central time includes also the time taken by intermediary processes, while time x of the delayed reactions corresponds to the time that allows a maximal facilitation of the pre-executive neural assemblies and requires one or more recurrent CCP according to the characteristics of the task (phonological or grammatical length and frequency of use).

(3) ACG latency at FP_x/ACG latency at FP_0, denominated intermediary process ratio, represents a further step as an absolute cue for intermediary processes. It is independent of individual psychomotor traits (like the *kinetic factor*) and, more generally, of cultural, educational and environmental characteristics (see 8.1).

Coming to the Point: What Do We Measure as 'Intermediary Processes'?

6.6.1
The Prefrontal Cortex Is Implied in Delayed Reactions: Memorizing Pyramidal Neurons and Specific Motor Setting Pyramidal Neurons Identified by Fuster

We assumed that afteractivity of earlier sensorimotor translation with facilitation of pre-executive neural assemblies may lead to shortened reaction times when a long interval is allowed to the subject between the task presentation and the 'go' signal. This principle is valid in as much as normal conditions are maintained, with reference to the intermediary brain processes. According to the results of Fuster's experimental work in primates [1993], the latent preparatory processes in delayed reactions can be related to the neural structures (particularly the frontal cortex) concerned with the temporal organization of behaviour [Winn, 1994].

If these structures were impaired, an alteration of the normal facilitation effect of foreperiods on reaction time would occur.

6.6.2
Changing Occurring in Delayed Response Tasks with Impaired Prefrontal Functions

It was found in primates that cooling of the prefrontal cortex leads to impairments in delayed response tasks, regardless of the modality in which the task takes place. The deficit reflects the fact that pyramidal neurons, not anatomically segregated but intermingled, might code for active memory and for motor set [Fuster, 1993]. Therefore we may identify two different brain processes involved in the control of purposeful actions, like speaking.

(1) A *first process* retains information on a perspective action. In Levelt's blueprint [1989], for natural fluent speaking, the first process is equivalent to the activity concerning the immediate coordinating processes at the level of the articulatory buffer. On the other hand, when the subject has to wait before giving an answer or formulate a question, i.e. when a delay occurs between conceptualization, formulation and execution, the afteractivity with recurrent circuits has to play a protracted role. This situation is artificially reproduced in the tests of delayed reaction, particularly the reactions with long foreperiods.

(2) The *second process* involved in the control of speaking is the preparation of a forthcoming action. This second process is a pre-executive process, equivalent to our concept of facilitation of corresponding neural assemblies. Anyway, one might state that this process is strictly linked to the beginning of the executive process and in this context it bears some relationship with a motor set function. The multiple denominations of these functional mechanisms clearly reveal the complexity of the underlying brain processes and the consequent difficulty of the psychologist who tries to

identify the most significant phenomena among many events probably occurring in parallel.

6.6.3
Classification and Interpretation of the Two Brain Processes Involved in Control of Speaking

Winn [1994] and Fuster [1993] named the first brain process we reported previously a mnemonic function and the second a motor set function. They also analysed these functions at the level of single unit activity and differentiated pyramidal neurons involved in mnemonic and in motor set functions, respectively.

In our blueprint of the dynamic succession of these 'core events', we recognize the following three different moments where the essential mechanism is represented by reverberating internal circuits of Hinton's internal feedbacks [Hinton et al., 1993]:

(a) The ongoing activity prolongs the early started process and remains at the disposal of the decisional process.

(b) If the execution process is planned, and then expected by the subject to be performed at a suitable (or conventional) moment (the so-called prospective action of Fuster [1993]), then the internal feedbacks facilitate a low-threshold neural assembly. This process presents both aspects of a mnemonic function[1] (i.e. inducing neuroplastic changes of lowered neuronal threshold of homogeneous synapses) and of a preparatory function for forthcoming actions.

(c) On the other hand, a specific motor setting represents in fact the initial executive process we have neurophysiologically analysed as a tuning effect on the executing motor units: in our methodology, it is experimentally recorded as the first phase of the EMG of the oromandibular district.

6.6.4
The Underlying Neural Machinery

Back to the single unit analyses, Fuster's memorizing pyramidal neurons represent the units that facilitate the hebbian assemblies, while the specific motor setting pyramidal neurons effect the tuning process.

Thus, one may agree with Fuster [1993] that, in terms of a delayed response task, 'the separate types of neurons have important functions, in that animals must retain information through a period of delay before a response is executed'.[2]

These mnemonic and *motor set functions* seem 'to lay a bridge from perception to action across time'. They are in fact crucial to the organization and planning behaviour, communicating with the premotor and motor cortices involved in collaboration with a variety of subcortical structures, in the execution of action that, in our case, is speaking.

---

[1] In other determined contexts we prefer to avoid the term 'memory' to name these processes for the reasons already given in the General Introduction and particularly for the semiological necessity to differentiate them from the short-term active memory. In contrast, the term 'mnemonic function' more correctly indicates an ongoing process of afteractivity with recurrent circuits.

[2] It is important to be aware of the fact that Fuster's experiment, at variance with our tests of delayed reactions, includes a short-term active memory since the task stimuli are not continuously perceived by the animal. In our tests, we deal with a process of *temporal bridging*.

Everitt [1994] outlined the general circuitry involved in the pavlovian conditions and more generally in behaviour. Certainly the actual natural performances require the activation of many brain structures organized in loops: prefrontal cortex, hippocampus (ventral subiculum) and basolateral amygdala with outflow via the ventral pallidum, mediodorsal nucleus of the thalamus (which returns also information to the frontal cortex), midbrain and pons. Moreover, the nucleus accumbens, interacting with other limbic structures, acts as a focus for several structures concerned with the gain of control by environmental stimuli over behaviour.

In our neutral tests for speech, the main parts of these neural structures are implied, but each at different degrees and under different conditions. Some are activated with a specific performance: this is the case for the grammatical and phonological translators and the corresponding articulatory executive coordinated movements. Wernicke's and Broca's cortical temporal and frontal areas are the most specific centres in this relation.

Also, attentional processes are certainly requested in the sequential purposeful actions of speech in both perceptual and motor performances.

Eventually the results of tests of picture naming (see Sections 7 and 8) will direct our analysis to the possible role of emotional factors in relation with some specific tasks: male and female images.

Findings and Evaluation of Slowing in the Aged Brain

Multiple-Delayed-Reaction Verbochronometry in Normal Aging: An Outline

7.1.1
The 1992 Investigation with 3-Second Foreperiods

Our investigations in young and old normal subjects with /clan/ and /cane/ reading reactions were carried out with 3-second delayed reactions. As we reported in Section 3, table 2, and in 6.4, we found that in the group of the youngest subjects (16–25 years old) the ACG latency decreases, in 3-second delayed reactions, from 483 ± 37 ms of the immediate reaction to 376 ± 48 ms, equivalent to a difference of –22%, and in the middle-aged group (26–35 years) from 443 ± 65 to 333 ± 64 ms, equivalent to –27% (these values represent the mean of those reported in table 2 separately for /mare/ and /muro/).

These findings prove that the 'mentally' carried out sensorimotor processes are repeated to produce a facilitated neural assembly that, at the 'go' signal, can be triggered immediately. It remained to ascertain which might be the shortest interval between the presentation of the target word and the 'go' signal in order to obtain the shortest ACG latency.

7.1.2
The 1993 Investigation with Multiple-Delayed-Reaction Verbochronometry

A study with multiple foreperiods was carried out with /mare/ and /muro/ in the year 1993. It was methodologically completed with respect to the study of 1992: we included an acoustic warning stimulus appearing 3 s before the presentation of the visual word stimulus. In subjects of older age investigated with the warning stimulus, the mean ACG latency was about 15% shorter than in those investigated without warning in 1992.

Immediate reactions and foreperiods of 0.1, 0.5, 1.5 and 4 s were used for three randomly mixed series of 12 reactions to two word pairs, with (a) 0, (b) 0.1 and 1.5 s, and (c) 0.5 and 4 s, respectively. The results with the 0.1-second foreperiod will be analysed in 7.4, whilst we will now discuss the results with long foreperiods.

In a few cases, beside the three mentioned foreperiods, 1-second instead of 1.5-second delayed reactions were performed.

As it has been reported in figures 55–57 in Section 6, in subjects 18–44 years old, ACG latency decreases with the 0.5-second foreperiod, from 376 ± 51 ms of the immediate reactions to 330 ± 49 ms, equivalent to a difference of –12%. With the 1.5 second foreperiod, ACG latency decreases to 308 ± 70 ms, equivalent to –18%. With the 4-second foreperiod, ACG latency is $+318 \pm 68$ ms, equivalent to –15%, a decrease slightly lower than that with 1.5 s. One could thus suppose that a 4-second interval marks the border between long and very long foreperiods.

A preliminary comparison of the results of the investigations carried out in 1992 with those carried out in 1993 must start by taking into account the methodological differences: first of all, the different task words and, secondly, the different foreperiods.

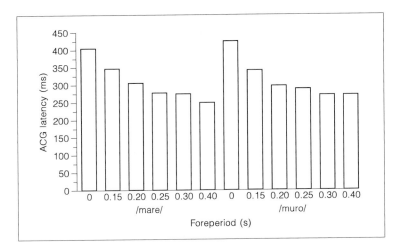

Fig. 58. Mean reaction times of 4 young subjects (aged 25–35 years).

With reference to the first point one must remember that the ACG latency of /clan/ and /cane/ in the immediate reaction is longer than that of /mare/ and /muro/. We previously analysed how this difference, apart from some specific articulatory connotations, might be considered as depending on a lower frequency of use, particularly for /clan/. Hence, one must consider the meaning of the effects of the foreperiods in the two different pairs of task words separately. There is no doubt that the decrease for /mare/ and /muro/ is already evident with the 0.5-second foreperiod, with a slightly larger decrease with 1.5 s. The decrease did however not reach the higher percentage found for /clan/ and /cane/ with a foreperiod of 3 s.

A research that is still in progress showed that for /clan/ and /cane/ the 0.5-second foreperiod produces a decrease in ACG latency of 9.5–10%, whilst only with 1.5 s does it reach a value of more than 20%.

Some evidence in the same direction has been given by a few investigations with trisyllabic nonsense words, like /ubavek/ and /ubamek/, with the result of a significant (–25%) decrease in ACG latency only with 1.5-second foreperiods.

7.1.3
Effects of 150- to 400-ms Foreperiods in Well-Trained Young Normal Subjects

Four subjects, 25–35 years old, who in the course of the previous 3 months had repeated 3 times the series of 36 /mare/ and /muro/ reactions with foreperiods of 0, 100 and 1,500, and 500 and 4,000 ms, were again investigated with 36 /mare/ and /muro/ reactions but with foreperiods of 0 and 200, 150 and 300, and 250 and 400 ms.

The results of these last series of reactions are given cumulatively in figure 58. The ACG latencies obtained in previous series from reactions with a foreperiod of 100 ms were 353 ± 27 ms for /mare/ and 359 ± 20 ms for /muro/. With a 500-ms foreperiod, it was 245 ± 18 ms for /mare/ and 242 ± 23 ms for /muro/; with one of 1,500 ms, it was 221 ± 22 and 216 ± 19 ms, respectively, and with 4,000 ms 228 ± 23 and 234 ± 25 ms.

With reference to the range of foreperiods from 150 to 400 ms, the most significant decrease in ACG latency occurred with 150 ms (–21% for /muro/). A further 16% decrease was observed with a foreperiod of 200 ms with a cumulative 150-ms decrease in ACG latency at FP_0, equivalent to –37%. No further significant decrease occurred with 250-, 300- and 400-ms foreperiods.

These findings prove that the latent processes of brain programming occurring during the foreperiod can directly continue just after the appearance of the 'go' signal. Hence we can explain how the ACG latencies at foreperiods of 100–400 ms appear to be shortened with respect to FP_0 reactions, in a time corresponding to the latent interval from the task word presentation to the 'go' signal.

A change of 50 ms differentiates the interval between two successive foreperiods from 150 to 250 ms; ACG latency decreases by 50 ms in the two intervals between 150 and 200 ms and between 200 and 250 ms. No further decrease occurs with foreperiods longer than 250 ms, which roughly corresponds to the duration of a single internal circuit of the neural systems involved in the cerebral programmation.

With 0.5- to 4-second foreperiods, a further decrease of –8% (total –45%) was observed at 0.5-second delayed reactions, and a more marked one, i.e. –12% (total –49%), at 1.5-second delayed reactions.

We have also observed after many repetitions (>5 times) an equalization between the decrease in ACG latency at foreperiod 0 and the decrease in ACG latency at an 'optimal' foreperiod.

7.1.4
An Evaluation of the Effect of 0.5- and 1.5-Second Foreperiods, in Relation to the Underlying Brain Processes for Differently Available Representations

The decrease in ACG latency induced by verbal reactions to long foreperiods might be explained by an analysis of the processes related to the buffer coding and decoding. This takes us back to the assumptions and presumptive calculations developed in the first chapters on the formation of hebbian assemblies. Thus, we will now shortly re-analyse the main steps of our considerations.

When asked to perform a reaction with a long foreperiod, the subject perceives the target word shown on the PC screen as a sequence of letters. We assumed for this process a time of 100 ms. In fact, immediately afterwards and while the latest phases of the word reading process are still in progress as PDP, the subject shifts his attention to the 'go' signal. This appears 500 or 1,500 ms, respectively, after the target words, /mare/ and /muro/ or /clan/ and /cane/, have been presented.

Meanwhile the CCP1 (see 3.1.2) related to the visuomotor transformation phase of programmation make their first cycle in the corticosubcortical loop: the time for the development of this internal circuit was calculated to be approximately 200–250 ms, a value that must be added to the previous 100 ms.

After the end of the first internal programming circuit (that lasts about 200 ms), one more CCP (i.e. a further 200 ms) develops for the most available representations, while a maximum of 6 CCP (i.e. 1,200 ms) is requested for the less available representations. Thus, the maximal shortening of ACG latency of the respective task words is reached with the corresponding periods of time (200–1,200 ms), according to the degree of availability of the representations.

We can assume the value of 1,200 ms as the period of time needed for less available representations to produce the best neural assembly facilitation, able to allow the invariant commands to reach the executive system.

Then we ask: what happens in these 1,200 ms? The answer can be given in both psychological introspective terms and in a likely neurophysiological interpretation. Waiting for the 'go' signal, the subject is mentally engaged to recall the task he must fulfil, that is the utterance of the word. How much this engagement implies an attentive, conscious process or can simply develop unconsciously is not a relevant question in this phase of our study.

In fact, during the 1,200-ms period, the internal programming circuit is repeatedly active. A flow of impulses running as an internal feedback exerts what Shallice [1988] named a *clean-up function*. In the hebbian language, one might think of a prompt alignment of the whole set of neurons in the assembly involved in the delivery of the commands for the executive coordinated muscles. In this way, the threshold of the entry layer to the assembly matches the enhanced responsiveness to the trigger impulses after the 'go' signal has been perceived. In the 1,200-ms period, the internal feedbacks should have been turned on about 6 times. The times taken by the alignment processes might be outlined in the following terms.

The perception of the target word has taken 100 ms, and the CCP visual-motor transfer starting the programme for the word utterance takes about 200 ms. After this first period of time, there are just the 1,200 ms left for repetition of the CCP internal feedback of 200 ms. Then, 1,200 : 200 = 6 is the number of repetitions of internal feedbacks required for the best matching of the low-threshold assembly that will be triggered for the last phases of speech control, after the perception of the 'go' signal.

With shorter foreperiods (500–1,000 ms), in most normal young subjects, we still observe a decrease in ACG latency in comparison with immediate reactions, when the task requires a rehearsal of the most available representations. This result proves that even a twice repeated internal feedback can trigger a responsive hebbian assembly for more available representations. A higher number of repetitions (2–6) can be sustained during longer foreperiods and may be needed to reach a triggering effect for less available representations.

On the other hand, longer foreperiods, starting from 4,000 ms, seem to decrease slightly the efficiency of the system. In neurophysiological terms, this means that a 20 times recurring internal feedback is an excessive performance that the central nervous system can hardly effect or that there is an upper limit for that individual subject to sustain the recurrent circuits, acting on the threshold of the particular hebbian assembly and corresponding buffer implied in that specific task (word stimuli).

Foreperiods longer than 4,000 ms seem to exert null or negative effects on ACG latency in comparison with immediate reactions. A psychological interpretation might take into consideration a fading of attention or the appearance of fatigue effects. In neurophysiological terms, one could hypothesize a time-dependent progressive decrease in the ability of the recurrent internal feedbacks to lower the threshold value after 4,000 ms.

7.1.5
A Recapitulation

As a conclusion of this chapter on verbal reactions with long foreperiods, we could summarize the events investigated with our methodology in the following blueprint: (1) the initial process is represented by the visual perception of the target word; (2) the recognized patterns of impulses are transmitted from the occipital to the frontal-subcortical loops where the first circuit of programming CCP takes place; (3) the CCP occur 2–6 times in recurrent internal feedbacks; we name them later CCP; (4) the 'go' signal is perceived; (5) a trigger stimulus activates the neural assembly; (6) the executive system is set in motion with its adapting feedback mechanisms.

Of course, one must be aware that in paraphysiological and particularly in pathological conditions first CCP time could be prolonged: let us take as an example a value of 400 instead of the normal 200–250 ms. The number of later CCP would then become 3 instead of 6 in an equal period of time. And, if under these conditions the hebbian assembly maintained its threshold and alignment within normal values, the facilitating optimal period would shift from 1,200 to at least 2,400 ms.

Delayed Reactions Are Relatively Preserved in Old Subjects

7.2.1
The Results

We refer again to tables 2 and 3 and the related figures in Sections 3 and 6, showing mean values and SD of ACG latencies of verbal reactions with two pairs of disyllabic words, with different long foreperiods, in middle-aged and old subjects.

In the groups of subjects who performed the verbal reactions with /clan/ and /cane/, only a 3-second foreperiod was chosen for delayed reactions. In the 36- to 60-year-old subjects, ACG latency decreased from 541 ± 53 to 432 ± 51 ms, equivalent to less than -20%. In contrast, in 61- to 78-year-old subjects, the decrease was from 570 ± 53 to 383 ± 47 ms, equivalent to -33%.

In the group of subjects investigated with reactions to /mare/ and /muro/ (Section 6, fig. 58), foreperiods of 0.5, 1.5 and 4 s were adopted. In the 45- to 59-year-old subjects, with a 0.5-second foreperiod, ACG latency decreased from 496 ± 69 to 423 ± 79 ms, equivalent to -15%. With the 1.5-second foreperiod, the decrease was from 496 ± 69 to 380 ± 91 ms, equivalent to -24%. In the 60- to 80-year-old group, ACG latency at $FP_{0.5}$ decreased from 619 ± 169 to 153 ± 64 ms, equivalent to -15%, and at $FP_{1.5}$ to 505 ± 131 ms, equivalent to -18%.

If we compare these last changes to those of the young subjects, one can observe that they are greater in the old individuals, at least in the oldest group. This difference suggests that the slow-down of brain processes in old subjects affects prevalently the programming CCP or the intermediary processes. The counterevidence should come from the comparison of the young-old differences of ACG latency in immediate responses in relation to those in 1.5-second delayed responses.

7.2.2
Evaluation of Differences in Acousticogram Latency between Immediate and Long Foreperiod Reactions

In order to critically assess the age-dependent increases in ACG latency occurring in immediate and in long foreperiod reactions, we analysed preliminarily the greatest differences in immediate and long foreperiod reactions. In the case of /clan/ and /cane/, they occurred between groups 2 and 4 for the immediate reactions and groups 2 and 3 for those with a 1.5-second foreperiod. In the case of /mare/ and /muro/, it was verified to occur between groups 1 and 3 in both types of reactions.

7.2.2.1
Latencies of the Acousticogram at Foreperiods of 0 and 3 s with /clan/ and /cane/

With /clan/ and /cane/, the mean young-to-old increase in ACG latency of immediate reactions was from 443 ± 56 to 569 ± 53 ms, equivalent to +29%. In 3-second foreperiod reactions, the young-to-old increase was from 333 ± 64 to 431 ± 51 ms, equivalent to +30%. This high increase in ACG latency of immediate reactions, which includes the distal phases of brain control, seems to confirm our previous interpretation of a peripheral negative factor present in the articulation of /c/, a factor that appears to increase in group 3. But if we look at the values of ACG latency as a function of age in immediate and 3-second delayed reactions (table 2), we observe the absolute values to increase in the immediate reaction from 483 ± 37 ms of the young group to 569 ± 53 ms of the oldest group, whilst with the 3-second foreperiod the values remain constant: 377 ± 41 and 383 ± 47 ms. Only in the third group is the ACG latency with the 3-second foreperiod increased (430 ± 50 ms), a value that remains anyway well below that of the immediate reaction (541 ± 53 ms).

7.2.2.2
Latencies of the Acousticogram at Foreperiods of 0 and 1.5 s with /mare/ and /muro/

Shifting now our attention to reactions to /mare/ and /muro/, mean ACG latencies in immediate reactions change from 376 ± 52 ms of the young group to 619 ± 169 ms of the old one, corresponding to +65%. In 1.5-second foreperiod reactions the increase is from 308 ± 70 to 507 ± 131 ms, equivalent to +65%. This result leads us to conclude that in old age there is a sort of generalized increased stiffness or viscosity in the system that decelerates all processes at an equal rate: the whole chain of cyclic circuits slows down so that the percentage of changes with respect to the activity of the young brain is equal in all kinds of reactions.

But let us look again at the curves of ACG latency as a function of age in the immediate and 1.5-second foreperiod reactions (fig. 34 and table 7). We observe the absolute values to increase in the oldest group in the immediate reactions from 376 ± 52 to 619 ± 169 ms (increase 243 ms), whilst in the 1.5-second foreperiod there is a smaller increase (197 ms), from 308 ± 70 to 505 ± 131 ms.

7.2.2.3
Comparing the Results of the Two Word Pairs

7.2.2.3.1
The Effects of Different Tasks

The mean ACG latencies of foreperiod reactions are relatively longer in old than in young subjects when people deal with /mare/ and /muro/ reactions rather than with /clan/ and /cane/.

This discrepancy recalls once again the role played by the peripheral constraints and their changes during aging, with different distributions of the level of the vocal tract. In the case of /mare/ and /muro/, a deterioration at the level of the oromandibular region might be involved.

Apart from these interfering constraint modifications, one can assert that the prevalent increase in ACG latency of old subjects occurs in immediate reactions.

7.2.2.3.2
A Comparison between Paired Young (up to 30 Years) and Old (over 50 Years)
Normal Subjects

Two otherwise homogeneous normal subjects, one 30 and one 55 years old, were investigated with MDRV (fig. 59–62).

A similar study was extended to 7 other subject pairs: the young men were 27–30 years old and the middle-aged ones between 50 and 62 years. The study of these cases showed a 15–20% longer ACG latency at FP_0 in the oldest subjects with a slightly larger increase at $FP_{0.1}$ (executive process ratio = 0.9–1). A decrease in absolute values was evident at $FP_{1.5}$, with similar values for young and old subjects (intermediary process ratio = 0.8). We could then conclude that the main stage that is slowed down in old subjects corresponds to the programming CCP, *whilst the intermediary internal feedbacks are preserved.*

We must also consider that ACG duration values were similar in the young and the old subjects, a fact that gives evidence of preserved timing and executive processes (diadochokinesis).

7.2.2.4
Latencies of the Acousticogram at Foreperiods of 0 and 1.5 s with the Multiple Task

A further step to better identify the most vulnerable level of processes and representations in old subjects can be made by adding a sentence to the mono- and disyllabic word stimuli (fig. 46–49; 6.2.1). The logic for this methodological modification is open to different arguments. If the grammatical task (the sentence) is specifically impaired, with increases in ACG latency and/or ACG duration, then one could infer that the alteration might involve the programmation of speech invariants [Peters et al., 1991].

However, a more differentiated analysis, taking into consideration many other variables, must be carried out in agreement with the clinical neurological physiopathogenetic procedure (see Section 8). Thus, the more exacting diadochokinetic performance required by the sentence task, even at the phonological level, cannot be ignored.

Secondly, one must be aware that the intermediary process including active memory, in a condition of short-term memory impairment, could be more markedly affected in the sentence task.

The ACG and EMG latencies of the triple task carried out by a young subject and an old one were reported in figures 50 and 51 (in 6.2.1). The ACG latency values are 15% higher in the old subject, but equal in the three tasks without any increase for the disyllabic word with respect to the sentence at FP_0. At $FP_{0.1}$ and $FP_{1.5}$, the increase from the disyllabic word to the sentence is moderate, whilst it decreases (nearly 20%) from FP_0 to $FP_{0.1}$ for the monosyllable. Altogether there is no consistent increase in ACG latency for the longest words or for grammatical tasks.

The latency time of the preparatory reaction, revealed by EMG latency, is relatively preserved in the old subject: the difference between ACG and EMG latencies at FP_0 is approximately 300 ms. (A more detailed analysis of this case will be carried out in 8.2, and it will be compared with the MDRV results obtained in one old subject of the same age but with an impairment of short-term memory.)

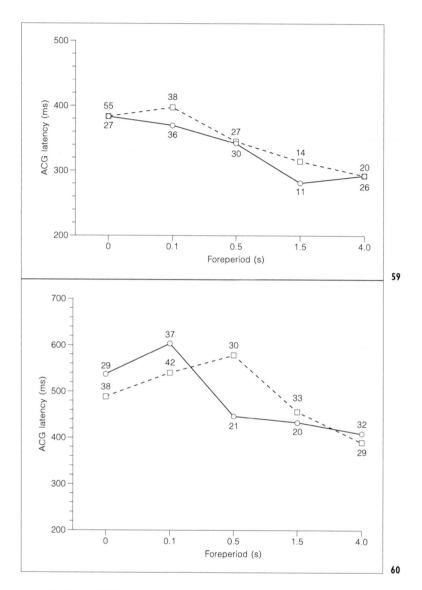

59

60

Fig. 59–62. MDRV of one young and one middle-aged subject. ○ = /mare/; □ = /muro/; figures near symbols indicate SD. **59** ACG latency, normal subject, 30 years old. **60** ACG latency, normal subject, 55 years old. **61** ACG duration, normal subject, 30 years old. **62** ACG duration, normal subject, 55 years old.

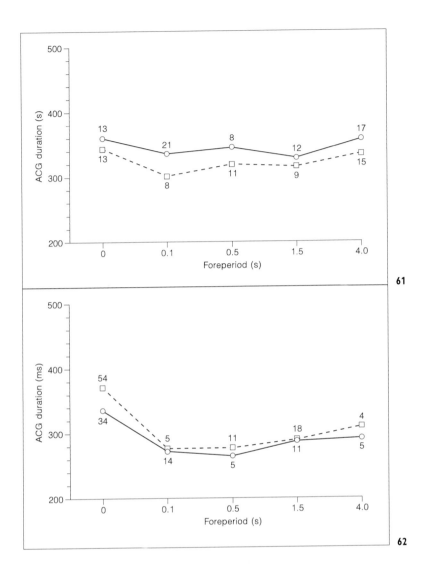

61

62

Formulating a Conclusive Issue

Up to this point and based on the present data, it seems correct to take into account
the slowing of verbal reactions in older subjects as a reliable clue for a slow-down of brain
function. Even if a small part of this slowing depended on a failure in attention (the introduction of the warning stimulus in the last series of research should have corrected this
interfering factor), we may assume that it essentially reflects an intrinsic information loss
[Myerson et al., 1990].

Starting from this assumption, we could proceed right now to evaluate the slowing
factors. The core problem concerns the identification of a central versus a distal vulner-

able point of the aging brain. At the distal level, it is particularly important to assess first of all the role played by the afferent and efferent peripheral pathways and receptors that are known to undergo some deterioration in the oldest subjects and could thus produce the age-related slowing of ACG latency.

As I mentioned previously, the data collected in the three series of research (1992, 1993, 1994–1995) with double and triple tasks confirm the preliminary results [Pinelli and Ceriani, 1992] of a prevalent slowing in early programming processes (CCP) with relatively preserved intermediary processes.

7.2.3
The Origin of the Information Loss in Old Age

The slowing occurring at the level of the CCP phase in old subjects is in agreement with the prevalent opinion among psychologists on the nature of the age-dependent information loss revealed by all functional mental tests [Capitani and Laiacona, 1988; Myerson et al., 1990]. Likewise, the most recent findings obtained with PET [Loesner et al., 1993; Paulesu et al., 1993a, b; Petrides et al., 1993; Decetry et al., 1994] showed a decrease in metabolic activity of the frontal lobes to occur in old subjects in comparison to younger ones, with relatively normal activity in the basal ganglia, cerebellum and brainstem. However, the relation between these results and those of the brain functional tests cannot be conceived as direct. The most meaningful correlation can be assumed to exist between the specific slowing phases in verbal reactions and the relatively preserved executive neural centres like the brainstem. On the other side, the more specific involvement of the frontal lobes suggests a prevalent impairment of the central CCP, independently of its primary or secondary origin. Anyway, a more precise and appropriate evaluation implies a better analysis of what pertains to an impairment of representation or to a process. This analysis will be treated in a separate chapter, dealing with more general principles of psychophysiology, according to the concepts elaborated by Plate et al. [1987], Levelt [1991] and Roelofs [1992].

....

Flashes in the 'Black Box': Processes, Representations and Their Role in the Temporal Development of Reading Reactions

The following considerations emerged when we were evaluating the results obtained in old people and comparing them to those of young subjects. The target under discussion was a slowing down in reaction times. Now we ask: does it depend on an impairment of dynamic active events or rather on an alteration modifying the more static conditions of stores?

The need for these premises to the analysis of aging effects is even more urgent when considering the fact that the two different alterations may interfere with each other, making our evaluation particularly intricate. Further research with suitable methodological modifications should be carried out. (1) A static or chronic impairment of the stores may increase their threshold with the consequence of an increased demand for active dynamic processes for decoding and coding tasks. (2) A specific primary impairment of the active dynamic processes – that are known to normally exert facilitating effects – may lead to an increase in the threshold of the related stores.

7.3.1
What Depends on Processes and What on Representation in Verbochronometry?

A further step in the evaluation of the pathogenesis of brain aging effects might be the identification of which of the two substrates of brain activities – *processes* and *representations* – is mainly affected by the impairment causing the information loss. Both terms are traditionally used in neurophysiology and science of speech [Pinelli and Ceriani, 1992], but the specific meaning of each, the relationship with experimentally investigated fields like coded patterns of impulses and neuroplasticity, and the interaction between the two are not always clear.

It seems that it is expedient to outline here a definition that intends to conform with the areas accessible by our methodology rather than to pretend to be definitive.

7.3.1.1
Processes

This term is used in neurophysiological publications in a broader sense than in science of speech. In fact, we prefer to underline its 'dynamic' nature as opposed to a 'static' one: it is an ongoing activity, a sequence of events in progress, the temporal dimension of the sequence being short, i.e. from seconds and minutes to 1 h. The term 'flow of impulses' used by McKay [1987] is not currently adopted in neurophysiology of speech, but it fits in well with the principles of psychophysiology analysed until now.

The process is constituted by a train of neural changes implying membrane depolarization leading to excitatory and facilitatory or to inhibitory effects at the level of synapses or presynaptically at the level of dendrites and axons. These effects may be autogenous (i.e. intrinsic) – developing on a unique neuron or group of neurons – or heterogeneous (i.e. extrinsic) when produced by adjacent or connected systems of neurons.

The effects of facilitation and inhibition are produced by a complex series of biophysical and biochemical events [Pinelli and Ceriani, 1992]. In a simplified view, one may describe the final effect as a change in the intracellular concentration of Ca^{2+} in the neuronal endings. In cases of inhibition, a depression in the conductance towards Ca^{2+} or an increase in the conductance to Cl^- are the most usual events.

These changes are affected in different lengths along the pathways from input to output, in our case from the retina to brain cortical-subcortical circuits and eventually to the brainstem, spinal anterior horns and to the muscles of the vocal tract. Thus, the processes include also conduction (along axons) and transmission (through synapses) events.

Volleys of impulse patterns are thus running in afferent and efferent pathways, synapsing in series, whereas 'reverberating' circuits in closed neuronal chains – where the component neural stations excite themselves reciprocally – maintain the flow of impulses to persist well after the short-term afferent excitation.

Several loops of such internal circuits are involved in the preprogrammation, programmation and timing processes developing in parallel (PDP). Particularly critical is the *distribution* of the activity in the population of neurons of specific channels or circuits *(the population code)* and the *intensity* in each component neuron that is represented by the internal frequency of each volley *(the frequency code)*. This codification secures the exact matching between the different stages, from programmation to triggering of neural assemblies.

All these different processes can be altered in pathological conditions by noxae acting at different levels: molecular, biophysical and neurofunctional. The level investigated with MDRV is just at the central area of the pathogenetic chain: the functional level in its temporal expression, including conduction velocity and synaptic transmission. From this central area, multiple effects arise acting in opposite directions, at the molecular (memorization and neuroplasticity) and the behavioural level implying the organization of complex systems.

7.3.1.2
Representations

This term is used with reference to its biological meaning, that is rather independently of the psychological term indicating the abstract images formed from perceptions. It is related to long-lasting neuronal changes implying *plastic* variations: when specifically concerning long-term memory they are called 'engrams'.

Relatively short-term neuroplastic changes are represented by events of synaptic potentiation (well known in the experimentally measured posttetanic potentiation) and presynaptic inhibition, which do not imply structural changes but rather regulate the Ca^{2+} concentration in the presynaptic endings. These functional levels of excitability and the threshold are related to the synaptic efficacy.

A determined number of neurons, specifically interconnected by well-defined (genetically and epigenetically) facilitating effects and lateral inhibition, form the so-called hebbian neural assemblies.

In the case of long-term representations, more deeply intracellularly located changes reach the nucleus of the cell body [Woody, 1982].

Broca's centre, Wernicke's centre, encyclopaedic memory, message mapping, all these terms indicate specific stores of representations, each containing representations with different accessibility according to the law of word frequency, phonological versus grammatical forms and eventually other factors included in Roelof's formulas [1992].

7.3.1.3
Intermediate Functions

As we previously stated, we define under this subtitle some terms dealing with events that take place between processes and representations: it is in fact a matter of processes which, on the other hand, are strictly connected with transport of representations.

The term 'buffer' is related to intermediary matching systems occurring to compensate and homogenize the descending patterns of invariant programming impulses. In fact, for their dynamic nature, we share the opinion that these events, too, belong to the domain of the processes.

Likewise the term 'formulator' is conceived by Levelt [1991] as the series of processes that map the message – a conceptual prelinguistic structure – onto a linguistic form; its final output is a phonetic plan that can be executed by the articulatory motor system. It seems then to embrace several phases that at a neurofunctional level we have analysed as visuomotor transfer or translation processes. 'The convertor operates in terms of linguistic elements, that is, items and the properties and relations by means of which they are characterized and related' [Roelofs, 1992].

Of course, *reading reactions,* investigated in MDRV, differ in many aspects from the formulation in language of prelinguistic messages and it becomes mandatory to clearly separate what is common in reading reactions, including the delayed reactions, and what is specific for each of the two forms of speaking. The following points deserve our attention: (1) to define the difference between reading aloud a word or a sentence and the verbalization and lemmatization of the conceptual preverbal message or translation of it into the semantic form of appropriate lexical entries; (2) to find out the specific activities occurring in reading aloud a non-word; (3) to differentiate the deficits of phonological lexical representations from deficits of translations.

7.3.2
Specific Processes in Reading with Respect to Spontaneous Speech

While in spontaneous speech the first operation is just to formulate the verbalization from the preverbal message, the first operation in reading aloud a written word or sentence, once the written word has been perceived, is a cerebral 'motricization' of visual representations.

The right question is then whether and how Levelt's convertor processes pass after the mental message to some kind of representation or visual-like representation and in a successive phase 'read' this representation. Even if this hazardous analogy held, we could at most rely on a 'beheaded formulator', and it would be more appropriate to indicate the second series of processes occurring in reading with the term 'convertor' rather than formulator: its main task, in fact, is just a transformation from representations to the final phonetic plan [Levelt, 1993].

A more definite nature of reading can be outlined by a series of observations and preliminary evaluations started since the golden age of studies on reaction times. Cattell [1980] conjectured that loud reading responses become automatic because of a strong association between written words and their pronunciation, caused by extensive practice, since they are repeated very often in everyday life. The influence of word frequency on word reading is expressed by a negative linear correlation between reading latency time and the logarithm of the word frequency unit [Levelt, 1993].

To better understand all the details of the progressing stages, we must take into consideration what we know about the internal word codes (logogens) necessary to produce the words. The study was carried out by comparing word reading and picture naming and led to the formulation of five different fundamental classes of hypotheses about the modality or the format of the internal codes and their transformation in reading [Levelt, 1993].

The most accepted hypotheses formulate a central, abstract, amodal and propositional internal code for long-term storage. The connection of this abstract code system with perception on the one hand and with language production on the other requires large recording systems with an extended processing capacity. Their long-term components contain morphemes of all words that an individual knows, together with their syntax and their phonemic and orthographic properties. Evidence was provided by Glaser and Düngelhoff [1984] for an extensive internal word processing without semantic components.

Many experiments proved that the mean latencies increase monotonically, from word reading over picture naming and picture categorizing up to word categorizing. The reading-naming difference was calculated as being approximately 90–160 ms. However, the word frequency effect is far greater in naming than in reading processes: the slope of the negative linear correlation between naming latency and the logarithm of word frequency is –254 ms per 10-log frequency unit (instead of –30 ms for reading).

Also, the results of priming studies [Bajo, 1988; Levelt, 1993] supported new evidence that the pathways of reading aloud do not contain a mandatory stage for semantic evaluation.

Studies of hesitations in reading speech showed that finite clause boundaries attract more pauses than non-finite ones [Levelt, 1993]. This sensitivity to surface clausal organization in reading speech is exactly what we could expect from Levelt's account of the assumption that reading involves the insertion of lemmas into a syntactic tree but not the creation of a propositional representation. However, we have previously commented how, with reference to word or very simple sentence reading, a syntactic phase is non-mandatory.

7.3.2.1
Reading Non-Words

Non-words are considered important methodologically [Levelt, 1993], as they permit us to assess whether brain damage has disturbed the translation processes themselves: in fact, phonological lexical representations are not implicated even in intentionally generated speech.

Typical tests include the reading of non-word stimuli. Students of this field assume that the processes of reading generate phonological information in the same format as phonological lexical representations – a list of segments, an outline of syllable structure and a stress pattern – which can be spelled out by the relevant systems and assembled by the phonological assembly subsystem.

7.3.2.2
Deficits of Phonological Lexical Representations versus Deficits of Sensorimotor Translation

Models of phonological encoding processes have been outlined that could help the examiner to better identify the subsystem impaired in consistent patterns of deviation from the phonological norm in the responses of patients with 'literal' or 'phonemic' paraphrasias. The model includes phonological encoding, phonological lexical representation or lexeme in the terminology of Kempen and Huybers [1983], processes translating the information stored in the phonological lexical representation into the phonetic representations appropriate to the current speech context that ultimately passes on to the articulators.

As a working hypothesis, it seems justified to assume that the most basic and apparently the most straightforward issue is whether the malfunction is due to some impairment in one of the translation processes.

In a detailed study of a patient with conduction aphasia by Plate et al. [1987], the item-specific consistency of errors was thoroughly assessed. The primary data come from tests of reading, and reading may involve the generation of phonological information by a non-lexical procedure, by mapping graphemes onto phonemes, and this may play a role in the generation and prevention of phonemic errors. Different reading contexts were used with multiple tasks of monosyllables, disyllables and sentences. The main factor in errors was the length of the target (as it was with Caplan's [1987] patient R.L.). Cross-word interaction errors did not occur.

According to Plate et al. [1987], these results reflect a constraint on the amount of phonological information, which can be programmed within a unit. That is to say, there is a kind of channel capacity limit to spell out apparently intact information in phonological lexical representations, which is perhaps combined with a loss of information in transmission, especially for unstressed material.

Information Loss in the Aged Brain Evaluated with Multiple-Delayed-Reaction Verbochronometry: The Impact on Early Processes and Relative Preservation of Intermediary and Executive Processes

7.4.1
A Tentative Interpretation of Information Loss in the Aging Brain: A First Step

With all these contributions and speculations in mind, we can now proceed to analyse which phases of brain processes, implied in reading reactions, are more significantly impaired in the aging brain.

7.4.1.1
The Input Layers Are Relatively Preserved in Old Subjects

That other processes besides CCP, particularly on input layers, do not play an important role in the increase in ACG latency of the immediate reactions of old subjects is proved by the following.

(1) Careful ophthalmic examinations were carried out, and visually impaired subjects were excluded from the group examined by MDRV. Dimensions and luminosity of the words on the screen, as well as the distance to the reader, were kept constant in all trials.

(2) The increase in visual-evoked potentials that is known to occur in old subjects is always relatively small (–6%) in comparison with that found in ACG latency.

(3) The methodological procedure in MDRV includes a visual perception time of the 'go' signal, occurring also in the delayed reaction. Therefore a possible increase in visual perception time of the word should not affect differently ACG latencies of immediate and delayed reactions, in as much as the visual perception time of the 'go' signal would be equal to that of the target word.

(4) As it was argued in many studies [Lieberman, 1991; Levelt, 1989], the brain central programming processes develop partly in a PDP modality, a point that will be better analyzed in the next chapter on very short foreperiods. I just want to stress here that partly simultaneous multiple functions can compensate a delay in one of their earliest lines of activity. An anticipation occurring as a corrective reaction in the second line of functions would in fact nullify a delay of the processes in the first line. Thus, an increase in time of perception of the target word would be completely masked by an earlier activation of the first CCP.

In conclusion, I can state that the verbochronometric methodology with delayed execution of choice reactions (MDRV) allows us to ascertain *CCP slowing* in old age.

At this point, the clear definition of the meaning of a functional change like the *slowing in CCP* we are dealing with becomes an important prerequisite. A fundamental law in neurology, which can be traced back to Huglings-Jackson [1884], states that a change in the parameters or development modality of a function, particularly in the centre levels that are characterized by redundancy and co-operative substitutive corrections, may either be primarily due to an intrinsic initial alterations or rather depends on upward repercussions and feedbacks (or top influence) from lower-level functional alterations.

There is experimental evidence of *overflow effects* affecting CCP under a condition of impaired final executors. In other words, an age-dependent impairment, in whichever part of the executors, might be reflected by a slowing of central CCP. Once again the rules of new-jacksonian [Swash and Kennard, 1985] physiopathogenetic analysis become paramount for a correct interpretation of our data (Section 6). Therefore an attribution of the cause of CCP slowing to 'information loss' [Myerson et al., 1990] can be taken into consideration only after having accounted for the possible role of backward influences from the executors or from changes in constraints.

7.4.1.2
Central Cerebral Process Slowing in Old Age Mainly Affects the Phonological Convertor

We examined the verbal reactions to three tasks (including a monosyllable, a word and a sentence) of 5 young normal subjects (21–37 years old) and for comparison those of 4 old normal subjects (70–78 years old). In all old subjects, we found a significant increase in ACG latency of immediate reactions in the order of +26% with respect to young subjects for the monosyllable /ma/ and of +19% for the word /mare/. No statistically significant difference was found for the sentence (/mare è bello/). A typical finding in 1 old subject (72 years old) is given in figure 63, with the complete diagrams for ACG latency in figure 64 and for ACG duration in figure 65.

Since the sentence reaction implies that the CCP is related to the grammatical convertor and latency time is only slightly increased in both immediate and delayed reactions in old age, one can assume that the CCP involved in the grammatical conversion are not markedly slowed in dependence on aging. It can also be inferred that the higher-level brain activity, which is more strictly connected to the linguistic operations, is not the specific target of the age-dependent neural deterioration in normal subjects.

The age-dependent slowing in central programmation seems to be localized at a second stage in Levelt's blueprint [1989] that is at the phonological convertor, as it is clearly indicated by the significant increase in ACG latency, particularly with the monosyllabic task. In the context of the total of the other previously reported results, we might also argue that the change responsible for this slowing does not seem to be linked to the velocity of the pattern flow in CCP. On the contrary, it appears more likely to hypothesize an impaired processing at the level of the articulatory buffer: *the threshold of the encoded representations is raised* in such a way that the decoding requires a higher number of impulses, eventually corresponding to an additional operative time.

Taking this hypothesis as granted, many related intricate questions emerge in the field of science of speech.

What is the relation of this increase in neural assembly decoding with the manifold aspects of operative memory and its substrates?

Would Broca's centre be specifically involved? Or are rather more generalized mechanisms of memory involved, like those provided by the hippocampal areas?

What are the biochemical and physicochemical processes reducing the neuroplastic efficiency of the brain? Is the glutamate-dopamine balance involved [Woody, 1982]?

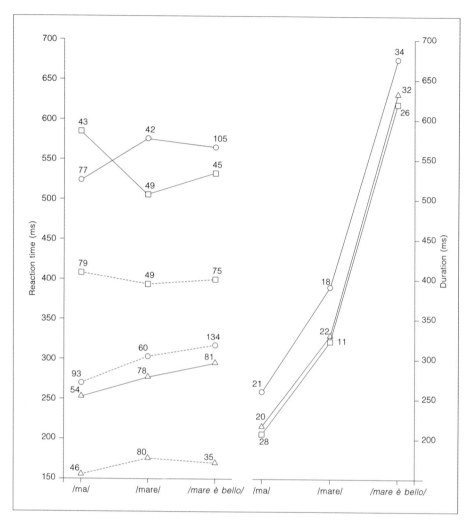

Fig. 63. Reaction times and durations of an old normal subject, P.P., male, 72 years old. —— = ACG values; ----- = EMG values; ○ = FP_0; □ = $FP_{0.1}$; △ = $FP_{1.5}$; figures near symbols indicate SD.

Certainly we should take into consideration all factors related not only to synaptic threshold but also to synaptic strength and efficiency [Linden, 1994].

7.4.2
A Further Methodological Approach – Reading Reactions with Very Short Foreperiods (0.1 s)

If the 'go' signal is presented when the first CCP are still in progress, the GO process of visual perception of the 'go' signal might not interfere with the ongoing neural pro-

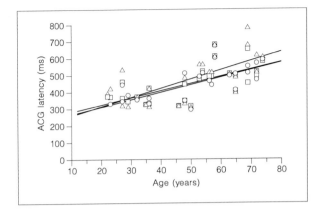

Fig. 64. ACG latencies at FP_0 obtained from normal subjects of different ages. $\bigcirc = $ /ma/ (r = 0.77, p < 0.0001); $\square = $ /mare/ (r = 0.78, p < 0.0001); $\triangle = $ /mare è bello/ (r = 0.75, p < 0.0001).

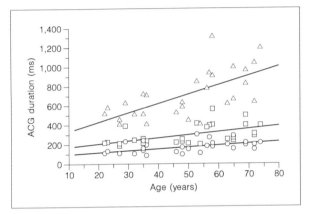

Fig. 65. ACG durations at FP_0 obtained from normal subjects of different ages. $\bigcirc = $ /ma/ (r = 0.61, p < 0.0003); $\square = $ /mare/ (r = 0.69, p < 0.0001); $\triangle = $ /mare è bello/ (r = 0.65, p < 0.0001).

cesses of speech control, if it could be independently processed on an available free channel. In an ideal normal situation of this type, the GO process of visual perception of the 'go' signal could even exert a speeding effect; one could think of a pressure-like stimulus. On the other hand, the occurrence of a limiting factor in the number of available channels is proved by the results of a less than 15% decrease in ACG latency of very short foreperiod reactions in normal adults.

It has been shown that the ACG latency of a very short foreperiod reaction is statistically significantly increased in old subjects. These results have been reported in figures 55–57. It appears from them that with /mare/ and /muro/ the 0.1-second foreperiod does not affect ACG latency in the two groups of subjects aged 18–44 and 45–59 years, respectively. In the first group, ACG latency of /muro/ seems even to diminish from 371 ± 48 to 345 ± 50 ms, equivalent to –7%. We can further observe that the ACG duration, too, has diminished in the same group of young subjects, with the 0.1-second foreperiod, from a mean value of 321 ± 78 to 285 ± 63 ms, equivalent to –11%.

On the contrary, in the group of the oldest subjects (60–80 years old), the 0.1 second foreperiod produces a statistically significant increase in ACG latency, from 619 ± 169 to 736 ± 168 ms, equivalent to +19%.

7.4.2.1
A Synopsis of Acousticogram Latencies with Different Foreperiods

A full comprehension of the heuristic value of the series of 0.1-second foreperiod re-actions can better be envisaged by considering its place among the whole series of immediate, very short and long foreperiod reactions. Two main sectors seem worth considering: (1) changes in all kinds of reactions occurring in relation with the aging process and (2) the criteria of evaluation to identify the programming processes with respect to the executive articulatory phase.

7.4.2.2
Multiple Foreperiod Reactions Applied to the Study of Aging Processes

It seems advantageous to re-examine our findings of the increase in ACG latencies in the older subjects (fig. 55–57). The study of 2 subjects of 30 and 55 years of age, submitted to systematic clinical, psychological and neurophysiological examinations, seems a particularly pertinent complement in this regard. The ACG values obtained are given in 7.2.2.3.2, figures 59, 61 and 60, 62, respectively.

The young and older subjects had the same social position, middle school education, and IQ (101 and 102, respectively). The mental deterioration of the older subject was 9 %. All physical and chemical examinations were normal. Visual acuity was 10/10; visual-evoked potentials had a +3% increase in latency time in the 55-year-old subject. Psycho-motor attitudes, evaluated as kinetic factor (see 8.1), were similar in the 2 subjects.

The central time of conduction from the frontal cortex to the orbicularis oris muscle (with transcranial electromagnetic stimulation) was 0.9 ms longer in the old subject, who was 2.5 cm taller than the young one. Both patients were not under any medical treatment; they were no hard drinkers and no smokers.

It appears from the diagram of the young subject (fig. 59–61) that ACG latency at FP_0 is nearly the same for the two word stimuli /mare/ and /muro/. Some differences occur at 0.1- and 1.5-second foreperiods, with a lower value for /mare/, in the order of –7 %. In the older subject (fig. 60, 62), the time difference in ACG latency for /mare/ and /muro/ is greater and inconstant between the two stimuli: the longest one occurs at 0.5-second fore-period reactions with a value of –25% for /mare/.

The SD are higher at the 1.5-second foreperiod in the older subject. In both subjects, there is a significant decrease in ACG latency from immediate reactions to 1.5- and 4-second foreperiods. The absolute value of the difference (ACG latency at FP_0 – ACG latency at $FP_{1.5}$ to FP_4) is greater in the 55-year-old subject: one must note however that the percent time difference is about the same in the 2 subjects. In accordance with this finding and in spite of a greater difference (ACG latency at FP_0 – ACG latency at $FP_{1.5}$) corresponding to $520–400 = 120$ ms, the older subject does not reach a minimal ACG latency as short as the one of the younger subject, being 400 and 300 ms, respectively.

The central brain processes are 20 ms slower in the old subject: however, a marked slowing seems to occur in the executive processes. In contrast, the analysis of ACG values reported in figures 60 and 62 appears to be similar at FP_0, with even lower values for reactions at $FP_{0.1}$ to FP_4 of the old subject. This behaviour proves that timing processes, even at the executive level (diadochokinesis), are not slowed down in old subjects with respect to young ones.

These results demand a comprehensive knowledge of all elements occurring as a mosaic in the chain of speech control. In relation to the just mentioned two subjects, but with a more general line of reference, we might propose the following argumentations.

7.4.3
Towards a Definite Interpretation of the Information Loss in the Aging Brain: Second Step

Since the peripherocentral afferent and centroperipheral efferent pathways (that is the input and output layers, operating as serial channels in topographically well-defined parts of the neural system) conduct the impulses at approximately the same velocity in young and old subjects, one might infer that the decrease in velocity, shown to occur in the executive processes of the old subject, should be localized at the interface between the internal output of the invariants and the process of adaptation representing exactly the first phase of the executive process.

We can now proceed to analyse this assumption in the context of the results obtained in the total population previously investigated and with the threefold task including the grammatical sentence.

(1) In a preliminary research [Pinelli and Ceriani, 1992], we relied on a dualistic conception with, on the one hand, the central programming and intermediary processes, corresponding to Levelt's formulators (or convertors in the domain of MDRV), and, on the other, the executive neuromotor processes. According to this view, the slowing of verbal reactions in older subjects, particularly in the 65- to 80-year class (i.e. in a more advanced age than that of the two paradigmatic cases), could be attributed to the involvement of the central processes rather than to the executive ones: the difference of ACG latency between the immediate ($= 600$ ms) and the 1.5-second foreperiod reactions was in fact of the order of >150 ms (ACG latency at $FP_{1.5}$ and FP_4 was in the range of 460–430 ms).

(2) In the more recent research we enlarged the previous dualistic conception with a more differentiated analysis of the intermediary processes that took the role of a third-order operation between the two: in line with this view, we adopted a more amplified methodology including both phonological and grammatical tasks.

The age-dependent slowing of verbal reactions (particularly in middle-aged people) was found to be confined to phonological rather than to even longer grammatical tasks. Therefore we inferred that the vulnerable point is localized at the level where phonology-related processes are specifically separated from the grammatical processes. This is represented by the corresponding phonological convertor and the corresponding functions between the programmer and the convertor.

7.4.3.1
The Initial Aging Process and a Factor of Correction

The last conclusion about the vulnerable point concerned normal middle-aged people. In these subjects, the vulnerable point is at the interface between the central and the second-level phonological processes. We will try to prove now that, when the age-dependent slowing is rather slight, it can be confined to this level; on the contrary, when it becomes more marked, it exerts backward top negative effects on the central process of the first level.

I want also to underline that, in the early phase, factors of correction occur to normalize the initial aging impairment as much as possible.

A normal, i.e. 'young', minimal ACG latency (at long foreperiod reactions) can in fact be obtained from old subjects by an ongoing process of correction. A process of this kind can appropriately be performed only under slightly impaired conditions, as in the case of our 55-year-old subject (fig. 60 and 62). When the slowing at the interface increases, as in our 60- to 80-year class, the correction process fails and a backward, or overloading, slowing effect impairs also the most early central processes.

Two other findings can offer a cue for this initial upwards spreading slow-down.

(a) The 0.5-second foreperiod of ACG latency is critical in the 55-year-old subject, since the increase in ACG latency that represents the usual finding at the 0.1-second foreperiod appears also with the 0.5-second foreperiod for the less easily pronounceable word stimulus /muro/. This may indicate that the codification-decodification at the buffer shows some difficulty as an initial sign of secondary impairment of the final phase of the central processes. In fact, the ratio between ACG latency at $FP_{0.5}$ and ACG latency at FP_0 will be >1. The exact identification of the increase in ACG latency at $FP_{0.5}$, limited to only one rather unusual task and anyway smaller than at $FP_{0.1}$, allows us to interpret this finding as a *secondary effect:* it is actually an extension of the 'early process impairment' detected with the very short foreperiod. This result is clearly different from the inversion of the ACG latency ratio $FP_{0.5}/FP_0$ that can be found in schizophrenics (see Section 9). In fact, it is *higher than the ratio $FP_{0.1}/FP_0$* and affects all word stimuli (including monosyllables, disyllabic words and sentences). This change, specific for schizophrenics, depends on an impairment detectable at the level of the intermediary processes (see Section 9).

(b) While in the 30-year-old subject (fig. 59 and 61) the decrease in ACG latency at delayed reactions becomes smaller from the 1.5- to 4-second foreperiod, this decrease becomes greater in the order of +8% for the 4-second foreperiod in the 55-year-old subject (fig. 60). This finding might be considered as a proof that a higher number of reverberating circuits is needed to obtain the best facilitated neural assembly and hence the minimal ACG latency.

7.4.3.2

Further Criteria for Differentiating Abnormal Articulatory Constraints from Brain Programmation Impairments

As outlined in 3.2, it appears highly appropriate to *carry out simple reactions* which can yield direct data on the functional state of the final executors and myo-articular movements of speaking.

A more extreme and intricate chain of bidirectional repercussions is offered by pathological conditions, i.e. cases with impairments of the articulators themselves at the peripheral reflex control. This condition of impairment can be named 'abnormal constraints'.

These cases require a differential analysis of central versus distal impairments. A paradigmatic condition is represented by the association of akinesia with hypertonia in Parkinson syndrome. A systematic study of parkinsonian patients, with reference also to bradyphrenia, will be reported later in section 9. Now only some methodological issues will be discussed, which are strictly related to the previous analyses of information loss in brain aging. What we have to evaluate is a motor disorder presumably depending on a central impairment (due to a nigral dopamine deficiency) but producing also an impairment of the articulators. The executors themselves are thus hindered in their cyclic movements by the hypertonic rigid state of the muscles. This constraint is in fact analogous to a primary anatomofunctional alteration occurring in the vocal tract [Pinelli et al., 1995]. A correct investigation of this situation requires the application of the following tests: (1) measurements of ACG latency and duration, electroglottogram and EMG latencies of chewing muscles for immediate and foreperiod verbal reactions; (2) measurement of the analogous EMG latency in specific immediate and foreperiod reactions of cyclic chewing movements.

Apart from these specific additional tests, the computational procedure of the central versus constraint-dependent increases in ACG latency and duration remains identical to that of central versus execution-dependent changes.

Two Individual-Trait-Independent Indices of Early and Intermediary Brain Processes

An Individual Factor of Variability in Multiple-Delayed-Reaction Verbochronometry: The Kinetic Factor

8.1.1
The Kinetic Factor

The search for an individual psychomotor personality trait, which can basically influence the speed of verbal reactions, is a core problem for an interindividual comparison of our test results. The problem concerns children as well as all adults and even pathological cases. Its analysis implies both theoretical and methodological considerations.

De Lisi [1940], in an enlightening study of extrapyramidal functions related to motricity, and Eysenck [1954, 1970], with his systematic investigations into the structure of human personality, pointed out that each individual subject has his proper level of activity, linked to an endogenous constitution. One can indeed identify an individual style of movement with varying degrees of motor easiness and accuracy, elegance, fitness and speed: some people are phlegmatic, some vivacious, some rather awkward and clumsy, others elegant and graceful; some are sluggish and slow, others, in contrast, rather prompt and quick.

Thus it seemed justified to identify a normal range of kinetic proneness, the so-called *kinetic factor,* from hypokinesia through eukinesia to hyperkinesia.

In the pathological field, the extrapyramidal syndromes represent the extreme variants with the akinetic complex on one side and the choreic and other frank hyperkinetic disorders on the other.

One can then argue that the system of the basal ganglia – that we have seen to be implied in CCP1 and CCP2 (see 7.1.4 and 3.1.2) for speech control – is endowed with different neurobiological properties in each individual subject.

The cause of kinetic factor variations could be the amount and distribution of neurotransmitters, neuromodulators and related enzymes and receptors: dopamine, acetylcholine, γ-aminobutyric acid, glutamic acid, serotonin, noradrenaline and neuropeptides.

The functional side of the individual kinetic variability should be represented by the hebbian neural assembly threshold and by the availability and speed of the internal reverberating circuits.

All these premises introduce new parameters that require an appropriate methodological approach. Hence, further research on brain motor control of speech should take up the tests for measuring the kinetic factor again. It is a very challenging task indeed that has never been faced specifically with consistent results.

At this preliminary stage of study, we can only quote a series of tests that seem to be more appropriate to our purpose.

In the section of psychomotor batteries, it is worth mentioning the Standford motor skill unit [Seashore, 1928], the rapid alternating movement tests with possible indices of performances [Fitts, 1954], the manual dexterity [Barnes, 1968] and steadiness tests [Boshes et al., 1960], some among the tests used by Potvin et al. [1981] for psychomotor changes in normal aging processes and those for alertness and vigilance [Potvin and Tourtelotte, 1985].

A subordinate way to better choose and apply a suitable test for the kinetic factor might be found if it could be related to a theoretical predication of the influences this fac-

Table 11. Evaluation of the kinetic factor

Accuracy (f)	R	L
0.3	>30%	>30%
0.6	15–30%	15–30%
0.1	<15%	<15%

R = Deformation of the square to a rectangular shape; L = length of lines exceeding the edges.
Kinetic index = t × f, where t = time taken by the subject to draw 10 squares.

tor might have on the chain of the brain process of speech control. (1) As far as the degrees of alertness, vigilance and attention are implied, the shortening in ACG latency could be expressed at the early phases of sensorimotor CCP1. (2) On the other hand, a more specific high level of activity might be related to the corticogangliobasal internal circuits and neural assembly threshold. A diminution in ACG latency correlated to a high kinetic factor could depend on a fast CCP2 and coding and decoding processes at the level of the invariant-variant interface.

8.1.2
Some Tests for the Kinetic Factor and Independent Indices

However difficult and intricate the quantification of the kinetic factor may be, it seems to be indispensable for the scientist intending to correlate and thoroughly analyse the results of word motor control tests.

At the present stage of our study, we rely on two different approaches: (a) an analytical supplementary short test and (b) the recourse to ratios of MDRV parameters where the effect of the kinetic factor is eliminated, being present in both the numerator and the denominator.

8.1.2.1
A Short Test for the Kinetic Factor

The subject is invited to draw 10 squares on a sheet of paper as quickly as possible. The time of the whole performance is measured with a stop-watch. The accuracy value is given with a factor of 0.3, 0.6 or 1.0 according to the degree of deformation of the square to a rectangular shape and the length of edge-exceeding lines, measured as mean values of the 10 squares (table 11).

8.1.2.2
Two Indices Independent of the Kinetic Factor

The ratios used are ACT latency at $FP_{1.5}$/ACG latency at FP_0, which represents an intermediary process inefficiency index, and ACG latency at $FP_{0.1}$/ACG latency at FP_0, which represents an early process inefficiency index. Their meanings and values will be discussed in 8.2, 8.3 and in Section 10.

....

An Early Process Index

8.2.1
How Speech Control by the Brain Can Be Evaluated with Multiple-Delayed-Reaction Verbochronometry

The outline of the evaluation of aging effects, developed in Section 7, can now be discussed as a point of reference for a correct inference from MDRV data to the activity of the brain machinery. Students familiar with neurological and neurophysiological diagnosis are well prepared to comprehend and apply these rules of inference. We think it useful to list them here as an agenda for the scientists working in the field of normal and pathological control of speech.

(1) All clinical conditions of the individual subject must be noted and 'measured' before selecting the verbal tests (see Appendix 1). (a) The anatomofunctional basic state of the vocal tract including its neuromotor condition must be assessed (electroglottogram, EMG or myogram). (b) Psychomotor abilities (the kinetic factor) should be evaluated with suitable psychometric tests. The variability depending on constitutional psychomotor ability can alternatively be ruled out with the resort to measurement of MDRV ratios with the kinetic factor influencing equally numerator and denominator at an equal rate.

(2) On the grounds of all preliminary data and the individual clinical syndrome, the examiner should outline a tentative scheme of the possible causes of increases in ACG latency time (at different foreperiods) and duration in the tests for that individual subject. This may be correctly performed if the following rules are respected:

(a) alteration or damage to buffers or to stores (hebbian neural assemblies) is consistent with an increase in the threshold and 'synaptic strength' [Linden, 1994] of the neural assemblies;

(b) demyelination could be a possible cause of central slowing and requires the central time with electromagnetic transcranial stimulation to be measured and brain MRI to be performed;

(c) two hierarchical orders of pathogenetic consequences must be remembered when selecting the tests and evaluating the results; the first (C_1) concerns the level of the lesion, i.e. from (1) the articulators, with reference to anatomical and functional constraints, to (2) the brain intermediary and executive processes and (3) the brain programming processes; the second hierarchical order (C_2)concerns the nature of the neural alterations, which can be a matter of (1) organic irreversible structural lesions, (2) organic reversible alterations, (3) functional irreversible or (4) functional reversible alterations.

It ensues from the analysis of these rules that we must know exactly all possible anatomical alterations in executive processes. Programming processes can then be impaired secondarily. In fact, we may attribute impairments of brain programming processes to *primary alterations only if no change is found at the two lower levels.*

8.2.2
An Experimental and Theoretical Analysis of the Heuristic Value of
0.1-Second Foreperiod Reactions

Let us evaluate, in more detail, the experimental condition preliminarily described in Section 6. After the presentation of the word stimulus, an expected visual 'go' signal is given while the subject is still mentally working, i.e. carrying out the verbal sensorimotor processes that develop in a diffuse parallel manner. Does the perception of the 'go' stimulus act as a negative interfering event that interrupts the brain activity started at the previous word stimulus, with a consequent delay or even a possible error or a block?

Our experience has convinced us that a negative interference of this kind is not all the rule, but that, on the contrary, the effects of the short 0.1-second foreperiod on ACG latency are quite varied, according to the age of the subject and possible abnormal conditions. The following changes were alternatively observed: (1) with the 0.1-second foreperiod, ACG latency becomes *significantly shortened*; this is the case for young normal subjects and some stutterers; it implies a PDP system with open collateral channels and self-adjusting hidden units; (2) the ACG latency at $FP_{0.1}$ becomes *significantly prolonged*; this is the case for old age, mental deterioration and some bradyphrenic disorders.

To better explain the meaning of these results it is worth clarifying how this method with short foreperiods differs from a test of simultaneous performances [Potvin and Tourtelotte, 1985; Baddeley et al., 1986].

8.2.2.1
Multiple Peripheral Diffuse Processes Are Not Equivalent to Simultaneous Performances

The condition of PDP with its individual limit of channels must not be confused with the number of tasks that an individual subject can perform simultaneously.

In the case of PDP, the pathway or each channel corresponds to the sequence of an input layer, an inner unit layer with multiple loops of CCP and an output layer, all involved in a one-goal operation. The result is a single purposeful complex coordinated sequential action. The question of an upper limit in PDP efficiency concerns the number of channels with inner unit layers in connection with specific input and output. The value of the upper limit reflects the degree of simultaneity and then of velocity of the operation.

In contrast, multiple simultaneous tasks involve *different separate* inputs and outputs and do not request a unique optimal performance. In fact, in multiple simultaneous tasks there are phases of prevalent attention on a single process and there are no precise parameters of the development time and of the executive duration along the unique chain of events.

It ensues that the examination of multiple simultaneous performances cannot be properly applied to obtain valid cues for the efficiency of PDP. However, a comparison of the two kinds of performances could be justified if we want to have some information on the number of different outputs and on the speed in central programming during interfering stimuli.

8.2.3
$FP_{0.1}$ Reactions in Normals and in Abnormal Deterioration

The short foreperiod reaction test was found to be a valid, reliable and highly sensitive method to detect abnormal mental deteriorations. The increase in ACG latency with

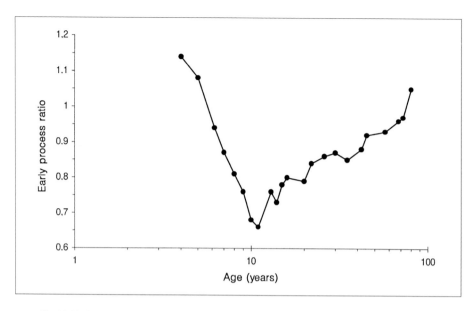

Fig. 66. Early process ratios of 202 patients of different ages.

0.1-second foreperiods can reach very high values in abnormal deterioration, as we will report in Section 9.

Actually, a ratio has been identified – i.e. ACG latency at $FP_{0.1}$ as numerator and ACG latency at FP_0 as denominator – that can be considered as an index of early process insufficiency in the sense previously defined. In normal subjects, aged from 7 to 60 years, this ratio is <1, whereas it increases to >1 in mental deterioration. The advantage of this ratio, with respect to the difference that we should calculate between the value measured in the subject under investigation for ACG latency at $FP_{0.1}$ and the corresponding mean value of the normal homogeneous population, is its independence from individual constitutional, cultural and educational features, the kinetic factor included.

Early process ratios were calculated in 202 patients of different ages, from 4 to 81 years, in 19 age groups, each composed of 10–11 subjects. The resulting diagram is reported in figure 66.

8.2.4
The Effects of Demyelination in Multiple Sclerosis

The investigation of demyelinating processes deserves particular mention. As we have already discussed, it requires an associated research of evoked sensitive potential and motor-evoked potential, which can provide essential information on the degree of slowing in conduction and transmission in input and output systems.

Secondary backward effects from an impaired executive corticospinal system to the CCP can play an important role in producing the paretic disorders of this disease. Its ascertainment is needed to plan a correct treatment for rehabilitation.

8.2.5
The Analysis of Acousticogram Duration

The heuristic value of the parameter ACG duration and its neurofunctional meaning have been analysed in previous Sections, in parallel with the evaluation of the other main parameter, ACG latency (6.4, table 10 for children and 3.2.3.3, table 7, 7.4.1, fig. 65 for adults). We will now analyse the values of ACG duration of /mare/ and /muro/ obtained from: (1) a systematic study of 26 normals, (2) 2 normal subjects of 30 and 55 years (7.2.2.3.2, fig. 61 and 62) and (3) some pathological cases with mixed, central and distal execution alterations.

8.2.5.1
The Values of Acousticogram Duration in Young and Old Normal Subjects

As previously reported in table 7 and shown in figures 61 and 62, ACG duration undergoes an increase in two age classes: (1) from the young to the middle-aged group and (2) particularly from the middle-aged to the old group. However, this increase is rather small, in the range of 7–14%, respectively.

The foreperiods give rise to a small decrease, particularly in the youngest and in the oldest groups (at variance with ACG latency). The decrease in ACG duration is more marked with the shortest foreperiod, but still in the range of 10%. It becomes insignificant at 1.5- and 4-second foreperiods.

8.2.5.2
The Two Paradigmatic Subjects

It seems worthwhile analysing in detail the behaviour of ACG duration in the 2 subjects we have thoroughly investigated with associated neurophysiological tests, as previously reported in section 7. As shown in figures 61 and 62, ACG duration is higher in the 55-year-old subject than in the 30-year-old one. On the other hand, at the 0.1-second foreperiod, the older subject shows a greater decrease in ACG duration than the younger one; this decrease reaches –25% for the word /muro/.

These findings show that the parameter ACG duration, at variance with the increment in ACG latency between young and middle age, does not yield statistically valid information for aging processes. One should infer that, in this limited span of aging at least, the timing CCP remains well compensated, while the peripheral diadochokinetic movements for speech of short words are still as quick as in young individuals.

8.2.5.3
The Values of Acousticogram Duration in Syndromes with Mixed Alterations
Affecting Central Programming Processes and Peripheral Executor Servo-Mechanisms

The parameter ACG duration acquires great importance in the abnormal conditions where the timing CCP are significantly impaired. This is, for example, the case in extrapyramidal akinesia. As it will be shown in 9.4, ACG duration undergoes a marked decrease from FP_0 to $FP_{1.5}$ reactions: from 625 to 446 ms, equivalent to −25%. These changes – related to slowing in timing processes – are greater than those found for ACG latency that are related to early programming processes.

8.2.6
A Comparison between a Normal Old Subject with High IQ and an Old Subject with Mild Deterioration of Short-Term Memory

8.2.6.1
Subject No. 1 (P.P.), Male, 72 Years Old, University Degree, IQ 121

As reported in figure 63 (7.4.1.2), ACG latency at FP_0 for /ma/, /mare/ and /mare è bello/ was 525 ± 77, 573 ± 42 and 560 ± 105 ms. The ratio ACG latency at FP_0 for /mare è bello/ to ACG latency at FP_0 for /mare/ was 0.49. The ratio ACG latency at $FP_{1.5}$ for /mare è bello/ to ACG latency at FP_0 for /mare è bello/ was 0.51. ACG duration was 220, 332 and 640 ms, respectively.

8.2.6.2
Subject No. 2 (P.C.), Male, 71 Years Old, Middle School Degree, IQ 92, Immediate Memory Deterioration Score 0.7

The results obtained from P.C. tested with the same verbal reactions as those performed by subject 1 (P.P.) were the following:

ACG latency at FP_0: 666 ± 94, 610 ± 76 and 560 ± 64 ms. The ratio /mare è bello/ to /mare/ was 0.81. ACG duration was 288, 486 and 788 ms.

ACG latency at $FP_{0.1}$: $1,051 \pm 128$, $1,010 \pm 100$ and 955 ± 76 ms, with an ACG duration of 417, 530 and 900 ms.

ACG latency at $FP_{1.5}$: 523 ± 75, 597 ± 127, and 574 ± 170 ms. The ratio ACG latency at $FP_{1.5}$ to ACG latency at FP_0 for /mare/ was 0.90. The ratio ACG latency at $FP_{1.5}$ to ACG latency at FP_0 for /mare è bello/ was 1.03.

8.2.6.3
Discussion

In both subjects, the reaction times for the sentence are never significantly increased with respect to those of the syllable or the disyllabic word. This confirms that even in slightly deteriorated subjects (No. 2), the grammatical convertor holds better than the phonological one. We had previously analysed the reasons for this behaviour and we can state now that they are valid also in old age.

On the contrary, only in subject No. 1, with well-preserved mental functions and high IQ, did the intermediary brain processes related to operative or dynamic memory allow a normal shortening of the reaction times with the 1.5-second foreperiod. In fact, the intermediary process index remains well below 0.9. This finding proves that Hinton's internal feedbacks are efficient in old subjects without impairments of short-term memory. Therefore the age-dependent slowing of brain function in non-deteriorated old subjects does not involve intermediary processes but is localized in the last phase of the CCP related to invariant patterns, just preceding the operative dynamic memory, decoding processes and the adaptive invariant-to-variant processes.

The analysis of the effects that impairments of short-term memory can produce on intermediary processes will be carried out in Section 9.

An Intermediary Process Index

8.3.1
0.5- to 1.5-Second Delayed Verbal Reaction: The Right Procedure and the Evaluation of Intermediary Processes

8.3.1.1
Rules for a Correct Application

In the analysis of the neural processes going on during intermediary foreperiods (0.5–1.5 s), one must be aware that they occur during a decision-making process implying an intricate series of states, psychologically defined by the following terms: expectation, preparation to pronounce a word, counterbalancing restraints while the programme of execution continues. Inhibitory processes may take place against an early tendency to respond immediately before the 'go' signal makes its appearance. The early tendency could express itself as an abortive EMG burst, just after a minimal latency time (of about 200 ms), shorter than that of the optimal foreperiod reactions. This interference might be avoided with a few preliminary trials, instructing the subject to moderately engage in high-speed reactions.

On the other hand, this psychological factor might play a significant role in pressed reactions, with a sort of short-circuit performances [Pinelli, 1964].

8.3.1.2
The Intermediary Process Ratio

As it was explained for the early process ratio, in relation to the early programming processes, the search for an index of the processes occurring during >0.4-second delayed reactions, independent of individual traits, represented an essential preliminary step towards a functional diagnostic application of our tests. It should provide reliable information about an insufficiency of the intermediary processes; they play a fundamental role in speech control by the brain and are particularly liable to impairment in specific mental disorders (Section 9).

With regard to the analysis of the intermediary processes, the reader must refer to the previous chapters on operative memory, verbal store and retrieval, in connection with grammatical and phonological convertors, buffer coding and decoding and adaptive processes. On the other hand, data concerning intermediary neuronal circuits are reported in Appendix 1.

The ratio ACG latency of $FP_{1.5}$ to ACG latency at FP_0 that we have called ratio of intermediary processes meets the requirement of independence of individual traits. It was measured in the same subjects as the early process ratio, the results of which are reported in figure 66.

The curve of the intermediary process ratio as a function of age (fig. 67) is rather complex as it could be guessed by the many different neurofunctional factors that may affect, at different degrees, its numerator and denominator.

8.3.1.3
The Factors Acting Homogeneously or Heterogeneously on Intermediary Processes

Here it becomes necessary to define the intrinsic and acquired psychomotor traits that act homogeneously on ACG latency at $FP_{>0.4}$ and on ACG latency at FP_0 of the individual subject. Secondly, I will point out how some neurofunctional factors can act asymmetrically on the two variables.

Dealing with the kinetic factor (8.1), I analysed the individually specific abilities to speak rather slowly [Lyberg, 1977] or more quickly. It seems right to state that these differences may depend on specific functional (structural and biochemical) organizations of the executive constraints, and we know that the values of these variables are equally expressed in immediate and delayed reactions. The same is true for the variables associated with the kinetic factor that are involved in programmation processes.

Likewise we can assume that working memory and the other associated intermediary pre-executive processes, including the triggering event, are proportionally as rapid as the previous early programmation and final executive brain activities. This assumption seems correct as far as normal intrinsic conditions are considered.

A dissociation between the temporal course of the early programming processes and the intermediary processes on one side and between these and the executive processes on the other could in fact occur only in the case of rather acute injuries affecting early or executive processes. In these cases, the intermediary processes could suffer the repercussions from the changes in early and/or in executive processes: they could in fact slow down or develop at a compensatory relatively increased velocity. This compensation could be achieved with a shorter wavelength of the reiterative internal feedbacks, i.e. with facilitated or shorter circuits in the corticosubcortical pathways (see also Section 9).

The same considerations seem to be valid for chronically acquired changes.

The situation is quite different in pathological conditions. An injury can affect the processes and representations involved in programmation, leaving working memory and executive processes intact: in this case, only ACG latency at FP_0 will be altered (increased). But it can happen that a different injury affects the executive processes without primarily involving early processes. In the first case (i.e. increase in early processes), the intermediary process ratio would decrease independently of a specific alteration in working memory. In fact, the supposed injury produces an increase in the denominator ACG latency at FP_0, while in this condition the numerator ACG latency at $FP_{>0.4}$ does not necessarily change: in fact, the increase in early processes is absorbed during the delay as far as the latter is longer than the increase in early processes.

The consequence is different under the supposed condition of an increase in ACG latency at $FP_{>0.4}$. In this case, the same increase occurs in ACG latency at FP_0, and the intermediary process ratio remains constant.

Let us now analyse how a change in the temporal course of working memory affects the value of the intermediary process ratio. If working memory slows down, the ratio will increase. The contrary occurs if working memory accelerates (and ACG latency at FP_0 is not affected by the injury): the ratio decreases. It ensues from these analyses that

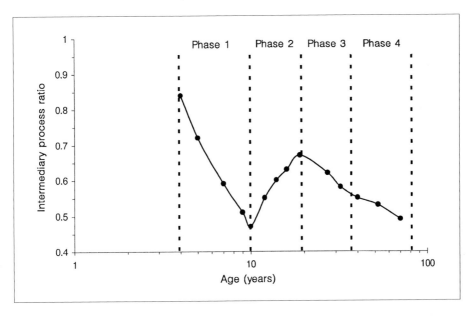

Fig. 67. The intermediary process ratio as a function of age.

changes of intermediary process ratio can be correctly evaluated and can then provide reliable information on working memory, only if we take also into consideration the values of the single variables ACG latency at FP_0 (the denominator) and ACG latency at $FP_{>0.4}$ (the numerator). The variations occurring in these single variables can be appreciated interindividually when compared, with cross-investigations, to the mean values of the normal population or intra-individually, in longitudinal investigations. The intra-individual evaluation provides the most precise information, since 'spontaneous, natural variations in normals, at long period repeated controls, are contained in a small range' (see Section 4).

8.3.1.4
The Curve of the Intermediary Process Ratio as a Function of Age

The curve presents four phases (fig. 67).

It seems logical to consider first of all the phase where ACG latency at FP_0 reaches the minimal value, and this has been found to occur at 18–32 years of age. In this third period of age, the difference of ACG latency at FP_0 – ACG latency at $FP_{1.5}$ can be taken as the best temporal measure of the intermediary processes. Thus, we might name this phase the 'intermediary-process-revealing phase'.

In the first period, from 4 to 10 years of age, the intermediary process ratio progressively decreases with a rather steep slope until the age of 10 years. The main factor responsible for this decrease is a progressively lower value of ACG latency at $FP_{1.5}$. On the other hand, this value is an expression of intermediary processes, and it is possible to assume that the corresponding corticosubcortical loops mature from 4 to 10 years of age.

In contrast, the neurological substrates of the visuomotor transformation and of the related elaboration of the invariants reach their full maturation later, at the age of 18 years, when ACG latency at FP_0 reaches its maximum.

Anyway the main cause of the relative immobility in time of the early brain processes, at the age from 4 to 10 years, can likely be attributed to a still failing parallel development in the different processes (PDP) from the visuomotor transformation, initiation and programmation to central timing and pre-adaptation.

In the second period, a reversal in the curve is observed that in fact increases until the age of 18 years. This increase could depend on the decrease in ACG latency at FP_0 with reference to an acceleration of the central programming processes and an optimal establishment of PDP.

In the third period, between 18 and 35 years of age, the decrease of intermediary process ratio may be produced by the best functioning of the intermediary processes.

A very slowly progressing increase in the intermediary process ratio occurs in the fourth period, from 35 to 86 years. This increase implies a dissociation between the two members of the ratio: ACG latency at $FP_{1.5}$ increases, or ACG latency at FP_0 decreases. Alternatively both members of the ratio could increase, but at a different slope, that of ACG latency at FP_0 being less steep. This assumption is in agreement with the previous analysis (see Section 7) of the effects of brain aging that do not specifically affect the early initiation and programmation processes but rather slow down some functions implied in the passage to the intermediary processes.

It must also be underlined that the increase in the intermediary process ratio occurring in the fourth period follows a logarithmic course: this means that the relative increase in ACG latency at $FP_{1.5}$ diminishes with the increase in age. In fact, in old age, the slope of the increase in ACG latency at $FP_{1.5}$ is relatively less steep, and this partially compensates for the increase in the early functional components of ACG latency at FP_0.

The occurrence of a relative compensatory acceleration of the intermediary processes with respect to early initiation and programmation can be considered as the main factor responsible for the decrease in the ratio in the fourth period, at the age of 35–86 years: ACG latency in fact increases at this advanced age.

In order to identify the real course of brain intermediary processes at the most advanced age, one can correct the value of ACG latency at FP_0: we subtract from the ACG latency, of the single individual subject, the difference between this value and the mean ACG latency at FP_0 of the population aged 20–35 years. With this normalization the curve of the intermediary process ratio takes the shape of a U (similar to that found for the early process ratio) showing that the intermediary processes are slowed down in the last period of aging, even if at a lower rate than the programming central processes.

In conclusion, in normal subjects, the intermediary process ratio (at $FP_{1.5}$) is ≤ 0.85 at all ages, from 4 to 60 years.

In subjects with mental decline and/or impairment of short-term memory, the ratio ACG latency at $FP_{0.1}$ to ACG latency at FP_0 increases, and one may find an increase, even if at a lower degree, also for ACG latency at $FP_{0.5}$ and more rarely at $FP_{1.5}$.

On the other hand, a marked specific increase in ACG latency at $FP_{0.5}$ and/or at $FP_{1.5}$, with a relatively normal ACG latency at $FP_{0.1}$, characterizes *mental dissociative disorders* (see Section 10).

A Study of Multiple Foreperiods May Differentiate the Location of Impairments in Intermediary Processes

A further more specific distinction of the above-mentioned intermediary processes may be attempted with several sets of supplementary criteria that we will now analyse.

(1) An impairment of the time course of internal reverberating circuits in frontobasal ganglia loops increases the intermediary process ratio by an amount independent of foreperiod length from 0.5 to 4 s.

(2) Buffer impairments with high neural assembly threshold increase the intermediary process ratio at relatively short foreperiods (0.5–1.5 s), while normal values are obtained at longer foreperiods (4 s).

(3) Specific impairments of grammatical rather than phonological convertors or vice versa produce a prevalent increase in the intermediary process ratio for sentences compared with monosyllables and disyllabic words, or the opposite.

(4) An impairment of the intrinsic mechanism of adaptive processes might increase the intermediary process ratio more specifically at middle foreperiod values (0.5, 1.5 s), but a significant difference occurs between phonological and grammatical tasks.

(5) An impairment of the pre-executive processes, dynamically transforming invariants into variant executive patterns of impulses, may increase ACG latency and even more so ACG duration without any change of the intermediary process ratio.

Primary as well as secondary increases in intermediary process ratios were found in *schizophrenics*, a topic that will be covered in Section 9.

8.3.1.6

Abnormal Increases in Acousticogram Duration and the Busy-Line Effect

Impairments of the articulatory movements in the vocal tract – of whichever origin, pyramidal, cerebellar or extrapyramidal, neuromotor or idiomuscular – may significantly increase ACG duration with a consequent repercussion on speech control. This repercussion can produce the following two kinds of effects:

(1) A *busy-line effect* occurs in delayed reactions with foreperiods longer than the first operative neuronal circuit of the reaction, that is with foreperiods >0.4 s when ACG duration is longer than the foreperiod: in the reactions with $FP_{0.1}$, the busy-line event does not take place since the brain is still engaged in the pre-executive processes and the articulatory motor performance has not yet been planned.

In order to avoid mistakes in the measurement of ACG latency in delayed reactions with foreperiods >0.4 s and shorter than ACG duration, we have to adopt a foreperiod longer than ACG duration. We can then speak of a 'constraint index' represented by the condition to be respected. If, in contrast, ACG duration exceeds the foreperiod, the pattern of the corresponding descending commands from facilitated neural assemblies to the executive system remains blocked; in fact, the recurrent internal feedbacks that should deliver the triggering process last as long as ACG duration. Therefore, the recurrent circuits that should trigger the executive system are unable to start working at the end of the foreperiod. Consequently, the value of ACG latency in reactions delayed for >0.4 s may be artificially prolonged with regard to the real reaction time. This has been just found to occur in a case of spastic dysphonia (9.2). Obviously, in this condition, ACG latency, at a foreperiod shorter than ACG duration, increases with an immediate process ratio apparently >1. As a counter-check, this artefactual increase in intermediary process ratio disappears with a delayed reaction at a foreperiod longer than ACG duration.

(2) *Neuroplastic effects* and possible kindling-like effects occur. Abnormal increases of ACG duration can exert a repercussion on the intermediary processes and slow them down, in line with the isochronal principle of functioning of the three main phases of brain control. These effects, when they persist for long periods, can induce neuroplastic changes, i.e. the receiving target in the intermediary processes, namely the system of the cortical-subcortical-basal ganglia, is not simply modified temporarily in its excitability but undergoes structural less reversible modifications.

Then the system, which becomes neuroplastically altered, might play a pathogenetic role in itself. By analogy with the generation of an epileptic focus by means of repeated subepileptic excitations – the so-called kindling effect – one could define the induced neuroplastic effect as a kindling-like effect.

8.3.2
Learning Effects

Repeating the same series of reactions to word stimuli (like /mare/ and /muro/) in at least 5 sessions in a 3-month period produces on the one side a decrease in ACG latency at FP_0 but on the other side reduces the difference between ACG latency at FP_0 and ACG latency at $FP_{0.1}$–FP_4 in comparison to the values usually observed in normals. This learning effect is consistent with our interpretation of the processes concerning facilitated neural assemblies, i.e. the facilitation exerted in the foreperiod by the recurrent internal feedbacks producing the shortest reactions.

In fact, learning corresponds to the creation of a facilitated hebbian neural assembly by the repetition of always identical tasks. In this case, we deal with an excessively long-lasting learning effect, whilst, in the 1.5-second foreperiod, the recurrent feedbacks unfolding in corticosubcortical loops produce the facilitated neural assemblies, a facilitation that corresponds to an internal short-term learning effect.

Therefore a general rule emerges in the evaluation of the intermediary process ratio: we must preliminary consider a possible previous learning effect. In one technician of our laboratory, who repeated the same multiple-delayed-reaction tests more than 4 times in a period of 5 months, the intermediary process ratio reached in fact a value of 0.95. It simply depends on a very markedly reduced ACG latency at FP_0. Hence the increase in intermediary process ratio, under this condition, cannot indicate a slowing of intermediary processes.

....

Maturational Phases of Speech Control in Normal and Some Abnormal Brains

> Although children need years of schooling to learn arithmetic, geometry or history, they effortlessly acquire the ability to use a system of communication that learned scholars cannot adequately describe.
>
> [Lieberman, 1991]

MDRV was used in children, with specific methodological adaptations and additional tasks. In 6.4, I have reported a general view on MDRV with /mamma/ and /papà/ in 8 children, and we have analysed in the last chapter of this Section the course of early and intermediary process ratio for reading reactions of /mare/ and /muro/ in 80 children.

I will report here, in more detail, the results of our investigations, with particular suitable tasks, in children from 4 to 9 years [Pinelli, 1993; Ceriani and Pinelli, 1994].

Two types of verbal reactions will be analysed: (1) word reading and (2) picture naming. I will then (3) discuss and evaluate the results obtained with the two types of reactions and (4) suggest the most suitable tests to be developed in the future.

8.4.1
Word Reading Reactions in 6- to 9-Year-Old Children

The results of word reading (/mare/, /muro/ and /mamma/, /papà/) are given in figures 68–70 and of picture naming (/mamma/, /papà/) in figures 71–73. All data are reported in table 12. The youngest children investigated with the verbal reading tests for /mare/, /muro/ and /mamma/, /papà/ were 6 years old.

8.4.1.1
Six-Year-Old Children

Two subjects were particularly bright with IQ 114 and 118, respectively. The child T.L. was investigated with /mare/, /muro/, G.I. with /mamma/, /papà/. The values of ACG latency in immediate reactions were twice longer than in adult young subjects. At foreperiod reactions, ACG latency showed a very marked decrease, without however reaching the mean normal values of young adults. The diagrams in figure 52 and table 10 (see 6.4.3) display the values of ACG latency at foreperiods of 0, 0.1, 0.5 and 1.5 s: for T.L. they are 918 ± 139, 944 ± 291, 625 ± 99 and 619 ± 87 ms, for G.L., 997 ± 62, $1,098 \pm 108$, 604 ± 74 and 639 ± 79 ms.

A 6-year-old child (N.S.) with Down syndrome (IQ 79) was investigated with /mare/ and /muro/. The ACG latency was long ($1,274 \pm 366$ ms) and no decrease was observed with foreperiods of 0.5–4 s. The results are in the range of normals, as it is for the case reported at the top of the diagram of figure 52 (6.4.3).

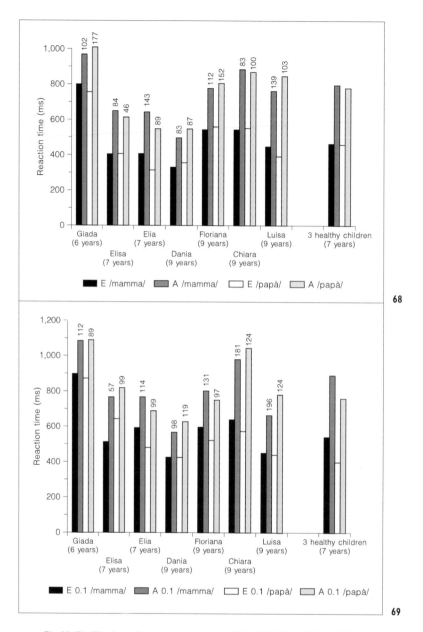

Fig. 68–70. Word reading reaction times at FP_0 (**68**), $FP_{0.1}$ (**69**) and $FP_{1.5}$ (**70**) of children. A = Acousticogram; E = electromyogram.

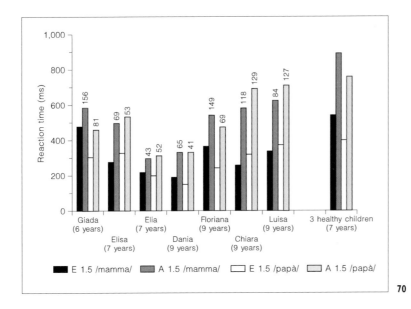

Seven-Year-Old Children

Seven-year-old children were investigated; 3 of them were classified in the middle intelligence range (IQ 102, 104 and 107); they performed the reactions to /mare/ and /muro/. The same reactions were carried out by 1 child (S.M.) with excellent ability in handling computers and with IQ 115, and in 1 less intelligent (C.P.) with IQ 94 and low scores in the subtest of verbal fluency and comprehension.

Two other children with hyperphenylalaninaemia were investigated with /mamma/ and /papà/ tests. One (ESA) had IQ 96, the other (ELA) IQ 76. The latter was characterized by a hyperkinetic syndrome that, as previously discussed (in 8.1), greatly influences the velocity of reaction. Hence we had to address the general problem of the effects of hyperkinesia on the temporal parameters of verbal reactions, not only in subjects with normal constitution but also in patients with pathological extrapyramidal syndromes. As previously reported, the psychomotor trait of the tendency to move more easily and quickly was termed by us (8.1) the kinetic factor and was considered as an interfering biasing neurobiological condition (a 'dirty' factor). In fact, the time taken by the sensorimotor computing processes involved in speech control can vary inversely to its 'rapidity'.

8.4.1.2.1
The Middle Intelligence Class
These 3 childrens had a mean ACG latency of 792 ± 104 ms in immediate reactions. The ACG latencies remained at about the same value at the 100-ms foreperiod but with a larger SD (140 ms). The decrease was very marked at the 1,500-ms foreperiod with a mean value of 547 ± 132 ms.

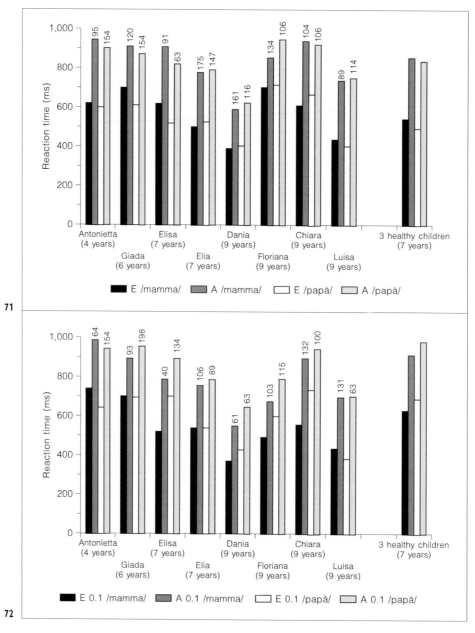

71

72

Fig. 71–73. Picture naming reaction times at FP_0 (**71**), $FP_{0.1}$ (**72**) and $FP_{1.5}$ (**73**) of children. A = Acousticogram; E = electromyogram.

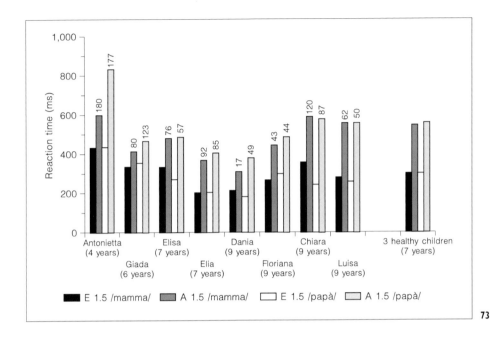

Values shown on bars (from left to right by subject group):

Antonietta (4 years): 180, 177
Giada (6 years): 80, 123
Elisa (7 years): 76, 57
Elia (7 years): 92, 85
Dania (9 years): 17, 49
Floriana (9 years): 43, 44
Chiara (9 years): 120, 87
Luisa (9 years): 62, 50
3 healthy children (7 years)

Legend: ■ E 1.5 /mamma/   ▨ A 1.5 /mamma/   □ E 1.5 /papà/   □ A 1.5 /papà/

Y-axis: Reaction time (ms), 0 to 1,000

8.4.1.2.2
The Most Intelligent Child (S.M.)

The results of the investigation of S.M. are reported in table 10 (see 6.4) while a single example of recording is given in figure 54 (6.4).

The ACG latencies of immediate reactions are in the order of the highest values of normal young adults. A small decrease in ACG latency is observed with 0.1-second foreperiod reactions, while the greatest decrease occurred at 0.5- and 1.5-second foreperiods, in the order of –20%. On the contrary, ACG latency increased at the 4,000-ms foreperiod, with +20% exceeding the ACG latency of immediate reactions. The EMG latencies showed a similar percent change, with a difference between ACG and EMG values of about 200 ms.

ACG duration was a little longer than in young adults (+15%) with a marked decrease in all foreperiod reactions, of about –30%.

8.4.1.2.3
The Less Efficient Subject (C.P.)

The values of ACG latency in C.P. were rather high, similar to those of G.I. (6 years old). The changes of ACG latency with different foreperiod reactions were moderate, in the order of $\leq 20\%$, approximately equivalent to those found in the child S.M. (7 years). The ACG latencies at FP_0, $FP_{0.1}$, $FP_{1.5}$ and FP_4 were the following: $1,012 \pm 119$, $966 \pm 132, 884 \pm 261, 753 \pm 127$, and $1,004 \pm 163$.

8.4.1.2.4
A Peculiar Ability of Hyperkinetic Children

The two 7-year-old children, ELA with IQ 76 and comprehension score 10 and ESA with IQ 96 and comprehension score 6.7, showed the best reactions, i.e. with the shortest ACG latency. This was particularly evident in ELA; the ACG latencies were lower than in 7-year-old children with a higher IQ.

Table 12. Picture naming reaction times (ms) of 6- to 9-year-old children

| | | Immediate reaction | | | | 0.1 s delayed | | | | 1.5 s delayed | | | |
| | | /mamma/ | | /papà/ | | /mamma/ | | /papà/ | | /mamma/ | | /papà/ | |
		E	A	E	A	E	A	E	A	E	A	E	A
Giada (6 years)	Mean	684.00	902.91	609.60	869.60	708.00	899.00	696.00	964.00	338.00	412.00	354.00	474.67
	SD	166.41	120.29	104.66	106.81	183.61	92.75	196.48	198.51	9.17	79.67	19.25	122.83
Elisa (7 years)	Mean	618.22	901.33	520.80	810.40	520.67	794.00	705.33	902.67	333.60	478.00	267.33	490.00
	SD	110.77	90.94	120.33	63.28	100.83	69.00	128.97	134.59	53.22	69.92	32.94	56.93
Elia (7 years)	Mean	493.71	770.40	526.18	792.18	541.60	760.67	541.33	787.00	204.00	377.60	202.00	411.33
	SD	173.67	175.09	127.02	147.02	192.26	105.87	118.31	89.24	40.32	92.07	24.90	84.99
Dania (9 years)	Mean	384.00	587.64	397.45	622.73	366.67	554.67	423.67	646.00	216.00	313.60	174.00	384.67
	SD	138.31	161.12	98.49	116.50	83.67	60.91	52.52	63.11	56.00	17.45	20.36	49.01
Floriana (9 years)	Mean	696.80	846.80	712.67	937.33	493.33	676.67	597.33	790.00	264.67	446.67	291.33	493.33
	SD	162.54	133.90	97.53	105.85	67.48	103.26	103.48	115.26	34.05	42.81	49.18	44.10
Chiara (9 years)	Mean	609.82	932.00	657.00	910.00	734.40	894.67	557.33	944.80	360.80	595.20	272.33	581.33
	SD	135.83	113.85	158.76	106.50	145.87	32.22	50.00	100.57	114.69	119.96	61.84	67.12
Luisa (9 years)	Mean	428.40	732.55	394.18	741.09	438.67	689.33	378.00	704.67	277.33	474.40	254.80	560.33
	SD	105.79	88.72	119.62	113.86	118.54	131.79	83.58	63.35	71.28	61.69	61.26	50.42

E = Electromyogram; A = acousticogram.

ELA obtained the following results: for /mamma/, 634 ± 143 ms, at FP_0, 776 ± 114 ms at $FP_{0.1}$ and 305 ± 43 ms at $FP_{1.5}$, for /papà/, 580 ± 89 ms at FP_0, 694 ± 99 ms at $FP_{0.1}$ and 318 ± 52 ms at $FP_{1.5}$.

For ESA we obtained: for /mamma/, 624 ± 84 ms at FP_0, 783 ± 57 ms at $FP_{0.1}$ and 490 ± 69 ms at $FP_{1.5}$; for /papà/, 605 ± 46 ms at FP_0, 807 ± 99 ms at $FP_{0.1}$ and 521 ± 53 ms at $FP_{1.5}$.

Now we ask: which parameter could be responsible for these short (i.e. good) ACG latencies, particularly in ELA, in spite of a poor cognitive score? A variable that could be taken into consideration in relation to this question was the high degree of hyperactivity.

A further argument to focus our attention on was the relation between extrapyramidal tremor and hyperkinetic movements of low degree and relatively normal verbal reactions in some parkinson-like syndromes (see Section 9).

An important issue emerging from these considerations is the necessity of adding an index of the kinetic state of the individual subjects for a correct evaluation of tachymetric tests. At the present stage of investigations, we rely on the counting of involuntary limb movements at rest during a congruent period of time. As discussed in chapter 8.1, we systematically evaluate different tests intending to give a measure of the kinetic factor.

However, a parameter independent of the kinetic factor is represented by the ratios ACG latency at $FP_{0.1}$ to ACG latency at FP_0 and ACG latency at FP_0 to ACG latency at $FP_{1.5}$.

8.4.1.3
Nine-Year-Old Children

Four children of 9 years of age were investigated with the word reading tests with /mamma/ and /papà/.

In the most intelligent child (D.A., with IQ 110), ACG latency of immediate reactions was the lowest (i.e. very good) in the group and clearly below that of 7-year-old children with an equivalent kinetic factor.

However D.A.'s ACG latencies (496 ± 83 ms for /mamma/ and 548 ± 57 ms for /papà/) were slightly longer than of young normal adults. The decrease in ACG latency at $FP_{1.5}$ was quite large, in the order of 220 ms. In contrast, the 0.1-second foreperiod gave a small increase in ACG latency (+30 ms).

8.4.2
Picture Naming Reactions versus Word Reading Reactions

A useful comparative model of picture naming and word reading was outlined by Roelofs [1992] (fig. 74). It may be used as a point of reference for the analysis of differences observed in the two kinds of tests.

We have previously reported that, according to the Nijmegen researchers, ACG latency in picture naming is longer than in reading the same words used for naming. This finding gives rise to two problems: (1) which are the origin and the functional meaning of this supplementary time? (2) which is the degree of discriminative sensitivity of the two kinds of tasks in relation with a clinical application?

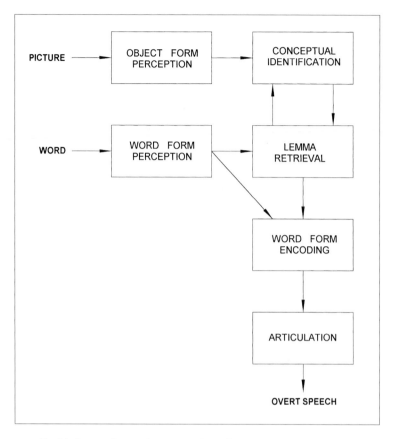

Fig. 74. Stages of mental processes (boxes) and relevant flow of information (arrows). From Roelofs [1992].

The Level of Investigation with Picture Naming

Picture naming reactions have been studied since 1885 [Cattell, 1980] with reference to adults perceiving concrete objects and have been compared with word reading. In spite of pictures being recognized slightly faster than words, the naming time was found to be prolonged 'due to particular difficulties to retrieve the name of recognized objects and to the fact that naming requires a voluntary effort'.

On the other hand, it was found that naming responses accelerated by 25.8% during 12 days of extensive training, but the time for naming remained 41% longer than that of reading; the latter was reduced by 16.8% due to the same amount of training. A constant reading-naming difference was present over age for all subjects who had learned to read, although reading times as well as naming times decreased from the first to the ninth grade among students.

More precise studies have taken into account the factor *compatibility*. Compatibility between a written and a spoken word is higher compared to a picture and its name.

A critical parameter is the number of response alternatives. The usual difference between reading and naming times disappear for two alternatives. In a picture naming task, response times are in the magnitude of the reading times for two alternatives.

A significant influence is exerted by the word and picture size with artefactual effects as high as 62 ms.

More sophisticated experiments including priming effects and Stroop-like interference (for the Stroop effect, see Glaser and Düngelhoff [1984]) were carried out, aiming to evaluate the role of semantic components in picture naming. It appeared to strengthen Levelt's hypothesis that the word entries of the lexicon have two separate components: (1) the *lemma* which contains syntax and naming; the latter refers to the semantic information that is necessary for the selection of (2) the *phonological form* governing the articulatory programming. This means that lemma retrieval and articulatory programme are two distinct processes which occur in strict temporal sequence.

On the basis of all these data, one can find some explanations of our results on an inverted reading-naming difference in reaction time, observed in most children. The following points must be taken into consideration: (a) we adopted only two alternatives; (b) the compatibility was very high; (c) the size of the pictures was markedly greater than that of the written words.

The relatively short naming reaction time led us to infer that under our conditions no symbolic process but only simple association processes occurred.

As for the youngest child showing a longer naming time, one could assume that the perceptual discrimination was quicker for the written words, while the intermediary processes of neural assembly facilitation and triggering had the same upper limit of speed in reading and naming reactions.

8.4.2.2
Picture Naming Reactions in 4- to 9-Year-Old Children

We resorted to the task of picture naming in verbal reactions to extend our research to children at preschool age. Two geometric designs, clearly explained to the subjects, were used to reproduce a female and a male. The words to be pronounced were the same used for verbal reading reactions: /mamma/ and /papà/.

A previous research carried out with different pictures in adults [Pinelli and Ceriani, 1992] had pointed out the relevance of the perceptual modalities for different geometric pictures, while the Nijmegen team had stressed the symbolic component implied in naming pictures rather than in word reading.

8.4.2.2.1
The Results in 4-Year-Old Children
The naming tests with immediate reactions required a longer ACG latency, in a range of +25 to +50%, an increase that occurred in EMG latency as well, in approximately the same time. On the other hand, the decrease in ACG latency in $FP_{1.5}$ was similar to that with word reading reactions, i.e. >200 ms.

In the same children, in reading reactions, ACG latency of immediate reactions is about 100 ms longer than in 7-year-old children. At $FP_{0.1}$, there is an increase in ACG latency but less than in older children.

Table 13. Reading and naming reactions (ms) of 9-year-old children

ACG latency	Reading	Naming
At FP_0		
/mamma/	772 ± 134	527 ± 62
/papà/	708 ± 88	606 ± 114
At $FP_{0.1}$		
/mamma/	581 ± 68	568 ± 121
/papà/	621 ± 93	616 ± 133
At $FP_{1.5}$		
/mamma/	466 ± 109	279 ± 24
/papà/	396 ± 83	301 ± 39

A peculiar finding occurred in a girl at $FP_{1.5}$. There was a >200 ms difference between /mamma/ and /papà/ ACG latencies, which corresponded to 615 ± 180 and 830 ± 177 ms, respectively. This can be due to a higher threshold (and then to a higher number of reverberating internal feedbacks) for /papà/ or to a retarded decoding of this neural assembly.

8.4.2.3
The Results in 6- to 9-Year-Old Children

In comparison to word reading reactions, ACG latencies in picture naming reactions do not show significant differences between different ages. In figures 71–73 and table 12, the cases ESA, ELA and, to a certain extent, D.A. (who have a short ACG latency in word reading reactions) have in picture naming reactions an ACG latency approximately equivalent to that of the other children with longer ACG latencies in both kinds of tasks.

This is also true for the increase in ACG latency at $FP_{0.1}$.

In the 1.5-second foreperiod too, the values of ACG latency are more similar for different children than at word reading reactions. Only the 9-year-old children show a decrease in ACG latency in naming reactions slightly greater than in word reading (table 13).

In comparison with the younger children previously discussed, one must underline: (1) the greatest decrease in ACG latency at $FP_{1.5}$ of the reading test in comparison with ACG latency at FP_0; the intermediary process ratio was 0.57 for /papà/ and 0.60 for /mamma/; (2) with ACG latency at $FP_{0.1}$, there is a significant decrease in reading reaction with respect to FP_0; the early process ratio was 0.76; (3) ACG latency for naming reactions is significantly shorter than for reading reactions except for ACG latency at $FP_{0.1}$ where the two ACG latencies become identical.

The difference is approximately 100 ms for ACG latency at FP_0 for /papà/, but it reaches 250 ms for ACG latency at FP_0 for /mamma/. The same differences are observed for ACG latency at $FP_{1.5}$. The intermediary process ratio (i.e. ACG latency at $FP_{1.5}$ to ACG latency at FP_0) is 0.53 for /mamma/ and 0.50 for /papà/. The early process ratio (i.e. ACG latency at $FP_{0.1}$ to ACG latency at FP_0) is 1.1 for /mamma/ and 1.02 for /papà/.

8.4.2.4

The Discriminative Sensitivity of Picture Naming Is Low

The differences in ACG latency for the different subjects appeared lower in the picture naming tests than in word reading. We have in fact reported a certain degree of reduction of changes in ACG latency of picture naming tests in comparison to word reading. For this reason, at the present stage of our research, we prefer to rely on the word reading reactions for routine investigations in children, as much as it would be possible to teach them to read the simplest words: according to the individual child one could choose /mamma/ and /papà/ or even two syllables like /ma/ and /pa/.

8.4.2.5

Can an Emotional Factor Be Identified in Speech Control Tests?

We have already reported how /papà/ pictures were named by young (4 years) girls, particularly in 1.5-second delayed reactions, with a significantly greater delay than those of /mamma/. This occurred also in 0.1-second foreperiod reactions, even though with a slightly smaller difference. Longer ACG latencies for /papà/ than for /mamma/ at 1.5-second foreperiods were observed also with word reading reactions.

The ensuing question is whether the difference in ACG latency for /papà/ versus /mamma/ may imply some emotional factors corresponding to fearful reactions or other unconscious inhibiting processes.

The assessment of emotional factors has been rather neglected in the quantitative examination of neurological functions. In contrast, Jung's test in psycho-analysis represents a milestone in this field. Moreover, psychogenic factors are considered in Rey's test [1964] and in the assessment of drive and motivation [Atkinson, 1954; Atkinson and Feather, 1966; Pfaff, 1981]. These tests may represent a useful complement of MDRV. Williams et al. [1988] have analysed how *emotional disorders* interfere with cognitive processes.

8.4.3

A Comprehensive Survey: Increase in Acousticogram Latency of Children with Respect to Young Adults

As it has previously been reported, a significant increase in ACG latency was found in both word reading (/mare/, /muro/; /mamma/, /papà/) and picture naming reactions in 4- to 6-year-old children in comparison with young adults. However, the difference seems to diminish in growing children: the highest ACG latencies of some cases (7-year-old S.M., ESA, ELA and particularly 9-year-old D.A.) were identical to those of young adults.

In fact, the correlation with age within the children's group was rather poor. On the other hand, neither IQ nor subtest scores appeared to be correlated with ACG latency.

We interpreted this incongruity as the consequence of some other interfering factors. A re-examination of all possible clinical aspects of the subjects with ACG latencies more largely scattered from the correlation line led us to verify that these subjects were characterized by a state of restlessness and sometimes by hyperkinesia. It ensued that the activity level, known to represent one of the main constitutional factors [Cattell, 1980], should also be included in our analysis.

Previous studies on personality structure showed that the general activity level is an inborn enduring temperamental feature that is more alike in identical twins than dizygotes [Plomin, 1987; Daniels and Plomin, 1985]. In the previous chapter, I addressed a particular field of investigation into the nature of this *kinetic factor* and its relation with the individual tendency to move at different degrees of speed and easiness. Its identification requires also the inversely connected factor of accuracy (analysed in 8.1).

Resorting to the result of higher ACG latencies in the total group of the children investigated, we can observe that the increase in ACG latency is quite evident in the immediate reactions, while in 1.5-second foreperiod reactions the ACG latencies decrease and approximate those of adults. In agreement with previous considerations, we might infer that the relative length of ACG latency in this group of children can be attributed to a high threshold of the hebbian neural assembly or to an incomplete development of the parallel organization of the diffuse processes involved in sensorimotor speech control.

8.4.4
A Study of Partially Reversible Mental Insufficiency (Phenylketonuria) and Its Differentiation from Attentional Deficits and Hyperactivity Disorder

MDRV appears a promising method to investigate children with neuropsychiatric disorders, with particular reference to the assessment of brain functionality. In fact, the results attainable with MDRV correspond to temporal parameters related to intrinsic cerebral representations and processes and do not necessarily equal the result of the neuropsychological tests. They may yield valuable data on the nature of brain functional impairments, with regard not only to primary alterations but also secondary repercussions and compensatory cortical remapping.

Recently, Gourovitch et al. [1994] have carried out a series of investigations with similar methodologies pivoted on reaction times that have close connections with MDRV.

8.4.4.1
A Transfer Time Study in Phenylketonuria and Attention Deficit and Hyperactivity Disorder

Gourovitch et al. [1994] assessed the interhemispheric transfer time with the procedure of Berlucchi et al. [1977] in 14 children with early treated phenylketonia of 6–16 years of age and with an IQ >80, 20 children with attention deficit and hyperactivity disorder aged 7–15 years and in 48 normal children of 6–13 years of age. Children with early treated phenylketonuria were significantly slower than those with attention deficit and hyperactivity disorder and normal children. The findings are summarized in table 14.

Interestingly, normals and subjects with attention deficit and hyperactivity disorder were slower under the uncrossed right-side target condition than the crossed condition. On the contrary, subjects with phenylketonuria had longer transfer time under the crossed right-side target condition.

We underline particularly the results obtained from children with attention deficit and hyperactivity disorder who were evaluated using international clinical DMS-III crite-

Table 14. Interhemispheric transfer time (ms)

Subjects	Right-side target		Left-side target	
	uncrossed	crossed	uncrossed	crossed
Normal	435	430	440	430
ADHD	425	420	435	425
PKU	470	495	490	485

ADHD = Attention deficit and hyperactivity disorder; PKU = phenylketonuria.

ria and Conner's rating scale [Goyette et al., 1978]. They showed a very similar reaction time pattern to normals with slightly, although non-significantly, faster reaction times than normals. This finding is in agreement with our observations leading to the concept of a kinetic factor.

Likewise the results in phenylketonuria are in agreement with our findings with verbal reactions: the slowing in those patients is 12 %.

8.4.4.2
The Nature of the Reversible Alterations

The pathophysiological causes of the functional impairment in phenylketonuria were correlated with the mental deficit and attributed to both biochemical and myelination abnormalities.

Investigation in specific cognitive processes carried out in early treated phenylketonuria documented impairments in attention, visuospatial functions, rate of linguistic development, short-term memory and academic skills [Craft et al., 1992; Gourovitch et al., 1994; Murdock 1990]. Deficits were observed also in executive factors [Welsch et al., 1990].

Most of these impairments are assumed to result from the destruction of catecholamine systems either at the time of testing or during brain development. Performances of tests of sustained attention were shown to fluctuate with changes in catecholamine or phenylalanine levels [Brunner and Berry, 1987; Gourovitch et al., 1994].

However, it was suggested that structural changes associated with abnormal myelination during development may also interfere with neuropsychological functions. In normals, myelination of the cortex occurs throughout infancy and childhood, with frontal cortical connections and tertiary association areas showing a prolonged course of maturation into adolescence [Dietrich et al., 1988]. Rourke [1988, 1989] hypothesized that developmental white matter abnormalities are related to a particular constellation of neurophysiological deficits, which he termed the non-verbal learning disability syndrome. On the other hand, in phenylketonuria, speech and language skills were found to be affected [Murdock, 1990].

The Brain Biological Cycle Tested with Early and Intermediary Process Ratios

8.5.1
From the Child to Adult Performances

At 12 years of age, the reaction times decrease and reach the adult values. The intermediary process ratio is practically the same as that of adults and the differences for /mamma/ with respect to /papà/ are markedly reduced. On the other hand, the reaction time for naming the corresponding pictures reaches with both 0- and 1.5-second foreperiods the lowest values measured for children.

The loss of the facilitation effect of the 'go' signal at the shortest foreperiod (0.1 s) observed in younger subjects might indicate that at the age of 12 years the brain processes for visual naming tasks involve all parallel channels; in this way, the operating time is markedly reduced, but it does not allow further reductions with the foreperiod of 0.1 s.

8.5.2
The Modular and Transmodular Brain Functionality in Relation to Aging

A general view of the variations of brain functionality in speech control for word reading (/mare/, /muro/) in the course of aging, in a logarithmic scale, has been given in 8.2 and 8.3, figures 66 and 67 reporting the values of early and intermediary process ratios of 202 normal subjects aged from 4 to 81 years.

The criteria of interpretation of these results have been analysed in 8.3. Now we will try to outline what they really tell us about brain functionality.

8.5.2.1
The General Meaning of Early and Intermediary Process Ratios

Individual psychomotor and educational traits, as well as variations occurring at the level of the final motor executors, are eliminated from the early and intermediary process ratios as far as they are present in both numerator and denominator. Therefore, with the integrated evaluation described in 8.3, these ratios may yield useful data on brain functionality related to available neuronal functional mass [Lashley, 1980], i.e. modular processes, message transmission and persistence in internal circuits, intermediary processes of working memory, buffer coding and decoding and adaptive processes.

On the other hand, it is important to stress again that the evaluation of the findings, with particular relation to the intermediary process ratio, is quite critical. The meaning it may have with respect to the intermediary processes can be correctly inferred only at the condition that the denominator of this ratio, i.e. ACG latency at FP_0, is normal or increased. Moreover, one must take into consideration also as a meaningful associated pattern the value of the early process ratio: an increase in intermediary process ratio, particularly at the relatively shorter foreperiod, may still depend on the same impairments revealed by an increase in early process ratio but has a completely different meaning when it is specifically found without a consistent increase in early process ratio (see previous Section 7).

If we were essentially interested in the study of *normal* brain functions, we should consider the early and intermediary process ratios with ACG latency at FP_0 as the *numerator:* thus, the ratios could really represent indices of *process efficiency*. However, in view of the aim of our investigations into functional assessment and diagnosis, we have inverted the terms. Both values must be read as indices of *process insufficiency* and the ratios will thus increase proportionally to the functional impairments of the brain (see Section 10).

In this Section, we deal with the brain functionality in normal subjects according to their age. It is convenient to look again at the curves of the early and intermediary process ratios reported in figures 66 and 67, but we will read them now upside down: the lowest values correspond to the best functionality. We should in fact rely on 1/R (respectively 1/early and 1/intermediary process ratio) as indices of process efficiency.

8.5.2.2
The Meaning of the Early Process Ratio

It can be inferred from the curve of figure 66 that the inverted early process ratio reaches a maximum, corresponding to 1.4 at 10–12 years. This is to say that the perception of the 'go' signal, appearing while the latent brain processes – elicited by the perception of the word stimulus presented 100 ms earlier – are still in progress, does not interfere negatively but rather accelerates the processes themselves. In order to have this acceleration produced, the modular activities must develop along well-isolated pathways at high speed: this requires a collateral inhibition to take place and conducting fibres as well as transsynaptic transmission to work best.

8.5.3
The Meaning of the Course of the Intermediary Process Ratio in Relation to Age

I have reported in 8.3 an analysis of the diphasic course of the intermediary process ratio as a function of age (fig. 67).

This diphasic course reveals the intervention of two different kinds of changes in the terms of the ratio, with a dissociation increasing along the maturation processes. Early programming and executive processes at the youngest age are still slow (and partly not perfectly organized to work in PDP). Until the age of 10 years, they improve a little and become only slightly shorter.

In contrast, working memory and intermediary processes develop at a higher rate and accelerate about twice as fast as the early and executive processes; in fact, the inverted intermediary process ratio becomes 2.08 at 10 years. The more marked acceleration in the intermediary processes could be attributed to a lower threshold of the neural assemblies that are triggered after the foreperiod, a condition that can be achieved through different mechanisms: (1) a more prompt and fast working memory; (2) a more efficient adaptive process that optimalizes the matching between descending invariants and ultimate buffers.

An inversion of this first slope takes place between 10 and 25 years, at least with reference to the phonological tasks requested by the disyllabic word choice reactions. Actually we observe an increase in intermediary process ratio that lets infer an acceleration in early and executive processes greater than in intermediary processes, possibly related to working memory. This greater acceleration could depend on a better intrinsic organization of the early programming system and of the executive systems. Moreover, the effects of previous learning and the best development of language in conversation and thinking may contribute, just in this period of 10–25 years of age, to a specific improvement of early processes.

The latest (from 35 to 80 years of age) decrease in intermediary process ratio corresponds to a working memory and associated intermediary processes relatively less affected than early and probably also executive processes, which undergo the deterioration of aging. In view of the prevalent slowing down of the programming processes, the less affected working memory allows a partly corrective function. Anyway, it must be underlined that the slope of this last part of the curve is significantly less steep than the first between 4 and 10 years of age. The low gradient of the slope is particularly marked if we take into consideration the fact that the abscissa is given in a logarithmic scale. The previous tentative analysis of the effects of information loss on the aging brain (Section 7) regards the more advanced phases of aging and might depend not so much upon impairment of working memory but rather upon other processes like short-term memory. A critical discriminative research is in progress with word presentation at a shorter time, aiming at differentiating the role played by deterioration of the active short-term memory with respect to specific intermediary processes and particularly working memory.

Eventually the occurrence of genetic alterations and developmental encephalopathy and their possible relationship with impairments of working memory in adolescence will be discussed in Section 9 and in the Conclusion (Section 10) with specific reference to *schizophrenia*.

8.5.4
A General View on Innate and Acquired Neural Endowments:
Universal Grammar, Maturation Involution and Neuroplasticity

(1) Brain processes develop at a short wavelength: innate mental organs, like the universal grammar, provide unconscious performances to be carried out in the order of a few hundred milliseconds.

(2) The parabolic course of maturation involution involves the brain at a longer wavelength. In the first 10 years genetic innate mental organs mature with the concurrence of epigenetic factors, whilst from the thirties to the most advanced age they slow down with a relative preservation of the working memory. This biological life cycle can be measured with MDRV, which can provide a large amount of integrated data: some models can be elaborated in a trial so that the 'scientist's brain may understand itself'.

(3) The epigenetic factor, by imitation and learning, exerts neuroplastic effects that reshape the neural assemblies. In the course of generation, the genes restructuralize the mental organs of the brain that forge the individual destiny in the impact with environment and human history.

9

Pathological Domains

Introductory Remarks

An important but rather aspecific abnormality revealed by MDRV in neuropathological conditions is the increase in latency time and duration of the response (ACG). We have also underlined that the significance of this parameter cannot easily be evaluated by the examiner as he must compare it with the mean values of matched normal subjects. In fact, the normal values greatly vary according to individual chronological, cultural and psychomotor characteristics.

We can easily realize how the early and intermediary process ratios, apart from the individual traits, may acquire the greatest importance in the investigation into pathological cases.

In Sections 3 and 7, I have tried to specify the evaluating criteria of these ratios, and I have explained that – however significant their changes may be – only an associated analysis of the variables ACG latency and duration can lead to a consistent interpretation of the nature and degree of variations in early and intermediary process ratios.

Primary alterations in the executive phases may produce *upward slowing effects* on the intermediary active short memories and earlier programming processes.

A consistent secondary slowing was in fact verified to occur as a consequence of impairment of the motoneural systems (motoneuron disease).

Proceeding from general pathogenetic considerations to the analysis of the single disease, we may assert that the more specific pathological sectors pertinent to MDRV investigation (related to *task-dependent processes*) are functional dysfluencies like *spastic dysphonia* and *stuttering*.

Spastic dysphonia represents a profitable area of research since it is advantageously treated today with botulinum toxin and the results of MDRV may be compared before and after the treatment.

Stuttering is a more complicated area, where many findings suggest that a higher-level neural alteration is involved with an oversensitivity to multichannel feedbacks.

Akinesia and plastic hypertonia (i.e. rigidity) alterations occurring in *Parkinson disease* can be reflected by increases in ACG latency and duration of immediate and delayed reactions. In contrast, early and intermediary process ratios are not significantly affected in these disorders. The akinetic impairment corresponds to an increased time taken by the corticosubcortical internal feedbacks that transmit the programming commands to the executive systems.

On the other hand, the impairment of motor servo-mechanisms responsible for rigidity seems to affect the final executive systems: the shortest attainable reaction time will be longer than that measured in matched normal subjects.

Delayed word reading reactions proved to be a promising detecting test in the psychiatric field, which is consistent with the fact that the delayed reactions allow us to measure a 'mental activity' occurring during the foreperiod and related to *task-independent processes*. In fact – however simple this latent mental process may be –, there is no doubt that it belongs to 'mentalese' [Pinker, 1995], developing in thinking and in the prognostic activities of the mind, in association with the memory of the future [Ingvar, 1985]. We can then realize how the delayed reaction tests are particularly pertinent to a study on mental disorders.

A special chapter will be dedicated to the *schizophrenic disorders,* where in fact the intermediary process ratio was found to be significantly higher.

On the other hand, an opposite finding, i.e. decrease in the intermediary process ratio, seems to characterize the *obsessive-compulsive disorders.*

In connection with these issues, it is worth mentioning the question arduosly debated by psychologists on the nature of bradyphrenia appearing in parkinsonian patients. Our data exclude a primary impairment of intermediary processes to occur in these patients, who actually show a normal intermediary process ratio. Their slowing of psychomotor performances seems rather related to impaired programming processes and executive servo-mechanisms.

On the basis of these results we might speak of secondary bradyphrenia in Parkinson disease, primary bradyphrenia or dysphrenia in schizophrenia and of tachyphrenia in some obsessive-compulsive disorders.

A different approach was made in the investigation of patients suffering from *affective psychoses.* Selective slowing was found in the verbal reactions to concrete words that are processed more specifically by the non-dominant hemisphere. The reaction time for abstract words remained relatively preserved within the normal mean values.

A particularly intricate and difficult question concerns the role played by short-term active memory in the phase of the intermediary processes. Its study requires appropriate methodologies for the display duration of the word stimuli in the foreperiod. Different individual modalities in executing the task must be taken into account.

Increases in the early process ratio mark the alteration found in *mental deterioration,* characterized by a remarkable slowing in the early processes of the brain.

Spastic Dysphonia

Spastic (or spasmodic) dysphonia consists in a complex movement disorder characterized by a disruption of vocalization: the patients lose the ability to speak quietly and fluently. The pathogenesis is still unclear; the absence of neuropathological data and the normality of laryngeal structures argued in favour of a psychogenic lesion. On the other hand, in the last decade, several neurophysiological and psychological studies addressed the hypothesis of an organic alteration, which raises the challenging question about the function of the subcortical motor control, i.e. the role of the basal ganglia.

As in other types of restricted dystonia, injection of botulinum toxin into the affected muscle of one vocal fold was attempted to provide a prompt and prolonged relief of the vocal disorder. Linguistic ability tests, vocal performance by means of laryngeal task-dependent reaction times and spectral voice analysis have been the most common methods to investigate this disorder.

Actually, MDRV seems the most suitable methodology to detect the temporal course of all the neural processes involved in visual perception, phonological planning, buffer encoding and articulatory execution. We have analysed in the previous sections the underlying brain activity and how it is modulated by facilitatory and inhibitory recurrent activity in the prefrontal and primary motor cortex, cerebellum and basal ganglion loops.

We applied MDRV to 4 patients affected by spastic dysphonia to quantify and monitor the changes induced by the local injection of botulinum toxin.

9.2.1
Methodology

Four Italian-speaking subjects (aged 33–58 years; 2 males and 2 females) were investigated.

The words /mare/ ('sea') and /muro/ ('wall') were displayed on the PC screen, in random order, and synchronized the signal acquisition. By means of dedicated hardware the following analogue signals were recorded: (a) the acoustic signal (ACG) transduced by a microphone; (b) surface EMG signals from the orbicularis oris and in some cases also from the digastric and masseter muscles; (c) the electroglottogram.

Reaction times were then automatically extracted for each recorded signal. Different phonatory reactions were tested in order to assess different cerebral processes: (a) immediate reactions: the subject had to pronounce the word as soon as possible after its presentation; (b) reactions with foreperiods: the subject had to wait for the presentation of a 'go' signal (asterisks) before pronouncing the word; the delays, referred to as the foreperiods, were 0.1 and 1.5 s.

Each test consisted of 12 random presentations of each item, i.e. /mare/ and /muro/.

To be sure that the mean values and SD were strictly related to the stochastic nature of neural processing and possibly unaffected by learning effects, the subjects were given a preliminary trial run.

Each patient was injected by 10 MU of botulinum toxin into the thyro-arytenoid or crico-arytenoid muscles.

MDRV was carried out under basal conditions and about 30 and 90 days after the injection of botulinum toxin. Statistical analysis included the paired Student's t test.

Table 15. Percent increases in ACG latencies and durations and absolute intermediary process ratios of patients with spastic dysphonia

Patient	Age years	Sex	Disease duration years		ACG latency		ACG duration		Absolute IR values
					FP_0	$FP_{1.5}$	FP_0	$FP_{1.5}$	
F. D.	57	F	1	before	56	62	157	142	0.87
				after	21	19	77	110	0.78
A. G.	30	F	3	before	143	440	433	388	+
				after	26	12	56	65	0.60
R. M.	46	F	18	before	65	54	155	119	0.74
				after	67	27	147	116	0.60
T. A.	58	M	20	before	53	46	65	74	0.75
				after	22	13	40	43	0.73
Normals	30–58			basal	0	0	0	0	0.78
				after 1 month	±7	±5	±2	±1	0.77

Results are percent increases compared to normals, before and after treatment with botulinum toxin. IR = Intermediary process ratio; + = no actual values could be measured because of a busy-line effect (4-fold increase in ACG duration).

9.2.2
Cases

The main features of the patients affected by spastic dysphonia, investigated before and after treatment with botulinum toxin, are reported in table 15.

9.2.3
Results

With reference to normal subjects, the series of 12 successive reaction times with randomly presented words appeared to give a reliable mean value of the actual performance times for both total brain speech control and single operations, from visual pattern extraction to motor articulation. Learning and fatigue effects were minimal. Because of the lack of statistical difference between the results obtained from /mare/ and /muro/, we considered the latency and duration times for the two words together.

The results of the reaction times before and after treatment with botulinum toxin are reported in table 15 and figures 75–79. The results were compared to the data of age-matched controls, collected in our laboratory.

9.2.4
Discussion

Before the botulin treatment, in all 4 patients with spastic dysphonia, all variables of ACG latency time and duration showed marked increases with respect to the corresponding mean values of a homogeneous normal population. The increase was particularly apparent in ACG duration that scored 200–300% more than normal mean values.

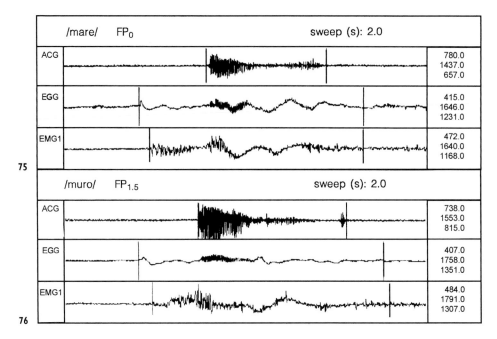

Fig. 75, 76. Patient A.G., female, 30 years old, with spastic dysphonia, before treatment with botulinum toxin. EGG = Electroglottogram; EMG1 = EMG of orbicularis oris muscle; figures on the right indicate latency time of response onset, latency time of response end and duration of the response (ms). **75** /mare/, FP_0 (3rd reaction). **76** /muro/, $FP_{1.5}$ (17th reaction).

The EMG of the orbicularis oris muscle (fig. 75, 76) showed a high-frequency recruitment of motor units, with a high amplitude in the first 150 ms, and with some bursts of a relatively high amplitude in the final period; *rhythmized patterns characterizing extrapyramidal disorders were never found.*

Contrary to normals and other pathological cases (even with severe disorders), the onset of orbicularis oris activity did not precede the onset of the electroglottogram, and it occurred, most times, some 10 ms later. This early onset of the electroglottogram may suggest a low activation threshold of laryngeal muscles, a condition that can be correlated with the 'spastic' or 'spasmodic' nature of their contractions.

No correlations was found between the duration of the disease and the increase in ACG latency and duration as far as it could be inferred from a comparison between the 2 cases with a short disease duration (1–3 years for F.D. and A.G.) and the other 2 cases with a long disease duration (18–20 years for R.M. and T.A.). In fact, the longest ACG duration was observed in case A.G.: it reached 1,665–1,987 ms, a value that exceeded that of the foreperiod (1,500 ms) of the delayed reaction. This condition actualizes a *busy-line phenomenon* dependent on ACG duration being longer than the foreperiod. As it was analysed in 8.3, a pseudo-increase in the intermediary process ratio occurs in this condition. In fact, in the 3 cases where it was correctly measured, the intermediary process ratio was found to be always in the normal range (0.84–0.87).

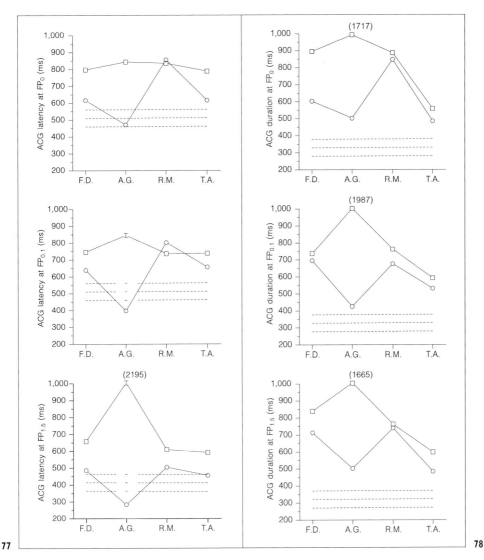

Fig. 77, 78. ACG latencies (**77**) and durations (**78**) of patients with spastic dysphonia before (□) and after (○) treatment with botulinum toxin, compared with those of normals (-----, mean and range).

The degree of normalization produced by the botulin treatment differs for ACG latency and duration. (1) ACT latency reached normal or nearly normal values in the 2 patients with a shorter duration of spastic dysphonia, and even in patient T.A. with a long duration of dysphonia. (2) In contrast, ACG duration remains always longer than in normals up to nearly 200 ms. The greatest difference from normals occurred in case R.M. with a deviation of more than 300 ms. This result suggests that: (a) the main primary alteration is represented by the sequence speed of the utterance; (b) the increase in ACG latency (and that of the electroglottogram, fig. 75, 76) might represent a secondary effect of the slowing in the utterance.

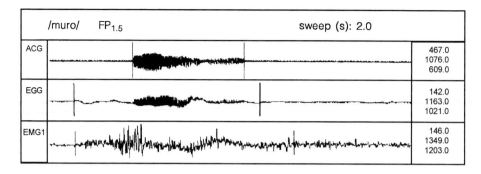

Fig. 79. Patient A.G., female, 30 years old, with spastic dysphonia, after treatment with botulinum toxin. For explanations, see figures 75, 76. /muro/, $FP_{1.5}$ (12th reaction).

On the basis of these facts, we may advance the following hypothesis. The core alteration of spastic dysphonia seems to be located in the executive timing process, producing a very marked increase in ACG duration. This alteration exerts a feedback slowing effect on the earlier processes of programming and intermediary brain activities. Therefore, if we searched for a model in an analogous motor disorder, we should take into consideration not so much the parkinsonian syndrome (affecting the programming processes) but rather a more distally located neuromuscular disorder with increased muscular stiffness at the level of the executing muscles. In fact, the slowed programming and intermediary processes – revealed by ACT latency at FP_0 and at $FP_{1.5}$, respectively – are quickly normalized after botulinum toxin has been injected into the muscles of the vocal folds. One could think that, as in a focal stiff-man syndrome, the reflex thresholds of these muscles is lower than normal, because inhibitory processes of excitatory descending commands in the brainstem are defective [Crucen et al., 1991].

The occurrence of the pseudo-increase in intermediary process ratio (ACG latency at $FP_{1.5}$ being >1,500 ms) can be attributed to the busy-line effect. In fact, the utterance of /mare/ or /muro/ is still in progress when the patient, perceiving the 'go' signal, should pronounce the next /mare/ or /muro/. To better analyse the sequence of the events, it seems useful to refer to single reactions taken as examples:

In a delayed reaction with $FP_{1.5}$ (reaction No. 6, /muro/ in the series /mare/, /muro/), before botulin treatment, ACG duration measures 1,993 ms with an ACG latency of 2,214 ms. This means that the 'line occupation' ends at 1,993 ms and it is only at this moment that the triggered neuronal assembly can elicit the impulses able to produce the vocal tract contractions producing the ACG. The difference ACG latency – ACG duration, i.e. 2,214 – 1,993 = 221 ms, corresponds to the duration of one recurrent internal circuit.

In a delayed reaction at $FP_{1.5}$ (reaction No. 1, /muro/ in the series /mare/, /muro/), after botulin treatment, ACG duration measures 608 ms, with an ACG latency of 467 ms; there is an interval of 1,500 – 608 = 892 ms, during which recurring internal feedbacks facilitate the neuronal assemblies; before that, at the 'go' signal, they will be triggered. The facilitation is proved to occur by the high value (738 ms) of the ACG latency at FP_0 with respect to the ACG latency at $FP_{1.5}$ (467 ms), corresponding to an intermediary process ratio of 0.63.

Stuttering

Stuttering can be seen as a paradigm of dysfunctions impairing internal feedbacks occurring in mental operations. One must underline that the same process may serve very different functions when inserted in hierarchically different neural systems (task-independent processes). Cortical-subcortical repetitive circuits allow the subject to perform delayed reading; analogous repetitive internal circuits allow the working memory to maintain the thought flow.

9.3.1
Verbal Reactions in Stuttering

The reader is to refer to the review by Pinelli and Ceriani [1992] on the basal theoretical concepts about the psychogenic versus neurogenic nature of stuttering, on the different hypotheses about a cerebral versus a neuromotor pathogenesis, the classification of developmental versus acquired symptomatic stuttering and on the large series of experimental research carried out in stuttering [Adams, 1982, 1987; Webster, 1985; Peters et al., 1991]. The application of feedbacks has been studied by Moore [1978], Lechner [1979], Garber and Siegel [1982] and Zimmerman et al. [1988]. A great amount of data has been gathered by the Nijmegen scientists, and we will analyse our actual data in the light of their most recent reports.

9.3.1.1
Blueprint of the Research

In the last 10 years, the identification of the activation order of the multiple executors involved in word utterance and of the duration of the different muscular movements constituted the main task of the scientists dealing with a quantitative semiological assessment of stuttering [Yairi and Ambrose, 1992; Yairi et al., 1993], a neuroscience model [Nudelman et al., 1989] and its possibly rational treatment [Molt, 1991]. On the other hand, more recently, the attention of the researcher has progressively shifted towards the level of the neural disorder responsible for this particular dysfluency. Likewise the methodology has developed progressively: kinematic and electromyographic multiple recordings included respirometry, electroglottography, electropalatography and more recently electromagnetic movement articulometry has been applied. On the other hand, MDRV represents a comprehensive set of functional chronometric tests.

In fact some authors, and particularly the Nijmegen Group, presented in 1991 some results suggesting a functional alteration of programming processes as the origin of stuttering. This alteration however can exert different effects on the final executors, with individually differentiated secondary adjustments and consequences, of positive or negative sign, on the resulting degree of speech efficiency. However, more recent investigations with new methodologies developed by the same authors did not confirm this view and brought evidence or a more 'distal' level of neural impairment [van Lieshout et al., 1993].

A relevant series of data showed that verbal utterances of stutterers are character-ized by an excessive feedback facilitation. Corresponding models of artificial speakers re-produced a disorder in the pronunciation of the second syllable of a word with repetitive incomplete low-amplitude utterances.

If our aim is the analysis of the CCP and their interface with the adaptive and execu-tive brain processes and their associated feedbacks, there is no doubt that the immediate and shortly or prolongedly delayed reading reactions – with multiple word stimuli of dif-ferent length, use frequency and phonological versus grammatical organization, carried out with MDRV – should represent the most suitable and reliable way to face the prob-lem. The previous theoretical and experimental analyses we developed with reference to normal subjects, under different physiological and paraphysiological conditions, will serve as an area of comparison and will provide the most pertinent criteria of evaluation.

9.3.1.2
A Paradigmatic Case of Stuttering

C.A., male, 24 years old, was affected by a form of stuttering. The task requested for reading reac-tions was /ma/, /mare/ and /mare è bello/ in all immediate, 0.1- and 1.5-second foreperiods.

As shown in table 16 and figures 80–83, there is a great increase in all reaction times with respect to normals. In the immediate reactions, the mean values of both ACG latency and duration are nearly dou-ble those of normals, particularly for /mare è bello/. The ACG feature can sometimes be continuous as in most normal people where one can observe a triple spindle-like pattern, each spindle corresponding to one lemma of the sentence, and the duration of the intervals (incomplete) being always below 20 ms.

Table 16. C. A., male, 24 years old, stutterer

			/ma/	/mare/	/mare è bello/	All
FP_0	Latency	EMG1	1,081 ± 586	940 ± 206	1,189 ± 300	1,061 ± 434
		EMG2	1,079 ± 594	953 ± 215	1,214 ± 291	1,071 ± 442
		ACG	1,099 ± 598	986 ± 208	1,221 ± 294	1,096 ± 442
	Duration	EMG1	205 ± 21	264 ± 67	2,025 ± 955	646 ± 842
		EMG2	199 ± 14	202 ± 55	1,916 ± 896	597 ± 804
		ACG	250 ± 24	405 ± 29	1,905 ± 912	679 ± 756
$FP_{0.1}$	Latency	EMG1	743 ± 131	762 ± 218	830 ± 99	835 ± 324
		EMG2	743 ± 120	738 ± 172	828 ± 99	818 ± 299
		ACG	761 ± 125	833 ± 207	874 ± 59	874 ± 305
	Duration	EMG1	180 ± 21	213 ± 23	1.186 ± 192	559 ± 529
		EMG2	154 ± 17	255 ± 112	1,151 ± 223	543 ± 499
		ACG	237 ± 27	378 ± 28	1,146 ± 166	557 ± 404
$FP_{1.5}$	Latency	EMG1	826 ± 363	671 ± 153	652 ± 166	715 ± 257
		EMG2	827 ± 368	653 ± 155	646 ± 159	818 ± 299
		ACG	868 ± 389	693 ± 153	707 ± 147	874 ± 305
	Duration	EMG1	193 ± 30	250 ± 41	1,364 ± 104	543 ± 512
		EMG2	177 ± 41	227 ± 38	1,248 ± 112	487 ± 462
		ACG	248 ± 59	392 ± 30	1,423 ± 123	612 ± 483

Results are indicated in milliseconds.

In contrast, the ACG of patient C.A. is most of the time divided into two (fig. 82d) or three (fig. 82a) parts, with intervals that could reach nearly 100 ms. In all /mare è bello/ reactions, the oromandibular EMG, even with continuous ACG, showed an initial burst with nearly null anticipation with respect to the ACG onset, whilst in normals the time latency of the onset of the EMG – that of the ACG was in a range of 130–210 ms. The loss of this anticipation represents a marked inversion in the order of activation of the different articulators: in the prevalent series of reactions in stutterers, the primum movens could be shifted to the vocal cords or the pharynx-tongue sector.

However, this was not the only pattern of oromandibular EMG observed in this patient, since, even exceptionally, a first burst could occur at about 200 ms before the remaining EMG, with a lower (about –50%) amplitude than those of the successive bursts. As shown in figure 80 for /ma/, in figure 81 for /mare/ and in figure 82b and c for /mare è bello/, the ACG was continuous in some rare reactions.

We must add that some blocks occurred during the series of reactions: at the 40th stimulus, the subject failed to react to 3 successive stimuli.

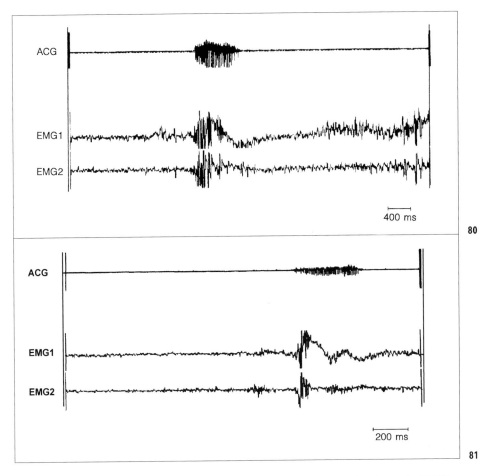

80

81

Fig. 80–82. Patient C.A., male, 24 years old, stutterer. EMG1 = orbicularis oris muscle; EMG2 = digastric muscle; figures on the right indicate response latency. 80 /ma/, FP_0. 81 /mare/, FP_0. 82 (page 232) /mare è bello/, FP_0 (2nd reaction, **a**), FP_0 (6th reaction, **b**), $FP_{1.5}$ (11th reaction, **c**) and FP_0 (16th reaction, **d**).

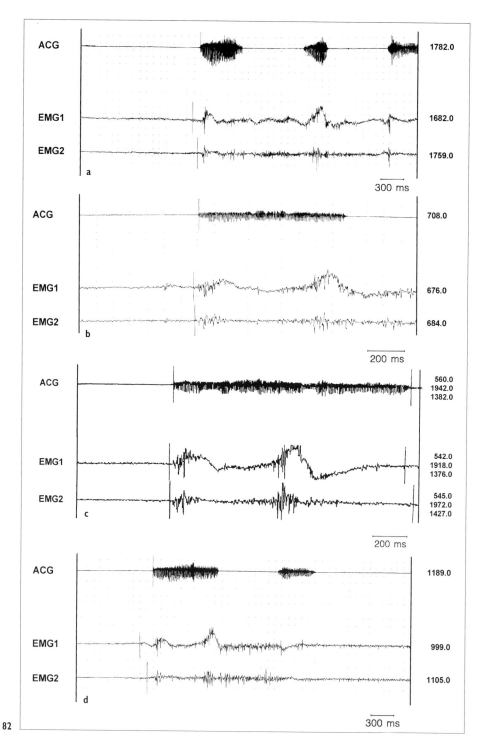

a

300 ms

b

200 ms

c

200 ms

d

300 ms

For legend see page 231.

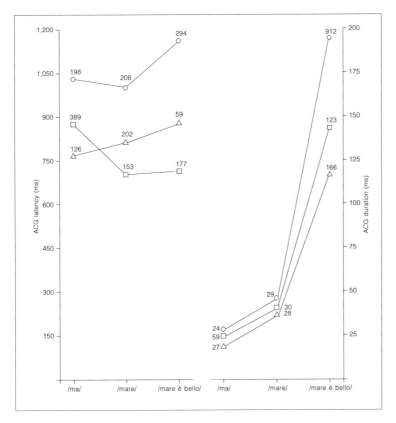

Fig. 83. ACG latencies and durations of patient C.A., male, 24 years old, stutterer. $\bigcirc$ = FP_0; $\triangle$ = $FP_{0.1}$; $\square$ = $FP_{1.5}$; figures near symbols indicate SD.

In delayed reactions, both ACG latency and duration were significantly reduced, with decreases that for /mare è bello/ at the 1.5-second foreperiod were in the order of 500 and 700 ms, respectively (table 16). But the most impressive difference with respect to normals was a 200- to 400-ms decrease in ACG latency at 100-ms delayed reactions (fig. 83). This marked facilitation with very short foreperiods has never been observed in normal people nor in abnormal and frankly pathological cases of different origin.

9.3.1.3
Heterogeneous Cases of Stuttering

Further cases were investigated with the same methodology.

Case 1, Z.L., 15 years, male. Developmental stuttering from 4 to 14 years; free interval until the age of 18 years when spasmodic stuttering occurred immediately after a right frontal trauma with transient signs of monobrachial and lower facial left paresis (for 48 h). The tasks were: /ma/, /mare/ and /mare è bello/ (fig. 84). Results for /mare è bello/: intermediary process ratio, 352/585 = 0.49; early process ratio, 589/585 = 1.01.

Case 2, G.M., 23 years, female. She began stuttering 14 months before the MDRV examination, after a frustrating psychological situation. Neurological examination: normal. The tasks were /ma/,

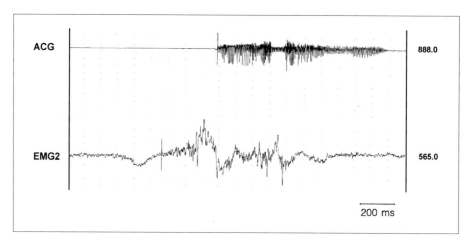

Fig. 84. Patient Z.L., male, 15 years old, stutterer. EMG2 = digastric muscle; figures on the right indicate latency times of response onset. /mare è bello/, FP_0. Means are given in the text (case 1).

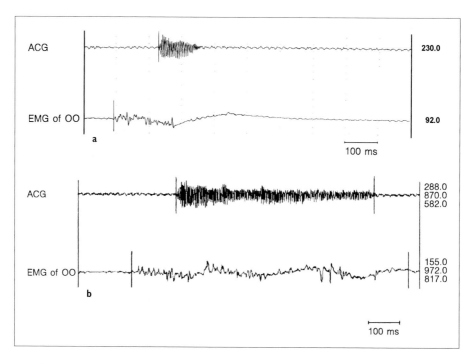

Fig. 85. Patient G.M., female, 23 years old, stutterer. OO = orbicularis oris muscle; figures on the right indicate latency time of the response onset (**a, b**), latency time of the response end (**b**) and duration of the response (**b**). **a** /ma/, $FP_{1.5}$. **b** /mare è bello/, $FP_{1.5}$. Means are given in the text (case 2).

Table 17. F.G.P., female, 24 years old, stutterer

	FP_0	$FP_{0.1}$	ER	$FP_{0.5}$	IR	$FP_{1.5}$	IR	FP_4	IR
ACG latency									
/ma/	562 ± 90	815 ± 47	1.45	776 ± 85	1.4	585 ± 124	1	702 ± 73	1.2
/mare/	587 ± 77	645 ± 94	1.1	813 ± 112	1.4	565 ± 68	0.9	646 ± 139	1.1
/mare è bello/	652 ± 97	734 ± 33	1.1	872 ± 53	1.3	687 ± 55	1	700 ± 130	1.1
EMG latency									
/ma/	371 ± 77	670 ± 77	1.8	606 ± 120	1.6	445 ± 133	1.2	527 ± 99	1.4
/mare/	355 ± 67	446 ± 101	1.2	569 ± 104	1.6	392 ± 105	1.1	460 ± 96	1.3
/mare è bello/	409 ± 70	483 ± 37	1.2	582 ± 60	1.4	434 ± 67	1	454 ± 127	1.1
ACG duration									
/ma/	235 ± 14	248 ± 8	1	236 ± 10	1	261 ± 15	1.1	238 ± 18	1
/mare/	448 ± 20	413 ± 16	0.9	411 ± 31	1	445 ± 25	1	429 ± 20	0.95
/mare è bello/	$1,025 \pm 50$	983 ± 24	0.95	907 ± 6	0.9	$1,016 \pm 52$	1	984 ± 36	0.9
EMG duration									
/ma/	333 ± 36	299 ± 37		345 ± 34		308 ± 28		297 ± 79	
/mare/	470 ± 54	401 ± 24		458 ± 46		409 ± 73		414 ± 23	
/mare è bello/	$1,494 \pm 78$	$1,481 \pm 59$		$1,407 \pm 67$		$1,483 \pm 57$		$1,462 \pm 51$	

ER = Early process ratio; IR = intermediary process ratio. Latencies and durations are expressed in milliseconds, the ratios are absolute values. EMG duration was measured from an EMG with > 3-fold amplitude of the eventual basal action potential to the end, identified at a > 300-ms interruption of action potentials.

/mare/ and /mare è bello/ (fig. 85a, b). Results for /mare è bello/: intermediary process ratio 371/440 = 0.80; early process ratio: 409/440 = 0.90.

Case 3, F.G.P., 24 years, female. She began stuttering at the age of 7 years. Neurological examination: normal. The tasks were /ma/, /mare/ and /mare è bello/. All results are reported in table 17, and some findings are given in figure 86a and b. For the sentence: intermediary process ratio, 687/652 = 1.07; early process ratio, 734/652 = 1.1.

Case 4, R.C., 37 years, female. She had been affected by stuttering for 1 month, with an acute onset. Cranial computerized axial tomography showed an arachnoidal cyst at the left hemicerebellum. A transient ischaemic attack (involving the vertebrobasilar arteries) was taken into consideration as a possible cause of the acquired stuttering. The tasks were: /ma/, /mare/ and /mare è bello/ (fig. 87). Results for /mare è bello/: intermediary process ratio, 360/423 = 0.85; early process ratio, 430/423 = 1.01; electroglottogram latency = 330 ms; EMG latency = 289 ms.

Case 5, T.A., 50 years, male. Persistent stuttering since he was 14 years old. Neural examination: normal. The tasks were: /ubavek/ and /ubamek/ (no examples of tracings are reported). Intermediary process ratios at $FP_{1.5}$, 433/650 = 0.57, at $FP_{0.5}$, 430/650 = 0.56; early process ratio, 481/650 = 0.7; electroglottogram latency = 391 ms; EMG latency = 325 ms.

Case 6, B.G., 40 years, male. Stuttering occurred acutely during a hypertensive arterial attack with no neurological impairments. The tasks were: /mare/ and /muro/ (no examples of tracings are reported). Intermediary process ratio, 482/735 = 0.55; early process ratio = 706/735 = 0.87; electroglottogram latency = 234 ms; EMG latency = 221 ms.

It can be seen from the above findings that 3 stutterers (No. 2, 5 and 6) show concordant results with the early process ratio relatively low: 0.90, 0.56 and 0.87.

In case No. 3, with stuttering persisting for 20 years, ACG latency at $FP_{0.1}$ increases (the early process ratio reaches the value 1.1). The same occurs in the patients with acquired symptomatic stuttering (cases 1 and 4).

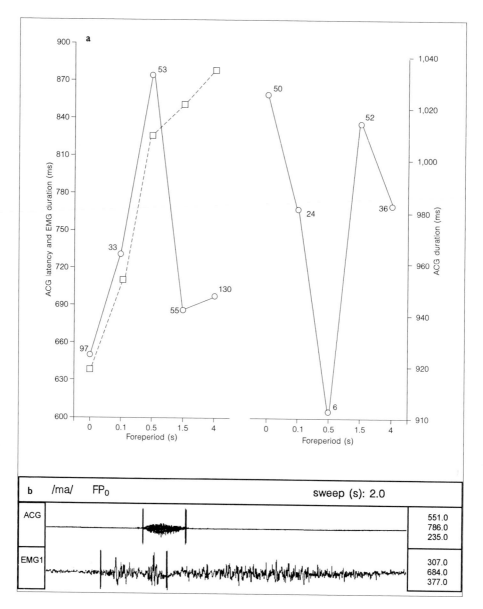

Fig. 86. Patient F.G.P., female, 24 years old, stutterer since the age of 7 years. **a** /mare è bello/; ACG values (○) and EMG (□) differences between the patient values and the mean values of normal controls; figures near symbols indicate SD. **b** /ma/, FP$_0$ (27th reaction). For explanations, see figures 75, 76 (in 9.2; text, case 3).

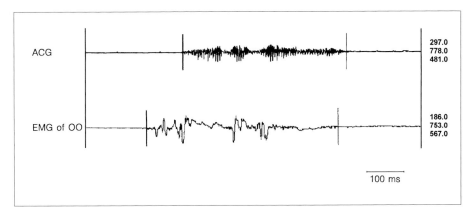

Fig. 87. Patient R.C., female, 37 years old, stutterer for 1 month. /mare è bello/, FP_0. OO = Orbicularis oris muscle; figures on the right indicate latency time of response onset; latency time of response end and response duration. Means are given in the text (case 4).

9.3.2
A Comparison between the Stutterers and a Patient Affected by Severe Dysarthria due to Systemic Motoneuron Lesions

A correct analysis of the result obtained from the stutterers in comparison with the normal mean values might provide more precise and specific cues if we developed a differential analysis of other types of impairments of speech control. A preliminary research was focused on a patient affected by a mixed spastic type of dysarthria, which might better resemble the functional 'dysarthric' disorder of the executive processes in stuttering.

B.A. was a 41-year-old subject with a severe pseudobulbar, bulbopontine syndrome due to amyotrophic lateral sclerosis with chronic course, dating 7 years back (fig. 88–90). ACG durations of /ma/, /mare/ and /mare è bello/ at FP_0 were 360, 910 and 2,140 ms.

In the stutterer P.T. (46 years, male, stuttering since he was 11 years old), ACG duration was shorter for /ma/ and for /mare/ and nearly equal for /mare è bello/: 255, 412 and 1,900 ms.

On the contrary, ACG latency was always longer in the stutterer: 1,140, 1,010 and 1,220 ms compared to 855, 910 and 850 ms of B.A.

Likewise, at 1.5-second foreperiod reactions, the decrease in ACG duration for /mare/ was only 60 ms (that is –8%) in amyotrophic lateral sclerosis, instead of –20% in the stutterer. Likewise, the decrease in ACG latency for /mare/ in amyotrophic lateral sclerosis was –20% in contrast to –30% in the stutterer.

9.3.3
The Level and Type of Neural Impairment in Stuttering

Our investigations of stutterers showed two main types of changes in verbometric tests that can help us to interpret the cause of the inverted order of activation of the articulatory executors and the marked slowing in latency times.

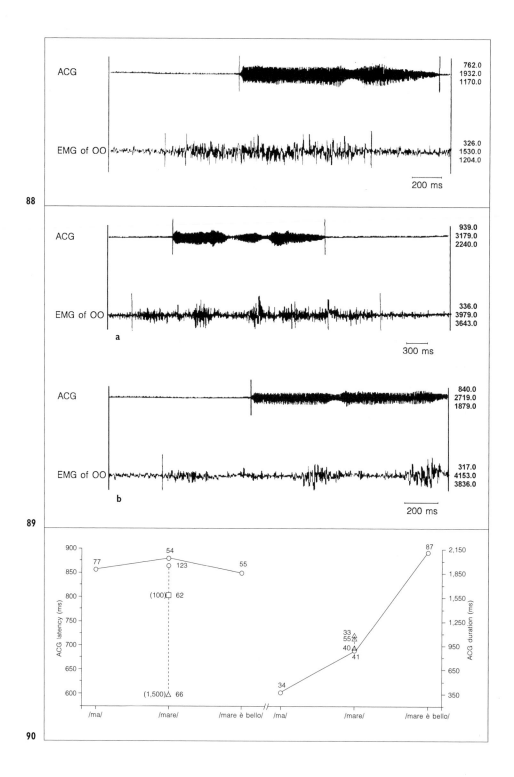

(1) The stutterer is able to greatly reduce ACG latency and duration in the delayed re-actions, much more than the dysarthric patient. This means that the final executors can be activated in nearly the normal time in stuttering, even if with an altered order.

(2) At immediate reactions, the stutterer's ACG latency for /mare è bello/ increases (about +10%) with respect to ACG latency for /mare/, while in amyotrophic lateral sclerosis it decreases (–4%) with respect to ACG latency of /mare/.

We remind that in normals, the grammatical sentence /mare è bello/ implies a certain reduction (–8%) in ACG latency with respect to ACG latency of /mare/.

If we consider separately a purely phonetic influence of the task /mare è bello/ to play a role with respect to /mare/, we have to calculate the influence of the component /è bello/: this is equivalent to an added accented letter and a disyllable with a rather high frequency of use. This has been found in *simple reactions* to correspond to 6 ms, i.e. +3% with respect to the 200-ms ACG latency of /mare/. But we can assume that in normals the grammar task applies a 'facilitatory effect' of a presumed –11%, with the result of –8% for ACG latency of /mare è bello/ with respect to ACG latency of /mare/.

In the stutterer, we have +10% of ACG latency for /mare è bello/, a result that im-plies a failure of the 'facilitating effect' of the grammar convertor. Moreover, we must take into account that ACG latency for /mare/ is remarkably longer, about 3 times, than in normals. Then the additional positive effect of /è bello/ may imply a $3 \times 3\% = 9\%$ in-crease in ACG latency of /mare è bello/. In all, the calculated added effect of /è bello/ will be: ACG latency of /mare/ +9%, that is very near the measured +10%.

We can summarize these evaluations by saying that the actual influence of length should be considered equivalent to the length of /è bello/ + the x due to *the facilitating ef-fect of the grammar convertor* that occurs in normals but *is missing in the stutterer.* The rel-atively more marked increase in ACG duration of /mare è bello/ supports the same inter-pretation.

With regard to the changes observed in patient B.A. with amyotrophic lateral sclerosis, we suppose that the –4 % instead of –8 % decrease in ACG latency can be attributed to the more marked decreasing effect of the phonological length, deducible from the value of ACG latency for /mare/: +7 % (if referred to the normal mean value of B.A. instead of +3%).

On the other hand, as previously reported, the increase in ACG latency is greater in the stutterer than in the severely dysarthric patient with amyotrophic lateral sclerosis and suggests that the alteration in 'flowing down' occurring in stuttering *is not primarily local-ized at the executive stage.*

(3) The paradoxical very great decrease in ACG latency at $FP_{0.1}$ could mean that the 'hesitating' brain of the stutterer (see the EMG initial burst) can efficiently be sup-ported by an early 'go' signal. On the other hand, at this 0.1-second foreperiod, a further small increase in ACG latency is still present for /mare è bello/. This facilitat-ing 0.1-second foreperiod effect occurs also in the dysarthric patient with amyo-trophic lateral sclerosis but at a lower degree than in the stutterer. Moreover, the EMG in the patient with amyotrophic lateral sclerosis shows a relatively normal

Fig. 88–90. Patient B.A., female, 41 years old, with amyotrophic lateral sclerosis for 7 years. **88** /mare/, FP_0. OO = Orbicularis oris muscle; figures on the right indicate latency times of the response onset and end as well as the response duration. **89** /mare è bello/, FP_0, 8th (**a**) and 12th (**b**) reactions. **90** ACG (—○—, latency and duration at FP_0) and EMG (-----; △ = EMG of orbicularis oris muscle at $FP_{1.5}$, □ = at $FP_{0.1}$, ○ = at FP_0) values, with figures near symbols indicating SD and figures in parenthe-ses foreperiods ($100 = FP_{0.1}$; $1{,}500 = FP_{1.5}$).

short latency with a continuous activity that starts >200 ms before the ACG onset. In fact we know well that, at the level of the vocal tract executors, no dyscoordination occurs in dysarthria, at variance with stuttering [Peters et al., 1991].

(4) In 1.5-second foreperiod reactions, the stutterer is able to perform the sentence in a shorter time than the syllable. The mean ACG latency values for /ma/, /mare/ and /mare è bello/ were 868 ± 359, 693 ± 153 and 707 ± 147 ms, respectively. This finding might suggest that the grammatical convertor is normal, but it requires a longer time for being activated in the immediate reaction. Therefore the failure of the facilitating effect of the grammar convertor argued in the discussion of the first point, must be interpreted as a relatively higher *threshold* of the neural assembly corresponding to the grammatical convertor, rather than as an intrinsic impairment of the convertor itself. The condition indicated with the terminology of the connective neural networks as relatively higher threshold could correspond, in a more traditional neurophysiological terminology, to less efficient internal circuits.

On the other hand, the term 'intrinsic' might rather suggest a transition from merely functional to frankly neurological aberrations. Taking into consideration both results of points 2 and 4, we can infer the following interpretation. The stutterer is unable to process the sentence when the phonological organization is required immediately. But if a certain period of time (1.5 s) is given to process it separately, the phonological organization is accomplished correctly in spite of an initially erroneously timed coordination, and the stutterer becomes able to exploit the lower normal threshold of the grammatical facilitated neural assembly.

Then the abnormal slowing should be localized at the interface between the commanded invariant patterns of descending impulses and the adapting pre-executive processes. According to the previously reported blueprints, the stutterer's disorder appears as a functional impairment of buffer retrieval and possibly of timing in sequential processes of working memory. This disorder implies an error produced in the order of the single articulators within the multiple elements of the vocal tract.

The ultimate origin of this error could be sought in an inborn impairment of the cortical scores or in a failure at the level of the neural pattern characteristic formation that might depend on a disruption in the course of central timing processes contributing to the control of speech. Thus, the stuttering abnormality might be conceived as a dissociaton event in agreement with the analysis developed in Section 4 on heterochronism. The temporal development of some earliest CCP (and particularly those connected to the phonological formulator) could be relatively faster in comparison to the interface executive processes: *overloading effects* could thus arise.

An impairment of timing central programming processes must also be taken into consideration, which can be completely compensated for when the subject is allowed a suitable period of time for performance (foreperiod 1.5 s). Under this condition, the greater improvement (decrease in ACG latency) for the sentence rather than for the syllable seems to support this view. Also the common experience of the marked improvement of speech in stuttering when a slower rhythm of utterance is allowed or promoted can be explained on the lines of the present theory.

9.3.4
The 'Diagnostic' and 'Functional' Meaning of the 'Facilitation' Found in Some Stutterers

The significant decrease in the early process ratio associated with a high increase in ACG latency of immediate reactions can be taken as a possible marker revealing a link of this kind of dysfluency. A decrease in the early process ratio can be observed in some young normal subjects but remains smaller in comparison to that observed in stutterers.

The only group of patients that may share some aspects of the same phenomenon is represented by those affected by obsessive-compulsive disorders. However, as we will see in 9.6, the cerebral dysfunction, demonstrated in obsessive-compulsive disorders by our tests, essentially differs from that of stuttering since in obsessive-compulsive disorders it is characterized by a marked decrease also in the intermediary process ratio. Concordant data prove that the abnormal facilitation exerted by frontogangliobasal circuits does not imply an enhanced feedback as it is represented in stuttering models [Mindus et al., 1990; Magno Caldonetto and Tonelli, 1993; Zvarich et al., 1994; Zovato, 1994].

At the present state of the research, we can outline the following draft for a physiopathogenic interpretation of stuttering. The decrease in the early process ratio in stutterers corresponds to a facilitating effect exerted by the 'go' stimulus perceived while the reaction is still in progress. This finding is consistent with the model of Ludlow [1991] of an increased sensitivity to sensory feedbacks occurring while the subject is speaking. That an enhanced sensitivity to afferent multimodal sensory feedbacks may play a relevant role in the origin of stuttering was also supported by Zimmerman [1980] and by Caruso et al. [1988] and Gracco and Abbs [1985, 1986, 1988]. This model is also in agreement with the well-known fact that letting the subject slow his utterances greatly reduces stuttering: slowing the pace in speaking provides longer delays, and then the recurrent facilitating feedbacks can also be slowed down.

Moreover, we found that overfacilitation occurs preferentially with monosyllabic words (like /ma/), more than with sentences (like /mare è bello/), and this fact can hardly be explained with an impairment of the 'suprasegmental sentence plan alignment' as the main causal factor of stuttering [Karniol, 1995]. This author presented several lines of evidence that stuttering is primarily a phenomenon at the sentence level; however, one cannot exclude that it may be the consequence of a functional neural organization implying a narrow and precise range of feedback facilitation. This organization may not be requested for the very simple utterances of children at the age of the 1-word or 2-word stage, but it is requested 23 months later, at the point in development at which children start incorporating the syntactic rules of language. Feedback facilitation could play a different role in spontaneous speech, with respect to reading: spontaneous speech may require a critical degree of involvement of feedback facilitation, as it is about 25% slower than reading.

We must also be aware that the increase in facilitation can occur through different channels with either the acoustic or the exteroceptive and proprioceptive afferences from the vocal tract. Eventually it must be borne in mind that each internal feedback can unfold at multiple levels in the neural hierarchical organization, the lowest level implying the shortest latency time.

9.4

Parkinson Disease: Akinesia, Hypertonia and Bradyphrenic Disorders

9.4.1
The Parkinsonian Triad

Since the beginning of the last century, the main functional disorder produced by idiopathic Parkinson disease was considered as a psychomotor impairment quite different from the central paralysis or paresis. However, its real nature has remained unclear until recently, because of scanty knowledge in the physiology of high motor control processes.

Meanwhile, the clinical neuropathological studies of the basal ganglia on the one side and the neurophysiological, pharmacological and biochemical research on the other developed with reciprocal integrations to explore this 'terra incognita'. Progressively more important data were discovered on the neural processes related to the unconscious mechanisms of the production of purposeful complex sequential actions.

Little by little the psychological terms were replaced by more precise and complete definitions of the related neurobiological substrates. This field of research became thus of paramount importance not only for the physiopathogenesis and treatment of Parkinson disease but also for the general problem of the brain processes involved in psychomotility and for the experimental approach to the PDP functioning in the central nervous system. An associated question considered also the interpretation of the kinetic factor as a constitutional personality trait.

The psychomotor impairment [Webster, 1968] at the core of the parkinsonian syndrome has been defined as a sort of loss of intentional movement, i.e. in the Greek scientific term, akinesia. The clinicians and neuropsychologists saw in it an impairment of the motor voluntary act, particularly in relation to the sequence of coordinated movements [De Long et al., 1984; McDowell et al., 1986]. The physiopathologists identified a deficit and/or a disorder in the neural processes of motor programming [Marsden, 1988] at a second level, i.e. after the translation from the conceptualizer and the purposeful eupraxic organization of action to the central initiating circuits.

The experimental models of homologous brain processes and the positive effects observed in the patients with dopamine, dopaminergic and central anticholinergic drugs on one side, together with the opposite negative role of antidopaminergic drugs on the other, yielded important cues for the comprehension of the functional meaning of the basal ganglia, their PDP functioning in the control of motor behaviour and the intrinsic biochemical machinery [Gayfield, 1994].

In spite of intensive clinical and neurophysiological studies on these patients [Hoehn and Yahar, 1967; Ceriani et al., 1993; Pasetti et al., 1994], there are many uncertainties about the actual role played by the centrally originated akinesia and the associated distal hypertonia in the actual motor impairment. Pallman et al. [1990] reported that in Parkinson disease movement amplitude and choice reaction time may be independent of dopaminergic status. The evaluation of the relevance of these two factors requires longitudinal assessments of single patients, in the spontaneous course and during the treatments. Parkinsonian defects in serial multi-articulator movements for speech have been analysed by Connor et al. [1989].

Even the connection with iatrogenic parkinsonian syndromes has not clearly been defined so far.

Moreover, in patients with idiopathic parkinsonism, the relationship between other symptoms – besides akinesia and hypertonia – like tremor, depression and mental deterioration is far from being completely understood.

In fact, even within the triad, the tremor superficially appears as a hyperkinetic movement, but physiopathogenetically it is completely different from choreic movements. The parkinsonian tremor can in fact be related to an enhanced myotatic reflex with rhythmically interrupted agonistic-antagonistic motoneuron hyperexcitability. However, a long series of experiments has shown that this is only a partial explanation, and one must also take into consideration a pacemaker which is disinhibited at the level of the supraspinal, brainstem and subcorticobasal ganglia and acts as a rhythmic generator. From this point of view, the occurrence of the extrapyramidal tremor, which affects a part only of parkinsonian patients and represents a favourable prognostic sign, could be related to an enhanced channel of executor processes that would produce a high tendency to motor activity. May it then exert a positive effect on the speed of reactions? Certainly it cannot be considered as equal to the *kinetic factor*, as the extrapyramidal tremor affects only the final servo-mechanisms at the executive brainstem-spinal system. Aiming to correctly address the question, we should first investigate the actual occurrence of the positive effect, with suitably modified MDRV, in a large material of well-classified subgroups of parkinsonian patients, with and without tremor, in comparison to other patients with essential tremor.

9.4.2
Application of Multiple-Delayed-Reaction Verbochronometry and Main Issues

MDRV seems to be a valuable method to measure, in the single patient affected by Parkinson disease, by ACG latency and duration, the time increase in the programming processes and in the sequential articulatory movements requested for uttering the word task.

The performance of delayed reading reactions besides the immediate ones should greatly help in differentiating the temporal slowing due to central processes from the negative interference of peripheral constraints in the final executive processes [Netsell et al., 1975]. Follow-up studies with these tests should allow a better evaluation of the course of the disease and the effects of drugs. The changes occurring in all these parameters could then be correlated with different clinical features and effects of treatments.

In light of the present results, the following four issues are open to further investigations and discussions: (1) parkinsonian tremor does not produce direct significant changes in the above-mentioned parameters; paradoxical facilitating effects were observed; (2) the akinetic disorder cannot be studied isolatedly from the repercussion that servo-mechanism impairments like hypertonia can exert on adaptive and other intermediary processes; (3) on the basis of differential measurements of changes induced in ACG latency and duration in our series of examinations with MDRV, it is possible to obtain reliable data on the functional impairments due to the central programming and those due to more distal alterations like hypertonia.

Table 18. Test (I) and retest (II) of /mare/ and /muro/ reactions with normals and T.E., male, 55 years old, tremulous patient No. 3

		ACG latency, ms		ACG duration, ms	
		normals	T.E.	normals	T.E.
FP_0	I	510 ± 45	548 ± 69	347 ± 46	293 ± 69
	II	$\pm 7\%$	477 ± 48	$<1.5\%$	271 ± 48
			-14%		-7%
$FP_{0.1}$	I	514 ± 70	511 ± 79	333 ± 57	324 ± 70
	II	$\pm 9\%$	451 ± 53	$<1.5\%$	353 ± 61
			-12%		$+9\%$
$FP_{1.5}$	I	406 ± 78	350 ± 93	342 ± 67	266 ± 80
	II	$\pm 4\%$	338 ± 92	$<1.5\%$	264 ± 72
			-4%		-2%

9.4.2.1
The Presence of Parkinsonian Tremor May Be Reflected by an Increase in Acousticogram Latency of Sentences

No doubt that most of the patients with tremor as the prevalent trouble, both at rest and during postural voluntary contraction, claim some impairment of fine motor abilities as using a spoon or writing. However, the clinical neurological examination does not show any evident motor impairment, whilst, at an elementary analysis, only mild signs of trochlea dentata may be noticed. The subjective ailments seem to emerge from the apprehension about a deterioration of the patient's own personal image among people, but, most of all, from the mechanical disturbance produced by intermittent involuntary movements that impair the fine and precise actions required in everyday activity.

A systematic research was carried out by us with parkinsonian patients whose main disturbance was tremor at rest and in postural attitudes.

Tremulous parkinsonian patients have been studied with /clan/ and /cane/ as word stimuli in 1992 in a study including for comparison akinetic parkinsonian patients and normal controls of old age. The results did not significantly differentiate tremulous parkinsonian patients from normals. The issues of this research are limited and will be analysed in the next paragraph together with a detailed analysis of the changes found in the akinetic patients.

More extensive studies, including triple stimuli (monosyllable, disyllabic word, sentence), have been carried out in 1993–1994, with investigations of patients not under pharmacological treatment and in different phases of the disease.

Four patients (55–67 years old) were investigated with /mare/ and /muro/ (tables 18, 19), 4 with monosyllable, disyllabic word and sentence and 1 with both, double and triple word stimuli.

Patient 1, G.E., female, 61 years (fig. 91), under moderate dopaminergic treatment (365 mg/day Madopar). The ACG latencies were normal. In contrast, the EMG latency (orbicularis oris) was longer than the normal mean values and could sometimes become equal to ACG latency.

Patient 2, M.T., male, 67 years (fig. 92), under 500 mg/day Madopar. Moderate increase in ACG latency at FP_0 and lower than normal ACT latency at $FP_{1.5}$. MDRV was repeated 1 month later (fig. 92, dashed line) without significant changes.

Patient 3, T.E., male, 55 years (table 18), under 125 mg/day Madopar. Normal ACG latency at FP_0 and lower than normal ACG latency at $FP_{1.5}$. A retest, 3 months later, did not show any significant change.

Table 19. Test (I) and retest (II) of /mare/ and /muro/ reactions with normals and C.M., female, 65 years old, tremulous patient No. 4

		ACG latency, ms		ACG duration, ms	
		normals	C.M.	normals	C.M.
FP_0	I	615 ± 137	595 ± 101	406 ± 69	409 ± 80
	II	$\pm 6\%$	-18%	$<1.5\%$	-6%
$FP_{0.1}$	I	684 ± 229	660 ± 133	399 ± 68	403 ± 66
	II	$\pm 7\%$	-20%	$<1.5\%$	-7%
$FP_{1.5}$	I	461 ± 127	355 ± 89	386 ± 74	299 ± 94
	II	$\pm 3\%$	-6%	$<1.5\%$	-1.5%

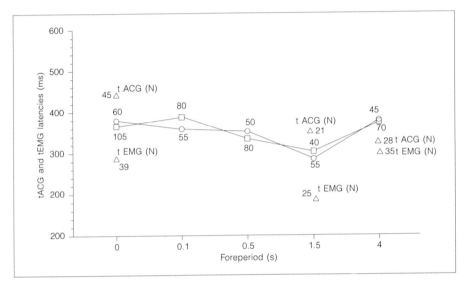

Fig. 91. Patient No. 1, G.E., female, 61 years old, with tremorigenous Parkinson disease. /mare/ + /muro/ mean values of ACG (○) and EMG (□) latencies (t). △ = Normal (N) mean values; figures near symbols indicate SD.

Patient 4, C.M., 65 years, female (table 19), under 250 mg/day Madopar. Normal ACG latency at FP_0 with a low ACG latency at $FP_{1.5}$. No significant change in a retest 5 months later.

Patient 5, M.M., 67 years, female, was examined 3 times. A first MDRV was carried out without any dopaminergic treatment, under 1 mg Tavor; word stimuli were /mare/ and /muro/ (fig. 93). Increased ACG latency at FP_0 with a normal ACG latency at $FP_{1.5}$.

A retest was done 3 months later under 250 mg/day Madopar and physiokinetic therapy including logotherapy. ACG latency at FP_0 was then normal, without any further decrease at $FP_{1.5}$.

A third examination was carried out 11 months after the second MDRV with different word stimuli (monosyllable, disyllabic word, sentence; fig. 94), with suspension of the dopamine treatment for 3 days: ACG latency at FP_0 was slightly increased, while ACG latency at $FP_{1.5}$ was relatively short. The ACG latency of the sentence was longer than those of the monosyllable and the disyllabic word.

Patient 6, A.C., 60 years, female, under 500 mg/day Madopar. Investigated monosyllable, disyllabic word and sentence. Relatively high values of ACG latency at $FP_{1.5}$ (table 20).

Three further patients (No. 7–9) were investigated with the 3 stimuli: T.O., 54 years, male; C.C., 68 years, male; G.P., 51 years, male. The mean values of the ACG latency of the 3 patients were: monosyl-

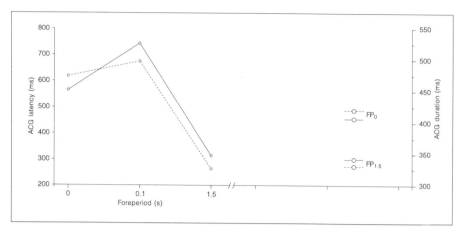

Fig. 92. Patient No. 2, M.T., male, 67 years old, with tremorigenous Parkinson disease. ACG latencies (t) and durations (D). —— = ACG1, first examination; ----- = ACG2, repeat examination 1 month later.

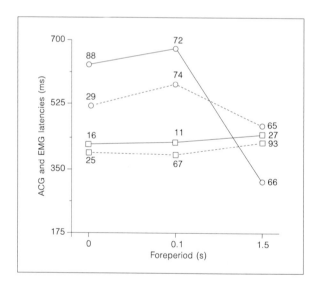

Fig. 93. Patient No. 5, M.M., female, 67 years old, with tremorigenous Parkinson disease. /mare/ + /muro/ mean values of ACG (——) and EMG (-----) latencies. ○ = First examination; □ = second examination 1 month later, under treatment.

lable, 518 ± 76 ms at FP_0 and 399 ± 61 ms at $FP_{1.5}$; disyllabic word, 588 ± 53 and 429 ± 40 ms; sentence, 633 ± 132 and 448 ± 101 ms.

The duration of ACG for the sentence was increased with a mean value (for the 3 patients) of $1,850 \pm 162$ ms at FP_0 and 907 ± 88 ms at $FP_{1.5}$.

A general evaluation of all these cases confirms a previous opinion [Pinelli and Ceriani, 1992] that tremorigenous Parkinson disease does not involve a slowing down of the cerebral functions of speech control. There are even some trends towards a higher speed of the executive processes and in some cases also of the intermediary processes.

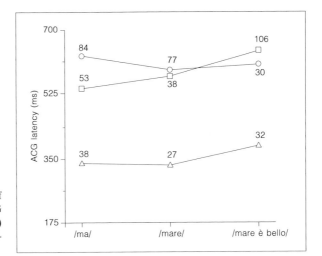

Fig. 94. Third examination of patient No. 5 (see fig. 93). ACG latencies at FP_0 (○), $FP_{0.1}$ (□) and $FP_{1.5}$ (△); figures near symbols indicate SD.

Table 20. ACG latencies (ms) of A.C., female, 60 years old, tremulous patient No. 6

	/ma/	/mare/	/mare è bello/
FP_0	530 ± 53	570 ± 38	612 ± 106
$FP_{1.5}$	390 ± 40	408 ± 32	439 ± 80

The findings of cases 5–9 showing a longer ACG latency for the sentence, at variance with the higher facilitation of grammar tasks of normal controls, might be interpreted as evidence of some central process impairment, related to the grammar convertor or more generally to the longest utterances. The partially normal ACG latencies at $FP_{1.5}$ rule out a negative interference of the abnormal rhythmization of motor unit recruitment on the executive-articulatory stage.

The delay observed in EMG onset (fig. 93) could be interpreted as an equivalent of the impairment in the preparatory processes clinically defined as block of the 'mise en train'. However, the absence of any negative effect in the ACG parameters makes a different distribution of the preparatory tuning among the oromandibular muscles a more acceptable interpretation.

A significant increase with respect to the mean values of normal controls occurs in the difference between ACG latency at FP_0 and that at $FP_{1.5}$ (table 20). Since the latter is not significantly increased with respect to normals, one might infer that the difficulty is localized at the programming and tuning central processes.

An additional finding can yield further cues for a better localization of the slowing event. In fact, the decrease in time of performance from FP_0 to $FP_{1.5}$ is greater for ACG duration than for ACG latency: the ACG duration of the sentence is 1,850 ms at FP_0, with a decrease to 900 ms at $FP_{1.5}$, i.e. a difference equivalent to –50% with respect to the difference of –25% that was found for ACG latency. On this ground, we may identify a prevalent impairment in timing processes when they develop continuously in immediate reactions. On the contrary, when an interval is allowed between the sensorimotor transfer and the timing of the executive phase, this process may improve significantly.

Table 21. /Clan/ and /cane/ reactions (ms) of normal (N), tremulous (TR) and akinetic (AK) subjects

	N		TR		AK		$p_{N/AK}$
	FP_0	FP_3	FP_0	FP_3	FP_0	FP_3	
EMG latency							
/clan/	300 ± 67	176 ± 28	334 ± 124	209 ± 79	424 ± 168	265 ± 159	<0,009
/cane/	279 ± 54	175 ± 19	309 ± 97	210 ± 89	422 ± 157	247 ± 79	
ACG latency							
/clan/	574 ± 67	401 ± 51	647 ± 122	603 ± 75	754 ± 197	527 ± 156	<0.03
/cane/	540 ± 54	411 ± 46	458 ± 100	463 ± 93	675 ± 178	411 ± 165	

N = 12 (mean 70 years, range 66–81), TR = 8 (mean 66 years, range 49–71), AK = 16 (mean 68 years, range 52–80). ACG duration showed significant increases only in AK subjects ($p_{N/AK} < 0.02$).

This means that 'the transfer from the initial central timing programming to the executive timing processes was impaired'. How can we relate this CCP transfer impairment to the abnormal pattern of tremor that has a more 'distal' origin? To answer this question, we must admit a feedback effect. We have explained in Section 2, with the example of the 'pipe in the mouth', how a preliminary functional change at the level of the vocal tract scheme (in the parietal cortex) provides the initial informations for the brain timing CCP. Furthermore, in a second order of mechanisms, the automatic sequence of tremulous grouped discharges interferes negatively with the adaptation process that becomes limited and rather stereotyped. This condition creates a sort of overloading effect (see 9.5).

9.4.2.2
Akinesia Is Characterized by a Significant Increase in Latency and Duration of the Acousticogram

As it is reported in table 21 showing the results of MDRV with /clan/ and /cane/, the comparison of the results of word reading reactions in normals, tremulous and akinetic patients shows that the results of the last group of patients are significantly different with a marked increase in ACG latency times at FP_0 and ACG durations. The analysis of these increases requires a double line of investigations since akinesia, which in itself represents a disorder of brain computing processes, is associated in patients with Parkinson disease with a disorder of the neuro-articulatory executors, namely extrapyramidal hypertonia.

Eight akinetic patients, 4 with hemiparkinson (fig. 95–98), 3 with generalized akinesia (fig. 99–101) and 1 with a mixed tremorigenous akinetic syndrome (fig. 102) were examined with /mare/ and /muro/. Five further akinetic patients underwent MDRV with the monosyllable, disyllabic word and sentence together with 3 tremulous patients (tables 22, 23).

Only 1 patient (fig. 100) presented normal MDRV values. He was the youngest among all patients investigated and was under treatment with 625 mg/day Madopar, under apparently normalized clinical conditions.

All other patients were characterized by increased ACG latency at FP_0 that could be more marked for /muro/ than /mare/ (fig. 95). ACG latencies were decreased at $FP_{1.5}$ but relatively less at FP_4.

The repetition of MDRV before and after dopaminergic treatment revealed a marked decrease in ACG latency at FP_0 but with a less evident decrease at $FP_{1.5}$ so that the intermediary process ratio could reach 1 or 1.1 (fig. 96).

The repetition of MDRV at 1- to 5-month intervals, under the same treatment (fig. 100), did not show any significant change. ACG latency at FP_0 was not systematically modified, while ACG latency at $FP_{0.1}$ and at $FP_{1.5}$ could show an increase not higher than 18 %.

The cumulative analysis of all parkinsonian patients investigated in the 1993 and 1994 study allows us to conclude that the corticogangliobasal CCP impairment, in connection with the dopaminergic failure, is reflected in MDRV. ACG latency and duration at FP_0 (table 21) are increased, while the difference between ACG latencies at FP_0 and at $FP_{1.5}$ is higher than in normal controls (tables 22, 24). These changes were statistically significant in 5 of 8 parkinsonian patients and precisely in 3 of 3 tremulous cases and in 2 of 5 akinetic hypertonic patients.

As we have previously reported, 3 patients were characterized by a relatively high intermediary process ratio at $FP_{1.5}$, a finding that seems to be specific for *schizophrenics*. In fact, as we will discuss in more detail in Section 10, this peculiar finding must be evaluated in the context of the other parameters. A first associated change to be pointed out in these 3 parkinsonian patients occurs in the value of ACG latency at FP_0 that is the lowest and which is never found elsewhere, particularly for the sentence: this low value makes the increase in intermediary process ratio a pseudo-increase as far as ACG latency at $FP_{\geq 0.4}$ is concerned. In fact, these patients were under treatment with rather high doses of dopamine with a marked clinical improvement and some iatrogenic *hyperkinetic movements* [Guy, 1976; Koshino et al., 1992]. The flattened shape of the curve of ACG latency as a function of foreperiod duration of these parkinsonian patients clearly differentiate it from the spiky (at $FP_{0.5}$ or $FP_{1.5}$) shape of the analogous curve of dissociative psychosis (see Section 10). On the other hand, it can be seen from table 24 that in these cases no difference was found for sentences with respect to simple syllables or disyllabic words. This result might be interpreted in favour of a still normal function at the level of preprogrammation connected with the grammatical operator, with reference to its threshold and its triggering.

9.4.2.3
Central and Distal Slowing Measured in Parkinsonian Patients

In Section 7, we have already discussed which investigations have to be carried out with MDRV to identify a slowing in CCP programmation versus a slowing due to an abnormal distal constraint like hypodiadochokinesia. The basic criterion is that ACG latency and duration are increased, at the level of both the minimal and total reaction times.

Under normal conditions and in parkinsonian patients, minimal reaction times can be measured with delayed reactions with long foreperiods. However, when delayed reactions are impaired (as it occurs in *dissociative psychosis*) and the reaction time cannot be reduced at $FP_{>0.4}$, we must make use of *simple reactions* that in any case reflect the final executive processes more faithfully.

The difference between ACG latency at $FP_{\geq 0.5}$ (3 s in fig. 103) of the single parkinsonian patient and ACG latency at $FP_{\geq 0.5}$ of normal controls corresponds to the effect of hypertonia (extrapyramidal rigidity due to the loss of control of shortening and stretch re-

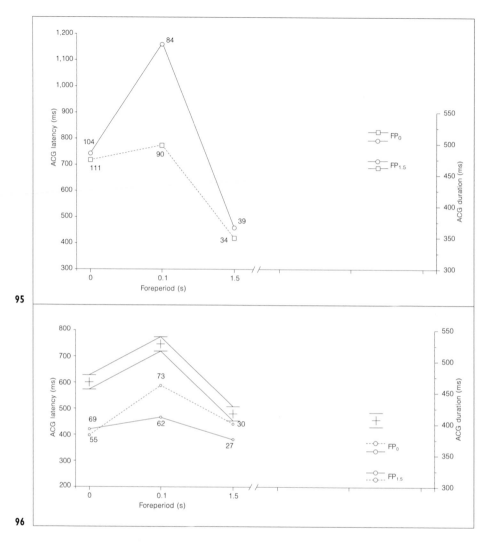

95

96

Fig. 95–98. ACG latencies (t) and durations (D) of patients with hemiparkinsonism. **95** Patient I.G., 68 years old, no treatment. ○ = /mare/; □ = /muro/. **96** Patient B.A., female, 68 years old. —— = First ACG; ----- = second ACG; + = before treatment. **97** Patient P., female, 54 years old. ○ = /mare/; □ = /muro/. **98** Patient C.P., 56 years old. —— = First ACG; ----- = second ACG.

flexes) on psychomotor reactions. Within certain limits, the same argument holds for ACG duration (fig. 104).

The difference between ACG latency at FP_0 and ACG latency at FP_3 (or of a *simple reaction*) can be taken as a reliable temporal measure of the early brain processes. The difference can be named the 'central time'. The difference between the central time of the individual patient and the mean central time of normal controls corresponds to the increase in reaction time of central programming processes due to akinesia. This akinesia-dependent slowing in central time can also be calculated as the difference between [ACG

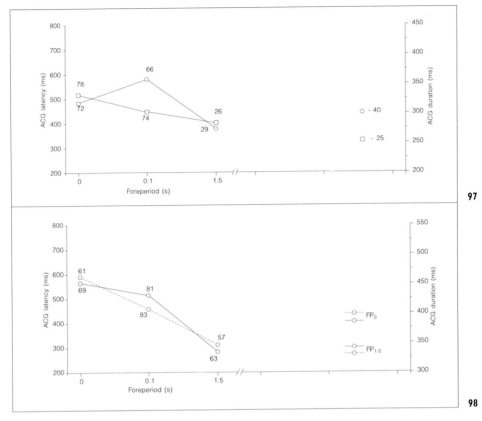

97

98

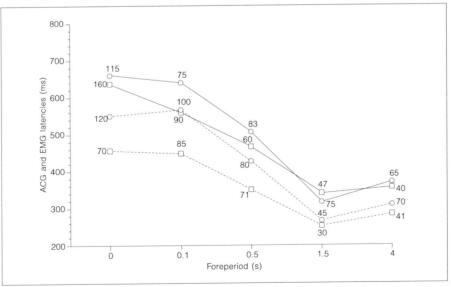

Fig. 99. Patient T.A., male, 53 years old, with akinetic Parkinson disease. ACG (——) and EMG (-----) latencies of /mare/ (○) and /muro/ (□). Figures near symbols indicate SD.

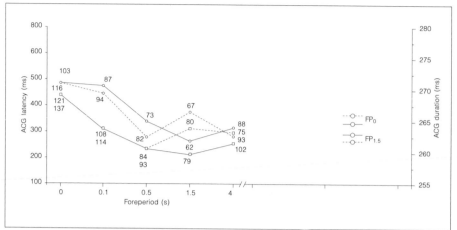

100

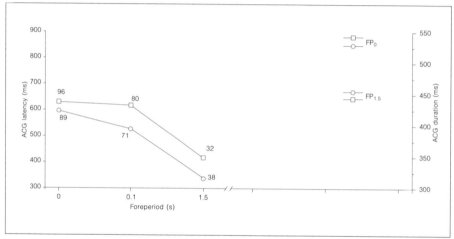

101

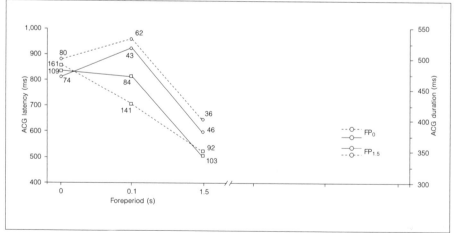

102

Table 22. ACG latency at FP_0 – ACG latency at $FP_{1.5}$ (ms)

	/ma/	/mare/	/mare è bello/
Tremor	224	246	287
Tremor	184	93	184
Akinesia and hypertonia	41	16	−54
Tremor	231	250	330
Akinesia and hypertonia	113	47	4
Akinesia and hypertonia	199	244	279
Akinesia and hypertonia	263	160	351
Akinesia and hypertonia	−64	45	60
Mean	149	138	180

Table 23. ACG latencies of tremulous (TR) and akinetic hypertonic (AK/HY) patients

Pa-tient	Age years	Sex	FP_0			$FP_{1.5}$			FP_3		
			m	d	s	m	d	s	m	d	s
J. (TR)	72	F	631 ± 85	653 ± 98	746 ± 84	791 ± 44	785 ± 87	734 ± 60	407 ± 29	407 ± 47	459 ± 28
L. (TR)	61	M	741 ± 100	683 ± 48	763 ± 93	838 ± 102	748 ± 100	762 ± 132	590 ± 65	557 ± 84	579 ± 70
C.R. (AK/HY)	67	F	590 ± 55	570 ± 78	595 ± 112	611 ± 99	497 ± 117	559 ± 95	554 ± 25	549 ± 54	639 ±106
M.E. (TR)	67	F	534 ± 53	552 ± 38	657 ± 106	612 ± 84	630 ± 30	566 ± 77	302 ± 27	303 ± 38	327 ± 32
G. (AK/HY)	55	M	491 ± 96	424 ± 55	403 ± 30	550 ± 50	534 ± 63	564 ± 33	377 ± 62	378 ± 31	399 ± 60
C.A.R. (AK/HY)	79	F	447 ± 29	470 ± 49	600 ± 137	542 ± 45	554 ± 60	546 ± 88	226 ± 33	248 ± 17	321 ± 46
M.A. (AK/HY)	81	M	856 ± 70	839 ± 72	977 ± 73	1,066 ± 323	912 ± 230	971 ± 131	679 ± 208	593 ± 109	626 ±211
C.R.I. (AK/HY)	55	F	532 ± 31	602 ± 74	607 ± 82	554 ± 24	571 ± 30	603 ± 30	557 ± 46	596 ± 31	547 ± 20
Mean			602 ± 136	599 ± 129	667 ± 167	695 ± 187	653 ± 145	663 ± 149	461 ± 156	453 ± 137	487 ±128

m = Monosyllable; d = disyllabic word; s = sentence.

Fig. 100. Patient C.P., male, 39 years old, akinetic. Latencies (t) and durations (D) of the first (○, March 3, 1992) and second ACG (□, April 7, 1993) of /mare/ (——) and /muro/ (-----). Figures near symbols indicate SD.

Fig. 101. Patient S.M., female, 67 years old, with generalized akinetic Parkinson disease for 3 years. ACG latencies (t) and durations (D) of /mare/ and /muro/ (□). Figures near symbols indicate SD.

Fig. 102. Patient F.A., male, 77 years old, with mixed tremorigenous akinetic Parkinson syndrome. ACG latencies (t) and durations (D) of the first (——) and second (-----) examinations. ○ = 'Off' state; □ = basal state; figures near symbols indicate SD.

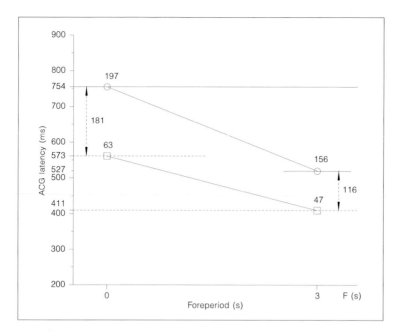

Fig. 103. ACG latencies (t) of /mare/ obtained from parkinsonians (○) and normals (□). Figures near symbols indicate SD.

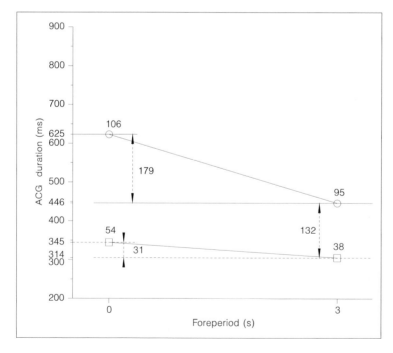

Fig. 104. ACG durations (D) of /mare/ obtained from normals (□) and parkinsonians (○). Figures near symbols indicate SD.

Table 24 A. Evaluation of ages of tremulous parkinsonian patients and normal subjects

Group	Count	Mean	SD	SE
A	14	67.07	9.4	2.51
B	26	65.15	5.38	1.05

Unpaired t test; X_1: column 21; Y_1: ETA 1; d.f.: 38; unpaired t value: 0.82; p (2-tailed): 0.415.

Table 24 B. Evaluation of ages of akinetic parkinsonian patients and normal subjects

Group	Count	Mean	SD	SE
A	17	68.82	7.89	1.91
B	26	65.15	5.38	1.05

Unpaired t test: X_1: column 21; Y_1: ETA 1; d.f.: 41; unpaired t value: 1.82; p (2-tailed): 0.0766.

Group: A = patients; B = normals; count = number of subjects; mean = mean age (years).

latency at FP_0 of the single patient – mean ACG latency at FP_0 of controls] and [ACG latency at FP_3 of the single patient – mean ACG latency at FP_3 of controls].

In the case of ACG duration, the analogous difference will reflect the timing processes that depend upon the brain control of cyclic excitatory and inhibiting (or de-activating) processes.

These series of measurements were carried out with the word stimuli /mare/ and /muro/ in 15 akinetic-hypertonic patients with primary Parkinson disease who were treated with a reduced dopamine dose 5 days before MDRV (250–375 mg/day Madopar). The results are reported for /mare/ in figures 103 and 104.

The increase in the executive processes for ACG latency was 116 ms and for ACG latency was 132 ms, which corresponds to +20%.

The increase in the initiation and early programming processes, which more strictly correspond to akinesia, was 65 ms (i.e. +10%) measured by the difference ACG latency at FP_0 – ACG latency at FP_3 and 132 ms (i.e. +30%) by ACG duration at FP_0 – ACG duration at FP_3. We can then assert that the more important negative factor in the akinetic hypertonic syndrome involves the timing processes at the most elementary level. It corresponds to an impairment of inhibitory processes in the cyclic sequence of the segmental control of motility. The negative factor exerted by the hypertonic alteration is in the order of a 20% slowing. The 10% change in initial and spatial programming processes could reflect some repercussion or upward effects of timing dysfunction.

9.4.3
Does Bradyphrenia Occur in Parkinson Disease as a Primary Disorder?

While akinesia and rigidity were analysed as factors increasing the time taken by central initiation processes and by executive processes, respectively, some authors wondered if some other functional impairments play a role in the psychomotor inability of patients affected by Parkinson disease.

Apart from depressive conditions (their effects on MDRV will be considered in 9.7) and mental deterioration with short-term memory impairments, bradyphrenia [Spicer et al., 1994] could play a significant role and cause an increase in ACG latency. The results of recent studies in this field deserve a particular mention for a correct evaluation also of the results of MDRV.

According to neurophysiologists and neuropsychologists involved in the study of Parkinson disease, bradyphrenia includes mental fatiguability, difficulty with focused attention [Downes et al., 1989] and inefficient decision making.

Some authors considered bradyphrenia to include also initiation of movement. An opposite view was shared by those who attempted to separate the mental and motor aspects of experimental cognitive tasks [Spicer et al., 1994]. The pros and cons can be summarized as follows:

(1) Data supporting a cognitive slowing in Parkinson disease: Hausch et al. [1982] found that patients with Parkinson disease had longer visual and auditory P_{300} latencies than did controls. This finding was assumed by some neurologists to support the hypothesis of a cognitive slowing in Parkinson disease.

(2) Data against the existence of a generalized bradyphrenia in non-demented Parkinson disease: The study of reaction time with Sternberg's [1969] memory scanning paradigm showed that, although non-demented patients with Parkinson disease were slower overall when untreated, as compared with their reaction times when optimally treated with antiparkinsonian medications, slowness was not proportionally greater when a larger memory set had to be scanned. Moreover, in tasks involving covert orientation of attention in the visual field, patients with Parkinson disease were equally fast in orientating themselves towards the attention cues under two treatment conditions [Rafal et al., 1984].

Performances of parkinsonian patients for processes that are effortful were investigated versus processes that are more automatic. According to Posner and Snyder [1975], an automatic attentional process is one that is fast-acting, occurs without intention or conscious awareness and does not interfere with other cognitive or behavioural processes. At variance, an effortful attention-demanding process is slow-acting, involves intention and conscious awareness and inhibits the performance of cognitive or behavioural processes that are unattended. Neely [1977] designed a lexical decision task requiring subjects to decide if a letter string was an English word, each letter string being preceded by a priming word. By varying the interval between the presentation of the primer and the presentation of the target, Neely was able to separate fast-acting from slow-acting processes involved in semantic activation.

With a variation of Neely's lexical decision paradigm, Spicer et al. [1994] determined the median reaction time, i.e. the time from presentation of the target (when the subject had to release button A) to the subject pressing a target button for word targets correctly identified as words. Parkinsonian patients responded more slowly than controls when responses were averaged over priming condition. Furthermore the priming condition altered reaction time compared with the neutral condition.

Expected-related and expected-unrelated versus neutral targets produced a greater degree of facilitation of reaction times for the parkinsonian group than for controls. That this was not simply a reflection of their relative slowness was proved by calculating the median reaction time of the neutral condition (median reaction time of the comparison condition/median reaction time of the neutral condition). As with reaction times, the par-

showed a significantly longer movement duration than controls under
s. Furthermore, the primer facilitated movement speed under the ex-
he expected-unrelated conditions and inhibited movement speed
d-unrelated condition.

ractive role for Parkinson disease and age as well as depression was
bradyphrenia. Parkinsonian patients were substantially slower for
movement times in choice reactions.

mains

The authors' conclusion is that patients with Parkinsonian disease are able to shift their attentional focus quickly and accurately. They do not appear to experience generalized bradyphrenia, even those aged 64 years and over. Moreover, the automatic and effortful components of semantic activation are not obviously impaired in Parkinson disease. An unanticipated level of facilitation (hyperpriming) was observed in the parkinsonian group. It could be produced by prelexical linguistic or postlexical decision impairments.

It was shown by many authors that patients with Parkinson disease have difficulty in setting up movement parameters prior to the act of moving [Pullman et al., 1990]. It is possible that lexical decision making and movement preparation are parallel processes that draw upon a common resource pool and therefore interact.

A greater facilitation of movement duration was found at short primer-target intervals in the parkinsonian group in the expected-related versus neutral comparison, as well as a trend towards decreasing movement duration with increasing primer-target interval in the expected-unrelated versus neutral comparison. These findings lend support to the idea that processing of the target influenced the preparation and execution of motor responses in the parkinsonian group.

Anyway Spicer et al. [1994] recognize that several additional questions are raised that 'leave the mysterious cognitive disorder of Parkinson disease still shrouded'.

In conclusion, the research carried out by Pullman et al. [1990], even if with simple hand movements as a response, presents many points of interest in relation to our study of Parkinson disease with MDRV. The following issues should be particularly stressed: (1) attentional processes are normal in Parkinson disease, including speed in shifting attentional focus; (2) reaction and movement times can be markedly influenced (with facilitatory effects) by collateral concurrent stimuli ('primers'), semantically related or unrelated, provided they are expected.

Consequently, proper experimental sets of multiple delayed reactions could be elaborated to identify factors of variability in motor performances of parkinsonian patients. The results could offer important cues for new ways to plan facilitating treatments.

9.4.4
Secondary, Iatrogenic Akinesia

We applied MDRV to 6 schizophrenics treated for different periods of time (10–20 years) with antidopaminergic drugs and affected by tardive dyskinesia with an associated Parkinson-like akinetic-hypertonic syndrome (table 25A).

A marked increase in ACG latency at FP_0 was found in 3 cases, with the greatest difference in case No. 1. The increase was not correlated with the mental condition, but only with the duration of the antidopaminergic treatment, which in case No. 1 was longest in comparison with the other patients.

On the other hand, in one case of schizophrenia with less marked akinesia, characterized by tardive dyskinesia of mild degree (case No. 4), in spite of a rather low IQ, the values of ACG latency were in the range of normals. Similar results were obtained from case No. 2, who was under rather high-dose antidopaminergic treatment and showed marked symptoms of tardive dyskinesia. These results raised the question if tardive dyskinesia, similarly to the kinetic factor, can exert in itself some kind of facilitation of motor reaction.

Table 25. Reactions of schizophrenic, parkinsonian and normal subjects

A. *Schizophrenic patients with extrapyramidal signs*

No.	Patient	Disease duration years	Age years	ACG latency, ms			IR	ER
				FP_0	$FP_{0.1}$	$FP_{1.5}$		
1	P.R. y	23	50	958 ± 133	985 ± 59	$1,058 \pm 152$	1.10	1.02
2	A.A.	15	43	425 ± 5	514 ± 51	364 ± 72	0.85	1.20
3	G.C.	17	58	747 ± 118	938 ± 45	729 ± 67	0.97	1.25
4	A.C.	10	43	576 ± 74	423 ± 54	376 ± 106	0.65	0.74
5	P.A. x	13	34	825 ± 217	$1,681 \pm 495$	$1,435 \pm 271$	1.73	2.03
6	D.M.	16	42	565 ± 76	765 ± 101	768 ± 154	1.35	1.33

B. *Comparison of schizophrenic patients with extrapyramidal signs, parkinsonian patients and normals (mean values)*

	ACG values, ms			IR	ER
	FP_0	$FP_{0.1}$	$FP_{1.5}$		
Schizophrenics					
Latency	643 ± 169	782 ± 335	720 ± 295	1.20 ± 0.31	1.19 ± 0.34
Duration	438 ± 78	447 ± 84	455 ± 96		
Parkinsonian patients					
Latency	747 ± 197	798 ± 136	527 ± 156	0.70 ± 0.22	1.00 ± 0.14
Duration	625 ± 106	656 ± 85	446 ± 95	0.71 ± 0.07	1.00 ± 0.10
Normals					
Latency	496 ± 69	541 ± 74	380 ± 91	0.76 ± 0.29	0.99 ± 0.17
Duration	371 ± 38	334 ± 46	337 ± 27	0.90 ± 0.90	0.90 ± 0.08

IR = intermediary process ratio; ER = early process ratio.

9.4.5
A Statistical Evaluation of Intermediary and Early Process Ratios of All Patients with Parkinsonian Syndromes

The intermediary process ratio was found significantly increased in iatrogenic akinetic patients, i.e. *schizophrenics* with extrapyramidal symptoms, versus patients with idiopathic parkinsonism and normals (table 25B). This finding instigated a series of investigations in schizophrenics that will be reported in the following chapter.

However, no significant difference in intermediary process ratios was found between normals and patients with idiopathic parkinsonism. The statistical evaluation of intermediary process ratios obtained from tremulous and akinetic patients, respectively, versus normals is reported in tables 26 and 27. The age distribution of idiopathic parkinsonian, tremulous and akinetic patients is given in tables 23 and 24, with a comparison to normal controls.

The statistical significance of early process ratios of tremulous parkinsonian patients versus normal controls is given in table 28.

Table 26. Evaluation of intermediary process ratios obtained from normals and tremulous parkinsonian patients

A. *Unpaired t test*

Group	Count	Mean	SD	SE
A	17	0.71	0.19	0.05
B	24	0.76	0.17	0.03

X_1: column 21; Y_1: intermediary process ratios of normals; d.f.: 39; unpaired t value: –0.96; p (2-tailed): 0.3442; for other explanations, see table 24.

B. *Anova*

1. X_1: *intermediary process ratios of tremulous parkinsonian patients*

Mean 0.709	CV 26.702	sum 12.054
SD 0.189	count 17	sum of squares 9.121
SE 0.046	range 0.459–1.051	number missing 46
variance 0.036	difference 0.593	

2. *One-factor Anova – repeated measures for X_1–X_2*

Source	d.f.	Sum of squares	Mean square	F test	p value
Between subjects	13	0.27	0.02	0.55	0.8522
Within subjects	14	0.52	0.04		
Treatments	1	0.09	0.09	2.67	0.1262
Residuals	13	0.43	0.03		
Total	27	0.79			

Reliability estimates for all treatments: –0.8, for a single treatment: –0.29. Note: 46 cases deleted with missing values.

Group	Count	Mean	SD	SE
Normals	14	0.84	0.13	0.04
Tremulous PD patients	14	0.72	0.19	0.05

Comparison	Mean difference	Fisher PLSD	Scheffé F test	Dunnett t
Normals vs. tremulous PD patients	0.11	0.15	2.67	1.63

PD = Parkinson disease.

Table 27. Evaluation of intermediary process ratios obtained from normals and akinetic parkinsonian patients

A.	Unpaired t test	Group	Count	Mean	SD	SE
		A	14	0.74	0.16	0.04
		B	24	0.76	0.17	0.03

X_1: column 21; Y_1: intermediary process ratios of normals; d.f.: 36; unpaired t value: –0.34; p (2-tailed): 0.7367; for other explanations, see table 25.

B. Anova 1. X_2: intermediary process ratios of akinetic parkinsonian patients

Mean 0.744	CV 21.066	sum 10.42
SD 0.157	count 14	sum of squares 8.076
SE 0.042	range 0.481–1.034	number missing 49
variance: 0.025	difference 0.553	

2. One-factor Anova – repeated measures for X_1–X_2

Source	d.f.	Sum of squares	Mean square	F test	p value
Between subjects	10	0.20	0.02	0.60	0.7828
Within subjects	11	0.36	0.03		
Treatments	1	0.05	0.05	1.59	0.2362
Residuals	10	0.31	0.03		
Total	21	0.56			

Reliabilty estimates for all treatments: –0.66, for a single treatment: –0.25. Note: 49 cases deleted with missing values.

Group	Count	Mean	SD	SE
Normals	11	0.82	0.15	0.04
Akinetic PD patients	11	0.73	0.17	0.05

Comparison	Mean difference	Fisher PLSD	Scheffé F test	Dunnett t
Normals vs. akinetic PD patients	0.1	0.17	1.59	1.26

For explanations, see tables 24 and 26.

Table 28. Evaluation (t test) of early process ratios obtained from normals and tremulous parkinsonian patients

Group	Count	Mean	SD	SE
A	14	1.04	0.17	0.05
B	24	1.08	0.28	0.06

Unpaired t test; X_1: column 21; Y_1: early process ratios of normals; d.f.: 36; unpaired t value: –0.43; p (2-tailed): 0.668; for other explanations, see table 24.

....

Schizophrenia

> To have forgotten that schizophrenia is a brain disease will go down
> as one of the great aberrations of twentieth-century medicine.
>
> [Ron and Harvey, 1990]

9.5.1
Introductory Remarks

An increasing number of experimental and clinical data proved a functional condition of 'hypofrontality' to occur in schizophrenic patients [Gur et al., 1983]. However, a suitable reliable methodology that could be applied in routine examinations to better identify and detect this dysfunctions has not yet been provided.

The window that neuropsycholinguistics can open on the processes developing within the mind was considered since the studies on the deep structure of syntax by Chomsky [1965], whilst Patricia Churchland [1986] in her book on neurophilosophy suggested how the analysis of the underlying brain functions could be advantageously performed with an investigation focused on purposeful actions like speech.

The importance of neuropsycholinguistic studies of patients affected by schizophrenia has recently been analysed by Crow [1993] and underlined by Thomas and Fraser [1994] in a general review on this subject (see also Appendix 2). Since 1978 Rochester had put forward the idea that disordered speakers might have particular problems in encoding and retrieval from short-term memory. However, this might be only the first step on the way towards specific experimental investigations. As pointed out in the same year by Sternberg et al. [1978], the studies of verbal motor control and vocal performance in normals showed that this methodology allows us to differentiate short-term memory from motor programme buffer versus retrieval of subprogramme for speech.

In fact, short-term memory concerns some items to be intentionally seized for a few minutes after their 'presentation'. It should be differentiated, at both conceptual and semiological levels, from the conscious processes taking place at an intermediary phase of the brain control of speech and allowing the invariant command to be transmitted to the executive system. These last unconscious processes correspond to the so-called active dynamic or working (according to Baddeley [1992]) memory.

Hoffman et al. [1986] carried out a discourse analysis in schizophrenics and discovered a failure of planning and general discourse proposition. In a further linguistic research, Harvey et al. [1986] stated that the alterations occurring in these processes could characterize schizophrenics with respect to manic patients. Further analyses of syntax in schizophrenics were performed by Thomas and by Fraser [1994], Hoffman et al. [1986] and by Thomas et al. [1993] who found consistent alterations.

An interpretation of the functional brain impairment underlying the mentioned language disorders in schizophrenics has been outlined since 1986 by Morice, who suggested that an alteration, like simplicity of speech, found in these patients could arise from a dysfunction in the dorsolateral prefrontal cortex. Both McGrath's studies [1991] and those of

Barr et al. [1989] suggested that the prefrontal cortex is the site that can be most likely associated with communication disorders in schizophrenia, given the importance of this area in planning. According to George et al. [1992], in autistic speech, both the frontal and the right temporal region seem to be implicated.

Eye tracking dysfunctions of genetic origin have been found in schizophrenic patients [Holtzman et al., 1988] to be associated with working memory deficits [Holtzman et al., 1995]. A consistent study of the deficiency in working memory and attention occurring in schizophrenics was published in 1993 by Thomas et al., who claimed that further research was necessary to better define the specific processes altered in these patients, particularly in the acute phase of the disease.

The newly developed methodology with verbal choice reactions including foreperiods after stimulus task presentation [Pinelli and Ceriani, 1992; Pinelli, 1993] named MDRV yielded promising data. It allowed us in fact to investigate the brain processes related to initiation [Gracco, 1987], psychomotor programmation, intermediary processes and execution of purposeful complex sequential actions like speech. Particular attention must be given to the evaluation of what pertains to task-independent processes (as mental delayed operations) rather than to task-dependent processes (more specifically speech).

The elaboration of the set of tests and criteria of evaluation in the specific area of schizophrenia required a preliminary definition of the functional mental impairment in this disease and the delimitation of the primary disorder. This requirement implies the reconsideration, on a more objective base, of the question formulated by Bleuler [1993] about the chain of deficits, secondary effects and tentative compensation that give rise to the symptoms of the schizophrenic dissociation, autism and reality distortion [Maier et al., 1992; Franke et al., 1994].

Hence two main points are discussed in this Introduction: (1) the hypofrontality hypothesis and (2) the results of experimental research carried out in the cases of selective functional prefrontal impairment.

9.5.1.1
Hypofrontality and Schizophrenia

A structural basis for schizophrenia has been theorized by recent progresses in neurochemistry and neuropharmacology [Crow et al. 1976; Snyder, 1981; Owens et al., 1982; Miller et al., 1992] and it has also been supported by neuroradiological findings of morphological brain abnormalities and alterations in cerebral regional blood flow [Gur et al., 1983].

In the context of the functional hyperactivity of dopamine in the brain of patients affected by schizophrenia, it has been argued that the mesocortical system may be the dopaminergic tract (to the A9 and A10 areas of the mesencephalon) most relevant to schizophrenia [Chiodo and Bunney, 1983; White and Wang, 1983]. Particular attention has been directed to the dorsolateral prefrontal cortex: psychometric testing suggests that this region may function quite poorly in schizophrenia and that its dysfunction may be correlated with mesocortical hyperdopaminergia [Weinberger et al., 1988]. A decrease in serotonin receptors in prefrontal areas has also been considered [Bleich et al., 1990].

On a neurofunctional and developmental related model, thanks to the sophisticated battery of experimental techniques in the laboratory [Alvisatos, 1992] and detailed visualization of functioning human brains, an increasing number of data was accumulated on the association of the frontal lobes (hypofrontality) with schizophrenia. The following are particularly consistent:

(1) blood flow in the dorsolateral prefrontal cortex is abnormally low following challenge with relevant cognitive tasks [Weinberger et al., 1992];
(2) there are reduced numbers of neurons in parts of the prefrontal cortex [Benes et al., 1991];
(3) the distribution of nitric-oxide-synthase-containing neurons is abnormal in frontal white matter in post-mortem tissue from schizophrenics [Akbarian, 1993a,b];
(4) molecular resonance spectroscopy suggested that there is an increased membrane breakdown in the frontal cortex of schizophrenic patients [Ebmeier et al., 1993; Ebmeier, 1994];
(5) PET revealed that the frontal cortex is functionally affected in schizophrenia [Andreasen et al.; 1992]; poverty of speech is associated with decreased flow in the left dorsolateral prefrontal cortex [Frith, 1995]. Limbic system abnormalities have been identified by Tanninga et al. [1992] with PET and by Weinberger et al. [1992] with MRI.

A critical involvement of dopaminergic neurons in the frontal cortex has been suggested to occur in developmental phases before signs and symptoms of psychomotor poverty [Bleuler, 1993] become evident. On the grounds of the most recent results of research with blood flow in the brain, other authors interpreted the prefrontal impairment in schizophrenia as a disconnection between the prefrontal and the temporal systems, where the reality distortion syndrome has been associated.

Rappelsberger and Weiss [1995] carried out systematic researches with electroglottogram coherence analyses during cognitive processes and found that some changes occur in schizophrenic patients, particularly in the *negative syndrome* [Andreasen, 1982; Klinidis et al., 1993].

9.5.1.2
Functional Investigation of Prefrontal Processes: Changes of Delayed Response with Impaired Frontal Function

It was found in primates that cooling the prefrontal cortex leads to impairments in delayed response tasks, regardless of the modality of how the task is performed. Neuropsychological research on prefrontal-dependent delayed reactions in man has been carried out by Kowalska et al. [1991]. The deficit in delayed responses reflects the fact that pyramidal neurons, not anatomically segregated but intermingled, might code for active memory and for motor set [Fuster, 1993].

We may thus agree with Fuster that, in terms of a delayed response task, 'the separated types of neurons have important functions in the animals that must retain information through a period of delay before a response is executed'. As we reported previously (5.2.2), these mnemonic and motor set functions seem 'to lay a bridge from perception to action across time'. They are in fact crucial to the organization and planning of behaviour, communicating with the premotor and motor cortices involved in collaboration with a variety of subcortical structures, in the execution of action, that is, in our case, of speaking.

Everitt et al. [1994] outlined the general circuitry involved in the pavlovian conditions and then in behaviour. Certainly the actual natural performances require the activation of many brain structures organized in loops: the prefrontal cortex, hippocampus (ventral subiculum) and basolateral amygdala with outflow via the ventral pallidum, mediodorsal nucleus of the thalamus (which also returns information to the frontal cortex), midbrain and pons. Moreover, the nucleus accumbens, interacting with other limbic structures, acts as a focus for several structures concerned with the gain of control by environmental stimuli over behaviour.

9.5.2
A Neurophysiological Model of Schizophrenia

Frith's [1992] model of the neurophysiological basis of schizophrenia (in particular the positive symptoms) places emphasis on an impairment of the prefrontal-cingular-entorhinal loops. It is known that these intermediary circuits normally interact between the limbic system and the basal ganglia, exerting a 'semantic' analysis or evaluation of the outcome of action [Gray, 1994]: such a recurring interaction appears as an internal feedback or working memory.

We can then wonder if the impairment of the intermediary processes, demonstrated with the investigation of the verbal control (MDRV), may represent an event of a more generalized failure of reverberating circuits in internal loops related to semantic and evaluating operations. The origin of this generalized deficit could be searched in the decrease found to occur in mesocortical dopaminergic innervation of the prefrontal dorsolateral cortex which, in its turn, produces [Gray, 1994] an enhanced dopaminergic activity of the mesolimbic system [Weinberger, 1987]. A decrease in *latent inhibition* with reference to attentional processes has been considered by Rawlins [1991].

9.5.3
Personal Investigations with Multiple-Delayed-Reaction Verbochronometry

9.5.3.1
A Serendipity: Investigation of Iatrogenic Parkinsonism Leads to the Discovery of a 'Schizophrenic' Impairment of 1.5-Second Delayed Reactions

The results of an investigation carried out in early 1994 [Pasetti et al., 1994] on iatrogenic parkinsonism have just been reported (see 9.4). The unexpected finding of significantly impaired 1.5-second delayed reactions made us investigate changes of intermediary process ratios in schizophrenia including patients without Parkinson-like iatrogenic syndromes, in acute and chronic phases, early phases of normal intervals with clinical recovery and residual state.

At the same time, the intermediary process ratio was evaluated in the material so far investigated, while patients affected by manic-depressive psychosis and obsessive-compulsive psychosis were expressly included in the new study.

Table 29. Schizophrenic patients

No.	Patient	Ext.	Age years	Sex	Disease duration	Active symptoms	Residual syndrome
1 (111)	P.R. x		41	M	18		×
2 (112)	P.R. y	×	50	F	23		×
3 (112)	A.A.	×	43	M	15		×
4 (106)	G.C.	×	58	M	17		×
5 (107)	P.A. x	×	34	M	13	×	
6 (105)	D.M.	×	42	M	16		×
7 (111)	P.A. y		43	M	18		×
8 (110)	V.M.		56	M	27		×
9 (108)	P.G.		50	M	25		×
10 (112)	R.P.		46	F	9	×	
11 (112)	P.F.		42	M	20		×
12 (109)	A.C.	×	43	F	10		×

Corresponding figures are indicated in parentheses. Ext. = Extrapyramidal signs.

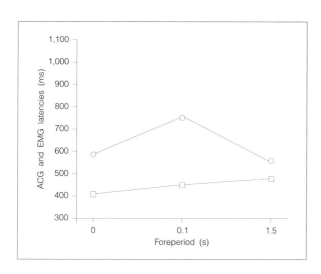

Fig. 105. ACG (○) and EMG (□) latencies of patient No. 6, D.M., male, 42 years old, with hebephrenic schizophrenia for 16 years, treated with Depo-Medrol at a medium-high dosage.

9.5.3.2
Primary Increases in Intermediary Process Ratio in Schizophrenia

9.5.3.2.1
Chronic Schizophrenia: Cases and Methodology

We have investigated 12 schizophrenic patients, with a duration of the clinical symptoms in a range of 9–27 years. Six of them presented extrapyramidal signs induced by the neuroleptic treatment, with a mean age of 50 ± 15 years, and 6 were free of extrapyramidal signs, with a mean age 46 ± 5 years.

The main clinical features of all schizophrenics are given in table 29 that includes a reference to corresponding figures of MDRV results of single patients (fig. 105–111) and one small group of patients

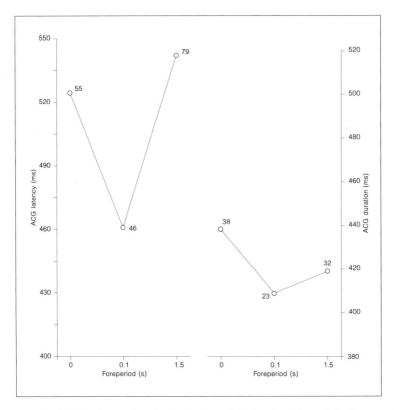

Fig. 106. ACG latencies (t) and durations (D) of patient No. 4, G.C., 58 years old, with chronic schizophrenia, treated with Akineton. Figures near symbols indicate SD.

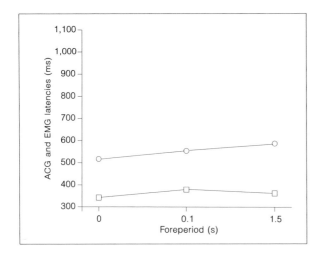

Fig. 107–110. ACG (○) and EMG (□) latencies of schizophrenic patients.

107 Patient No. 5, P.A. x, male, 34 years old, with chronic paranoid schizophrenia for 13 years, treated with Depo-Medrol at a medium dosage and chlorpromazine (25 mg/day).

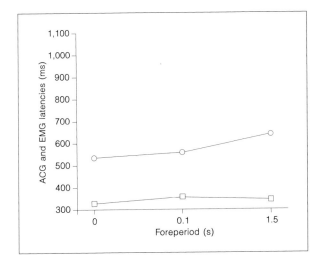

108 Patient No. 9, P.G., male, 50 years old, with chronic paranoid schizophrenia with acute attacks for 25 years, treated with haloperidol at a medium dosage.

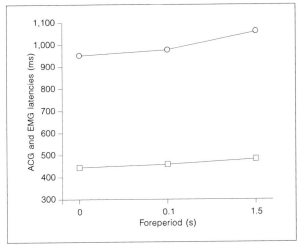

109 Patient No. 12, A.C., female, 43 years old, with chronic paranoid schizophrenia for 10 years, treated with haloperidol at a medium dosage for 7 years.

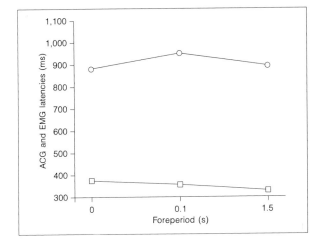

110 Patient No. 8, V.M., male, 56 years old, with chronic paranoid schizophrenia for 27 years, treated with haloperidol at a medium-high dosage for 28 years.

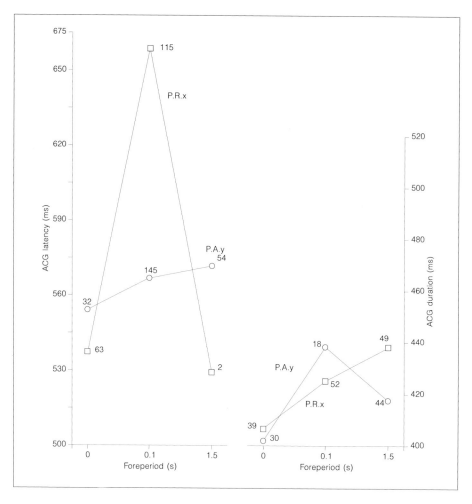

Fig. 111. ACG latencies (t) and durations (D) of schizophrenic patients No. 1, P.R. x, male, 41 years old, and No. 7, P.A. y, male, 43 years old. Figures near symbols indicate SD.

with similar results (fig. 112). Ten out of these patients were classified as having negative syndromes, and they were in the residual state. The other 2, at the moment of the examination, still presented positive symptoms with delusions and acoustic hallucinations.

Reaction times of ACG and EMG from the orbicularis oris muscle were recorded with the methodology previously reported. The equipment consisted of two computer-based units: the word presenter and the signal acquisition system [Colombo et al., 1993].

The stimulus in this first group of cases consisted in reading two words presented at random in a series of 12 each – /mare/ and /muro/ – with two different modalities of reaction: (1) an immediate reaction and (2) delayed reactions with foreperiods of 0.1 and 1.5 ms. Some patients were tested with the triple task /ma/, /mare/ and /mare è bello/. The subject was instructed to give the response as soon as the asterisks were added to the word stimulus displayed on the screen.

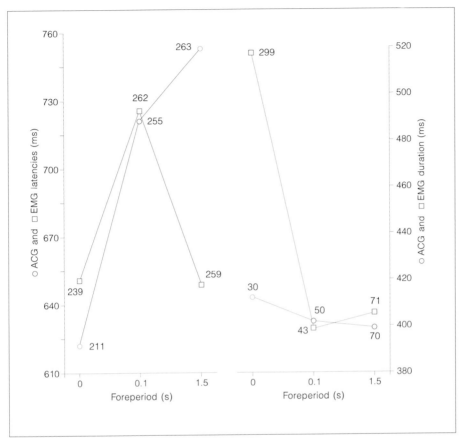

Fig. 112. Mean values of ACG (○) and EMG (□) obtained from 4 schizophrenic patients with dysarthric mannerisms, 42–52 years old: No. 2, P. R. y; No. 3, A.A.; No. 10, R. P., and No. 11, P.F. Figures near symbols indicate SD.

9.5.3.2.2
Results

9.5.3.2.2.1
Normal Controls

The mean values and SD of normal controls are included in table 30. The intermediary process ratio at FP$_{1.5}$ is <0.9 in the 41 normal controls, 16–45 years old, with a mean value of 0.61 ± 0.16. The intermediary process ratio was evaluated in these subjects also for FP$_{0.5}$: 0.89 ± 0.17 for /muro/, 0.83 ± 0.11 for /mare/. The early process ratio was 0.89 ± 0.11. In the older group (n = 55; 46–81 years old), higher values were found for both intermediary (0.76 ± 0.29) and early process ratios (0.99 ± 0.17).

Table 30. Neurological patients

	n	IR	ER
Normals			
16–45 years	41	0.61 ± 0.16	0.89 ± 0.11
46–81 years	55	0.76 ± 0.29	0.99 ± 17
AP	7	0.68 ± 0.09	0.97 ± 12
HMSN	14	0.69 ± 11	0.91 ± 12
ALS	52	0.73 ± 0.08	0.94 ± 10
MFCV	16	0.80 ± 12	1.08 ± 0.13
TNPI	9	0.88 ± 13	1.22 ± 0.14
FD	13	0.76 ± 0.14	0.97 ± 12
PD	14	0.87 ± 0.13	1.32 ± 0.26
AD	18	0.92 ± 0.14	1.51 ± 0.35

IR = Intermediary process ratio; ER = early process ratio; AP = acquired polyneuropathy; HMSN = hereditary motor-sensory neuropathy; ALS = amyotrophic lateral sclerosis; MFCV = multifocal cerebrovascular disease; TNPI = traumatic neuropsychiatric impairments; FD = focal motor disorder; PD = Parkinson disease; AD = Alzheimer disease.

Table 31. Schizophrenic patients without extrapyramidal signs

No.	Patient	Disease duration	Age years	ACG latency, ms			IR	ER
				FP_0	$FP_{0.1}$	$FP_{1.5}$		
7	P.A. y	18	43	513 ± 82	530 ± 71	567 ± 47	1.10	1.03
8	V.M.	27	56	879 ± 91	936 ± 176	848 ± 285	0.96	1.06
1	P.R. x	18	41	585 ± 92	716 ± 93	555 ± 90	0.94	1.22
9	P.G.	25	50	549 ± 134	563 ± 88	644 ± 202	1.17	1.02
11	P.F.	20	42	632 ± 133	711 ± 147	590 ± 101	0.93	1.12
10	R.P.	9	46	473 ± 47	633 ± 43	707 ± 60	1.49	1.33

IR = Intermediary process ratio; ER = early process ratio.

9.5.3.2.2.2

Patients with Chronic Schizophrenia

In schizophrenic patients, the main change is represented by the values of ACG latency at $FP_{1.5}$ with respect to those at FP_0. The mean values of ACG latency at FP_0 and at $FP_{1.5}$ in schizophrenics without extrapyramidal signs are 605 ± 145 and 651 ± 111 ms, respectively (table 31).

The analogous values in schizophrenics with extrapyramidal signs (table 25, 9.4.5; fig. 113) are 673 ± 180 and 772 ± 177 ms. The intermediary process ratio at $FP_{1.5}$ was >1.00 in 3 patients without extrapyramidal signs and in 3 with extrapyramidal signs. The mean values of these 6 patients in comparison to normal controls and other neuropsychiatric patients are given in figure 113. The remaining 3 cases without extrapyramidal signs have intermediary process ratios ≥ 0.93. One of the patients with extrapyramidal signs had a ratio of 0.97, one of 0.85 and one of 0.65. The mean intermediary process ratio at $FP_{1.5}$ for all schizophrenics (22–52 years old) was 1.11 ± 0.28, while the early process ratio was 0.87 ± 0.12.

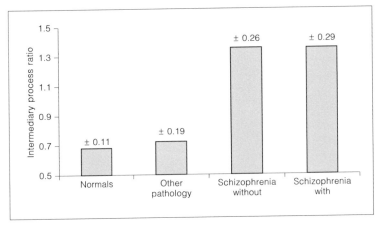

Fig. 113. Intermediary process ratios ($FP_{1.5}$ vs. FP_0) of normals, schizophrenics with and without extrapyramidal signs and patients with other pathologies.

The intermediary process ratio at $FP_{0.5}$ was also found to be significantly increased in 10 out of the 12 patients with a mean value of 1.04 ± 0.22.

The highest intermediary process ratios at $FP_{1.5}$ were observed at a duration of the disease of 13 (1.35) and 15 years (1.73).

One patient (P.R.) with a ratio of 0.94 was retested with double and triple tasks at an interval of 3 months, while he was under antidopaminergic treatment; the intermediary process ratio at $FP_{1.5}$ increased from 0.94 to 1.02 (table 32A, B).

9.5.3.3
Findings in Recent Schizophrenia with Positive Syndrome

A complete investigation with MDRV (including both double and triple tasks) was carried out in 5 young subjects affected by schizophrenia for 6–19 months. Two of them were under a moderate-high dose of Valium. The other 3 had been free from antidopaminergic treatment for 48 h.

9.5.3.3.1
Description of the Clinical Syndrome and the Result of Multiple-Delayed-Reaction Verbochronometry

A complete description of the clinical syndrome and the result of MDRV is given for 1 patient of the last group of 3 recent cases, without Valium (table 33).

C.S., male, 22 years. Introverted, asthenic personality. Since 1993 (19 months before the present MDRV) he had experienced verbal acoustic (from known people), visual (strange images on the walls of his house) and somato-aesthetic hallucinations, depersonalization, pseudo-hallucinations and a feeling of 'having in his hands some people who were not seen by the bystanders'. In the following month, he left the family house for half a day, without any information to his parents, wandering without any apparent purpose (a 'fugue'). More recently, he had been affected by manierisms with iterative flexions of his knees. Episodes of pseudo-anxiety and psychalgias occurred often in the week. Haloperidol was

Table 32. Test and retest of patient P.R. with chronic schizophrenia

A. *ACG latencies and durations (ms)*

	/mare/	/muro/	/ma/	/mare/	/mare è bello/
First examination					
Latency at FP_0	582	582	–	–	–
Duration at FP_0	430	414	–	–	–
Latency at $FP_{0.1}$	750	669	–	–	–
Duration at $FP_{0.1}$	463	451	–	–	–
Latency at $FP_{1.5}$	555	535	–	–	–
Duration at $FP_{1.5}$	467	451	–	–	–
Second examination					
Latency at FP_0	458	365	464	484	534
Duration at FP_0	498	440	412	510	1005
Latency at $FP_{0.1}$	707	597	597	534	602
Duration at $FP_{0.1}$	521	597	444	590	932
Latency at $FP_{1.5}$	466	509	539	396	490
Duration at $FP_{1.5}$	526	521	443	532	991
Latency at $FP_{0.5}$	571	605	–	–	–
Duration at $FP_{0.5}$	485	524	–	–	–
Latency at FP_4	369	412	–	–	–
Duration at FP_4	560	541	–	–	–

B. *Early (ER) and intermediary (IR) process ratios*

	/mare/, /muro/		/ma/	/mare/	/mare è bello/
	first examination	second examination			
ER	1.25	1.5	1.3	1.1	1.1
IR					
ACG latency	0.96	1.02	1.16	0.87	0.91
ACG duration	1.24	1.35	1.16	1.12	0.93

Table 33. Patient C.S. with acute schizophrenia

	/mare/, /muro/	/ma/	/mare/	/mare è bello/
ER	1.09	1.3	1.25	0.92
IR				
ACG latency at $FP_{1.5}$	0.99	0.96	1.01	1.13
ACG duration at $FP_{1.5}$	1.05	1.00	1.09	1.20
ACG latency at $FP_{0.5}$	1.1	–	–	–
ACG duration at $FP_{0.5}$	1.2	–	–	–

ER = Early process ratio; IR = intermediary process ratio.

administered at moderate doses for short periods at the beginning of 1994 and again in the last month before the MDRV, associated with tricyclics in the latter period.

The treatment was interrupted by his physician 24 h before the present investigation. On the day of the investigation, the patient was well oriented and compliant. He complained only of some abnormal sensations in his body.

The results of the MDRV are reported in table 33. The intermediary process ratio is increased not only for the ACG latencies (0.96–1.13) but also for the ACG duration (1.09–1.2).

The values of ACG latency at $FP_{1.5}$ were practically unchanged for /mare/ in the triple task and in the double task, being 509 ± 98 and 532 ± 36 ms, respectively.

The ACG latency was shorter for the sentence than for the monosyllable and disyllabic word in immediate as well as in delayed reactions: the ratio ACG latency for the sentence to ACG latency for the monosyllable is 0.9 in spite of a very high ratio of ACG duration for the sentence with respect to ACG duration for the monosyllable which reached 3.4.

It is worth underlining that in double-task reactions, the ACG latency of /mare/ (and analogously of /muro/) reaches the highest value at $FP_{0.5}$ (619 ± 121 ms) with an ACG latency at FP_0 of 532 ± 36 ms; at $FP_{1.5}$, it was 583 ± 97 ms. We note also the same to occur for ACG duration that at $FP_{0.5}$ was 367 ± 17 ms, at FP_0 300 ± 21 ms and at $FP_{1.5}$ 330 ± 121 ms.

9.5.3.3.2
Recent Schizophrenics Who Present an Increase in Intermediary Process Ratio Limited to $FP_{0.5}$

The intermediary process ratio at $FP_{1.5}$ was normal in 2 young patients (17 and 20 years old) who were investigated with MDRV, free of drugs for 48 h. The values of ACG latency at FP_0 were in the normal range and shorter for the sentence with respect to the monosyllable and disyllabic word. The value of ACG latency at $FP_{0.1}$ was also slightly diminished with an early process ratio <0.88.

In contrast, ACG latency greatly increased at $FP_{0.5}$ with a high intermediary process ratio (>1.01), particularly for the sentence with values of 1.27 and 1.33.

9.5.3.3.3
Recent Schizophrenics under Valium

In 2 patients who were examined with MDRV without antidopaminergic treatment but under a high dosage of Valium, we found a 16–21% increase in ACG latencies in immediate reactions, with a decrease, even if moderate, in the delayed reactions particularly at $FP_{1.5}$. The intermediary process ratio at $FP_{1.5}$ remained in the normal range (0.60 and 0.74) and was only slightly higher at $FP_{0.5}$ (0.81 and 0.89). In one of these patients, MDRV was repeated after 2 months, without Valium, under antidopaminergic treatment; the intermediary process ratio at $FP_{1.5}$ rose from 0.60 to 0.84, that at $FP_{0.5}$ from 0.81 to 0.93.

9.5.4
Statistical Evaluation of Intermediary Process Ratio in Schizophrenia with Respect to Normals and the Other Neurological and Psychiatric Patients

The increase in intermediary process ratio found in schizophrenics is highly significant as it is reported in tables 34–39 by Student's t test and Anova evaluated for schizophrenics versus normal controls (ACG latency, early and intermediary process ratios) and versus tremulous and akinetic parkinsonian patients.

Table 34. Evaluation of ages of normal subjects and schizophrenic patients

Group	Count	Mean	SD	SE
B	16	44.25	9.26	1.64
A	13	43.85	9.22	2.56

Unpaired t test; X_1: column 23; Y_1: ETA1; d.f.: 43; unpaired t value: 0.13; p (2-tailed): 0.895; group: A = schizophrenics, B = normals; count: number of subjects; mean: mean age (years).

Table 35. Evaluation of intermediary process ratios obtained from normals and schizophrenic patients (positive + negative syndromes)

A. *Unpaired t test*

Group	Count	Mean	SD	SE
B	32	0.807	0.133	0.024
A	13	1.110	0.286	0.079

X_1: column 23; Y_1: intermediary process ratios of normals; d.f.: 43; unpaired t value: –4.887; p (2-tailed): 0.0001; for other explanations, see table 34.

B. *One-factor Anova – repeated measures for X_1–X_2*

Source	d.f.	Sum of squares	Mean square	F test	p value
Between subjects	9	0.64	0.07	0.79	0.6321
Within subjects	10	0.90	0.09		
Treatments	1	0.44	0.44	8.49	0.0172
Residuals	9	0.46	0.05		
Total	19	1.54			

Reliability estimates for all treatments: –0.26, for a single treatment: –0.12. Note: 50 cases deleted with missing values.

Group	Count	Mean	SD	SE
Schizophrenics	10	1.12	0.32	0.10
Normals	10	0.82	0.13	0.04

Comparison	Mean difference	Fisher PLSD	Scheffé F test	Dunnett t
Schizophrenics vs. normals	0.3	0.23*	8.49*	2.91

PLSD = A Fisher's test of evaluation.
*Significant at 95%.

Table 36. Evaluation of early process ratios obtained from normals and schizophrenic patient

Group	Count	Mean	SD	SE
B	16	0.98	0.1	0.02
A	12	1.2	0.31	0.09

Unpaired t test; X_1: column 19; Y_1: early process ratios of normals d.f.: 42; unpaired t value: –3.56; p (2-tailed): 0.0009; for other explanations, see table 34.

Table 37. Evaluation of intermediary process ratios obtained from normals and schizophrenic patients

Group	Count	Mean	SD	SE
B	16	0.81	0.13	0.02
A	13	1.11	0.29	0.08

Unpaired t test; X_1: column 23; Y_1: intermediary process ratios of normals d.f.: 43; unpaired t value: –4.89; p (2-tailed): 0.0001; for other explanations, see table 34.

Table 38. Evaluation of intermediary process ratios obtained from tremulous parkinsonian patients and schizophrenics (positive + negative syndromes); one-factor Anova – repeated measures for X_1–X_2

Source	d.f.	Sum of squares	Mean square	F test	p value
Between subjects	11	0.55	0.05	0.32	0.9656
Within subjects	12	1.86	0.16		
Treatments	1	1.07	1.07	14.90	0.0027
Residuals	11	0.79	0.07		
Total	23	2.41			

Reliability estimates for all treatments: –2.12, for a single treatment: –0.52. Note: 48 cases deleted with missing values.

Group	Count	Mean	SD	SE
Schizophrenics	12	1.13	0.29	0.08
Tremulous PD patients	12	0.71	0.20	0.06

Comparison	Mean difference	Fisher PLSD	Scheffé F test	Dunnett t
Schizophrenics vs. Tremulous PD patients	0.42	0.24*	14.9*	3.86

PD = Parkinson disease; for other explanation, see tables 34 and 35.
* Significant at 95%.

Table 39. Evaluation of intermediary process ratios obtained from akinetic parkinsonian patients and schizophrenics (positive + negative syndromes); one-factor Anova – repeated measures for X_1–X_2

Source	d.f.	Sum of squares	Mean square	F test	p value
Between subjects	11	0.61	0.06	0.54	0.8407
Within subjects	12	1.24	0.10		
Treatments	1	0.75	0.75	17.08	0.0017
Residuals	11	0.48	0.04		
Total	23	1.85			

Reliability estimates for all treatments: –0.85, for a single treatment: –0.3. Note 48 cases deleted with missing values.

Group	Count	Mean	SD	SE
Akinetic PD patients	12	0.72	0.16	0.05
Schizophrenics	12	1.08	0.27	0.08

Comparison	Mean difference	Fisher PLSD	Scheffé F test	Dunnett t
Akinetic PD patients vs. schizophrenics	–0.35	0.19*	17.08*	4.13

PD = Parkinson disease; for other explanations, see tables 34 and 35.
*Significant at 95%.

A critical question is raised by non-schizophrenic patients who show an increase in intermediary process ratio. Our studies reveal that these cases are exceptional with MDRV and can be classified in the following two areas: (1) cases with moderate frontal lesions; (2) cases with impairments of short-term memory interfering with the normal activity of the working memory. A detailed analysis of these cases will be given in the next chapters and particularly in 9.8.

9.5.5
Inversion of the Intermediary Process Ratio in Schizophrenia and Its Relation to Impairment of Working Memory and Hypofrontality

The meaning of the inversion of the intermediary process ratio can be evaluated correctly if we follow the principles and criteria reported in Section 7.

The inversion is specifically due to an increase in ACG latency at $FP_{1.5}$, while no increase is found in most cases (particularly with positive syndrome) in ACG latency at FP_0. Therefore its dependence upon an alteration of the intermediary processes, and more likely upon working memory, can be inferred beyond any doubt.

Short-term memory was not impaired at the neuropsychological examinations. The executive processes and related parameters (threshold, sensorimotor conduction evaluated by visual-evoked potentials and electromagnetic muscle responses) were found to be in the normal range.

An analysis of the neural processes that can produce marked impairments of working memory will be carried out in 9.8 dealing with the interpretation of the psychophysiological data collected with MDRV in the whole psychiatric area.

Particular attention must be given to two issues: (1) the increase appears to be limited to the short foreperiod of 0.5 s in the early phases of the positive syndromes in young patients; (2) Valium administration, at variance with the antidopaminergic treatment, seems to exert a 'making effect' on the failure of acceleration of the delayed with respect to the immediate reactions.

(1) The normal reaction time at a very short foreperiod cancels the role of alterations affecting early programming processes. As a cause of the increase in delayed reaction times, we may consider a factor linked to an increase in the threshold of the neural assemblies that must be facilitated to trigger the executive systems. Likewise it could be a matter of slowed internal reverberating circuits that are normally involved in this facilitation process. One can infer that these impairments are slight in the first phase of the disease so that a longer delay is sufficient to compensate for the abnormal retarding factors.

(2) A masking effect of pharmaceutical agents like Valium that exert inhibitory effects in frontosubcortical synapses could be explained if we take into account the hypotheses of a failure of de-activation processes as a main functional alteration in schizophrenia. This has been inferred from a systematic PET and functional MRI investigation in schizophrenic patients by Frith [1995].

···

Obsessive-Compulsive Disorders

According to Gray [1994], the obsessive-compulsive disorders might be due to a hyperactivity of the septohippocampal comparative system. The primary impairment is hypothesized by this author to affect the descending directive control normally exerted by the prefrontal cortex on the hippocampal system. Moreover, on the grounds of anatomo-clinical evidence, with particular evidence of the Gilles de la Tourette syndrome, Gray, in agreement with Model et al. [1989] and Rapaport and Wise [1988], considers an associated hyperactivity of the corticogangliobasal system for the physiopathogenesis of obsessive-compulsive disorders.

Since this alteration could involve the temporal development of the intermediary processes that are investigated with MDRV, we submitted to this a patient affected for many years by a chronic form of obsessive-compulsive disorder and who had not responded to treatment with serotonergic drugs.

Since his adolescence, P.L., male, 53 years, had shown an introverted character and attended to his jobs painstakingly, with a sometimes rather exaggerated diligence. For the last 20 years, he had complained of some difficulties in his professional work because of more persistent, disturbing mental rumination. For the last 6 years, he had been affected by rather severe psychosomatic disturbances and particularly belching, with anxiety and a tendency to sleepiness during some hours of the day.

The results of the MDRV are given in table 40. Both early and intermediary process ratios at $FP_{1.5}$ were extremely low with respect to normals, a result that is just contrary to the changes found in schizophrenia. Also the intermediary process ratio at $FP_{0.5}$ presented low values of 0.6–0.71.

This marked alteration emerging from MDRV spurred us to investigate another chronic case of obsessive-compulsive disorder (patient R.M.), and we found a similar decrease in early and intermediary process ratios. The values are reported in table 41 that includes 4 other cases with anxiety, 2 of them with associated phobias and 2 with secondary sensitive delusions ('Beziehungswahn', delusion of reference).

It can be seen from the table that, at variance with the marked decrease found in the 2 cases with obsessive-compulsive disorder, the 4 other patients affected by severe anxiety, phobias and sensitive delusions have intermediary process ratios within the normal range, even if at the lowest limit (see case B.A.).

We can thus stress the following two points.

(1) The marked decrease in early and intermediary process ratios represents a specific finding of obsessive-compulsive disorders and can be related to a situation of abnormal tachyphrenia involving both early programming parallel processes (as reflected in the decrease in early process ratio) and intermediary processes (as reflected in the decrease in intermediary process ratio).

One must underline that ACG latency at FP_0 was significantly increased in patient P.L. (table 40), and certainly this increase can play a role in the decrease in the intermediary process index. However, this is not the main cause of its low value: the most marked decrease was found in ACG latency at $FP_{>0.4}$.

Table 40. ACG latencies and durations (ms) of patient P.L., male, 53 years old, with obsessive-compulsive neurosis

	/ma/		/mare/		/mare è bello/	
	latency	duration	latency	duration	latency	duration
FP_0	473	191	509	358	657	947
$FP_{0.1}$	404	201	357	381	398	835
$FP_{0.5}$	293	215	300	350	337	992
$FP_{1.5}$	214	186	234	381	294	996
FP_4	284	222	302	403	371	1,155
ER	0.40	0.60	0.60			
IR	0.46	0.46	0.40			

ER = Early process ratio; IR = intermediary process ratio.

Table 41. Obsessive-compulsive disorder (OCD) and anxiety (ANX)

Subject	Age years	Sex	Syndrome	Intermediary process ratio		
				monosyllable	disyllable	sentence
R.M.	49	M	OCD	0.61	0.48	0.48
P.L.	53	M	OCD	0.45	0.46	0.46
M.G.	61	M	,ANX, phobia	0.86	0.86	0.75
B.A.	39	F	ANX, phobia	0.64	0.66	0.68
G.L.	58	M	ANX, delusion	0.88	0.80	0.84
P.L.	64	F	ANX, delusion	0.75	0.73	0.71
18 patients affected by schizophrenia				–	1.21*	–
10 controls	45–59	6 M, 4 F	normals	0.69	0.73*	0.74

*$p < 0.001$.

Moreover, the increase in ACG latency at FP_0 was somewhat smaller than in some schizophrenics who nevertheless showed an increase (see 9.5).

The increase in ACG latency at FP_0 was not found in patient R.M. affected by obsessive-compulsive disorder and it seems not to represent a specific change of this group of patients. Anyway, the increase in ACG latency at FP_0 found in P.L. was not associated with a higher accuracy of the response: a spectrographic frequency analysis of the ACG (see Sections 2 and 3) did not reveal any difference in comparison to normals.

(2) The absence of significant changes in MDRV in patients with severe anxiety but no obsessive-compulsive disorder is in line with the classical interpretation of the Italian and French school that clearly separated obsessions from phobias. In contrast, our findings are at variance with the opinion of some psychiatrists who ascribe the pathogenesis of both obsessive-compulsive disorders and severe incapacitating anxieties to a common impairment of corticosubcortical internal feedbacks that may be corrected by selective capsulotomy [Mindus and Nyman, 1991].

In conclusion, our findings are in agreement with Gray's hypothesis [1994] of a hyperactivity of the comparative corticogangliobasal systems. The consistency of our results with the neuropsychological investigations systematically carried out by Galderini [1995] is also intriguing.

With regard to the specificity of the decrease in the intermediary process ratio, it must be noted that it can be exceptionally observed in young subjects in the phase of recovery from traumatic injuries to the brain: in such cases, there is a marked increase in ACG latency at FP_0, in the order of 50% (from 400 to 600 ms), while ACG latency at $FP_{1.5}$ is relatively less increased. In other cases, the increase in ACG latency at FP_0 was very marked, in the order of 300%, with a rather high increase also in the delayed reactions so that the intermediary process ratio increased moderately. In these cases a great number of errors is made during MDRV, in a range of 17–28%; clinically, marked bradyphrenia is observed.

Depressive Psychoses

9.7.1
Stimulus Tasks with Concrete and Abstract Words

In previous investigations with MDRV of some depressive patients with pseudo-dementia we adopted different double tasks with pairs of concrete words and of abstract words [Pinelli et al., 1994]: /mare/, /muro/ and /virtù/, /vizio/, as we mentioned on page 102 (table 42).

We continued our research with 3 other patients in order to prove the previous result of an increase in reaction time to the concrete words: we compared the responses to /mare/, /muro/ and to /male/, /mito/. The results of normal controls are included in tables 42 and 43.

Table 42. Immediate and delayed verbal reactions (ms) to concrete and abstract words of the first two patients

		/mare/	/muro/	/virtù/	/vizio/
FP_0					
Healthy subjects	EMG	305 ± 39	289 ± 42	328 ± 46	322 ± 51
	ACG	541 ± 55	528 ± 65	560 ± 68	554 ± 51
Patient 1	EMG	312 ± 49	303 ± 51	346 ± 59	343 ± 63
	ACG	705 ± 81	686 ± 94	552 ± 74	563 ± 98
Patient 2	EMG	370 ± 58	349 ± 53	312 ± 38	307 ± 51
	ACG	790 ± 104	761 ± 90	573 ± 81	597 ± 87
$FP_{0.1}$					
Healthy subjects	EMG	313 ± 69	295 ± 73	360 ± 76	353 ± 90
	ACG	554 ± 109	548 ± 114	588 ± 164	591 ± 179
Patient 1	EMG	406 ± 78	376 ± 90	342 ± 84	361 ± 88
	ACG	785 ± 191	707 ± 159	571 ± 123	598 ± 160
Patient 2	EMG	378 ± 64	381 ± 86	322 ± 76	348 ± 83
	ACG	845 ± 204	786 ± 184	611 ± 140	645 ± 132
$FP_{1.5}$					
Healthy subjects	EMG	190 ± 36	174 ± 38	236 ± 36	231 ± 40
	ACG	420 ± 58	407 ± 63	486 ± 54	463 ± 59
Patient 1	EMG	204 ± 42	180 ± 47	211 ± 30	203 ± 35
	ACG	493 ± 83	501 ± 77	478 ± 51	482 ± 58
Patient 2	EMG	176 ± 39	149 ± 40	242 ± 46	222 ± 46
	ACG	475 ± 69	464 ± 60	447 ± 70	480 ± 63

Healthy subjects: n = 7; 60–66 years old.

Table 43. Depressive psychosis

A. *ACG Latencies (ms) of /male/ and /mito/*

		FP_0	$FP_{0.1}$	$FP_{1.5}$	IR	ER
Case 1	/male/	546 ± 55	564 ± 60	325 ± 51	0.59	1.02
	/mito/	555 ± 59	540 ± 69	312 ± 40		
Case 2	/male/	602 ± 59	615 ± 57	384 ± 58	0.61	1.01
	/mito/	590 ± 44	586 ± 50	375 ± 43		
Case 3	/male/	568 ± 46	577 ± 66	365 ± 42	0.63	1.02
	/mito/	572 ± 53	594 ± 67	365 ± 46		
Normals (n = 4, 47–70 years old)						
	/male/	578 ± 81	594 ± 89	340 ± 76	0.59	1.02
	/mito/	595 ± 78	593 ± 80	329 ± 73		

B. *ACG Latencies (ms) of /mare/ and /muro/*

Case	/mare/			/muro/			ER	IR
	FP_0	$FP_{0.1}$	$FP_{1.5}$	FP_0	$FP_{0.1}$	$FP_{1.5}$		
1	705 ± 81	785 ± 191	493 ± 83	686 ± 94	707 ± 159	501 ± 77	1.07	0.79
2	790 ± 104	845 ± 204	479 ± 69	761 ± 90	786 ± 184	464 ± 60	1.09	0.66
3	754 ± 90	778 ± 119	719 ± 81	711 ± 84	725 ± 105	708 ± 68	1.03	0.84

IR = Intermediary process ratio; ER = early process ratio.

We measured also the early and intermediary process ratios to allow a comparison with the findings of patients with obsessive-compulsive disorders (that some psychiatrists consider similar to depressive disorders both due to a common type of response to serotonergic drugs) and of schizophrenics (who nosologically border on schizo-affective disorders, a group of patients who are in between depressives and schizophrenics).

9.7.2
Results of the Last Three Cases

Case 1, A.F., female, 39 years, had a first episode of retarded depression at the age of 23 years. At that time she was successfully treated with electroconvulsive therapy (6 applications in 3 weeks). At 31 years of age, she showed a hypomanic episode that required treatment with major tranquillizers for 6 weeks. The last episode started 9 months before the MDRV examination, with mixed symptoms of logorrhoea, fugue of ideas, evanescent delusions of poisoning, abnormal interpersonal reactions and a pessimistic 'Grundstimmung'. She underwent MDRV while still treated with moderate doses of antidopaminergic drugs.

Some tracings and a diagram of the results with double tasks of the concrete words /mare/ and /muro/ are given in figure 114a–e. The corresponding values of /mare/, /muro/ and /male/, /mito/ of a normal control are given in table 44.

Table 44. P.F., male, 47 years old, normal subject

	FP$_0$				FP$_{0.1}$				FP$_{1.5}$			
	EMG		ACG		EMG		ACG		EMG		ACG	
	latency	duration	latency	duration	latency	duration	latency	duration	latency	duration	latency	duration
/mare/												
	471	559	501	301	371	606	455	291	213	654	304	338
	±91	±72	±74	±18	±39	±31	±42	±23	±31	±35	±46	±21
/muro/												
	300	674	456	301	292	670	459	286	160	621	312	304
	±21	±23	±48	±16	±44	±31	±65	±13	±442	±42	±29	±10
/mare/ + /muro/												
	350	623	475	300	333	634	458	298	184	637	309	320
	±86	±76	±66	±19	±65	±36	±56	±19	±42	±39	±41	±22
/male/												
	362	538	435	341	526	504	458	317	207	271	271	336
	±28	±57	±36	±41	±45	±33	±50	±11	±9	±17	±17	±8
/mito/												
	343	610	437	301	388	550	351	348	187	261	261	363
	±40	±68	±31	±89	±54	±52	±21	±8	±5	±11	±11	±19
/male/ + /mito/												
	351	569	436	321	320	519	398	332	193	269	269	353
	±38	±76	±37	±69	±75	±55	±62	±20	±15	±23	±23	±25

Latencies and durations are indicated in milliseconds.

Case 2, B.A., male, 62 years, had suffered from classic migraine since his childhood and from a duodenal ulcer since the age of 28 years. A first episode of depression occurred at 19 years and lasted 4 months. A second episode at 41 years required tricyclic drug treatment during 2 months. The last episode started 7 months before the present MDRV examination, with severe anxiety, early morning insomnia and taedium vitae. The pharmacological treatment (with tricyclics) was interrupted 8 days before MDRV.

Case 3, M.G., male, 65 years, had suffered from moderate blood hypotension since he was 7 years old. A first episode of depression occurred at the age of 51 years, when he decided to resign from his office. A moderate improvement was observed 2 years later, but the patient still complained of persisting psychosomatic sufferings. The last episode started 2 months before the MDRV examination, with severe symptoms of retarded depression and suicidal intentions. MDRV was carried out with the patient under a moderate treatment with tranquillizers.

The findings of MDRV in all 3 cases are reported in table 43A and B.

The 3 patients are characterized by a significant increase in reaction time for concrete words that are known to be processed by the non-dominant hemisphere. These results are in agreement with those of depressive patients published in a previous paper [Pinelli et al., 1994].

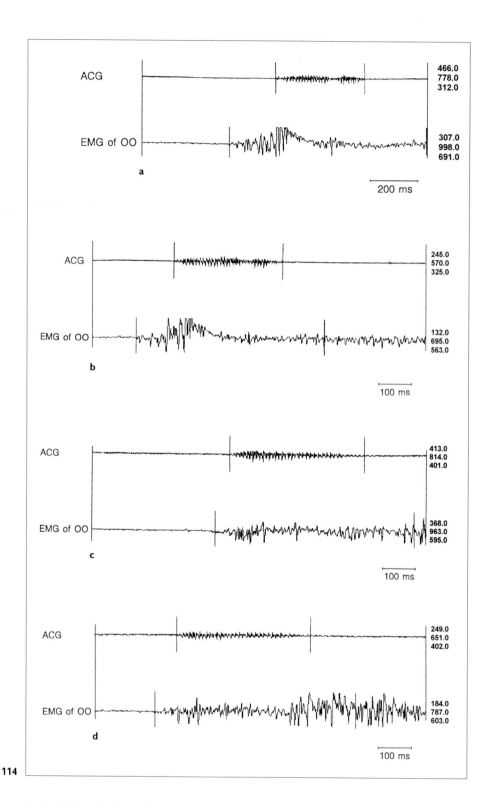

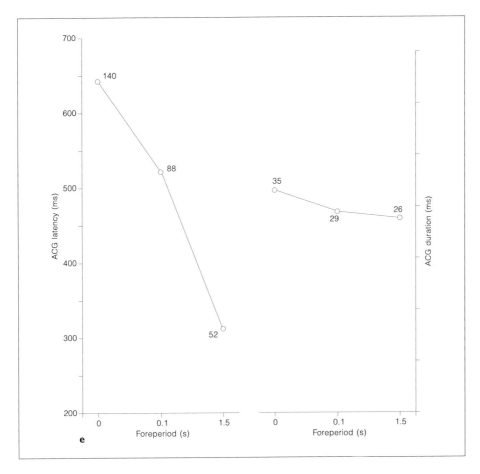

Fig. 114. Patient A.F., female, 39 years old. OO = Orbicularis oris muscle; figures on the right indicate latency times of response onset and end as well as response duration. /muro/, FP_0 (20th reaction, **a**) and $FP_{1.5}$ (8th reaction, **b**), and /mare/, FP_0 (22nd reaction, **c**) and $FP_{1.5}$ (**d**). **e** Mean (n=9) ACG latencies and durations of /mare/ and /muro/. Figures near symbols indicate SD.

On the other hand, intermediary process ratios were in the normal range.

We may add here that selective impairment of abstract word reactions was found in cerebrovascular lesions of the dominant (left) hemisphere. An example will be reported in the next chapter.

···

Mental Deterioration and Selective Short-Term Memory Impairments

9.8.1
Mental Deterioration

Mental deterioration represents one main area for fruitful investigation with MDRV. The early process index increases significantly: values up to 2, in association with a high number of errors, appear as a usual finding in the early phase of dementia.

The increase in ACG latency at $FP_{0.1}$, which is responsible for the increase in the early process ratio, can be attributed to neuronal loss in frontal and temporo-occipital associative areas leading to reduced availability of PDP. Intermediary processes may also be involved, but the change of the intermediary process ratio remains at a lower range than that of the early process ratio.

The MDRV findings for /mare/ and /muro/ of a single patient with early symptoms of Alzheimer dementia are reported in figure 115 and cumulatively of 3 other patients in figure 116. In figure 117, the MDRV findings of /ma/, /mare/ and /mare è bello/ are reported for a patient affected by olivopontocerebellar disease with mental deterioration.

Some consequences of aphasic impairments may also be fruitfully investigated with MDRV. This investigation can be added to the neuropsychological tests in relation to well-defined questions of controversy. With specific reference to paraphasias (see Section 3), it was demonstrated that temporal parameters of speech control may be significantly altered. The same author showed the great difficulties of identifying the site of a defined speech error and suggested that non-word reading tests can be used to eliminate, in the functional diagnosis, lexical and hence potential storage deficits. One must bear in mind that aphasic patients, especially those with conduction aphasia, may suffer problems at the input and end of such tests, which will affect repetition of such stimuli.

9.8.2
Selective Deficits: The Impairment of Active Short-Term Memory

The investigation with MDRV of the effects of a selective impairment of active short-term memory on reading reactions is particularly wanted to better analyse the repercussions it can exert on the temporal development of the intermediary processes and more precisely on working memory. The influence of impairments of 'intentional' short-term memory on the intermediary process ratio appears to be extremely critical for the evaluation of an aspecific increase in the intermediary process ratio independent of a failure of 'unconscious' working memory.

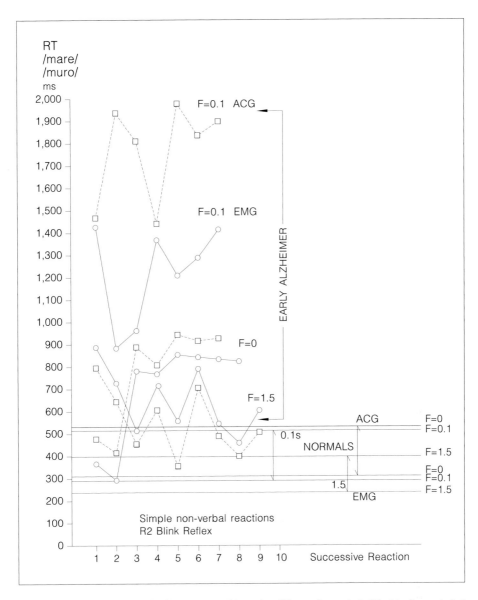

Fig. 115. Reaction times (RT) of /mare/ and /muro/ at different foreperiods (F). At a foreperiod of 0.1 s, blocking effect from parallel to serial processes. R2 = Polysynaptic response.

9.8.2.1

Differentiating Short-Term Memory from Working Memory

The term 'active short-term memory' is used by some authors in a rather broad sense [Pinker, 1995] so that working memory is sometimes considered as a component of short-term memory or as being, at last, closely associated with it.

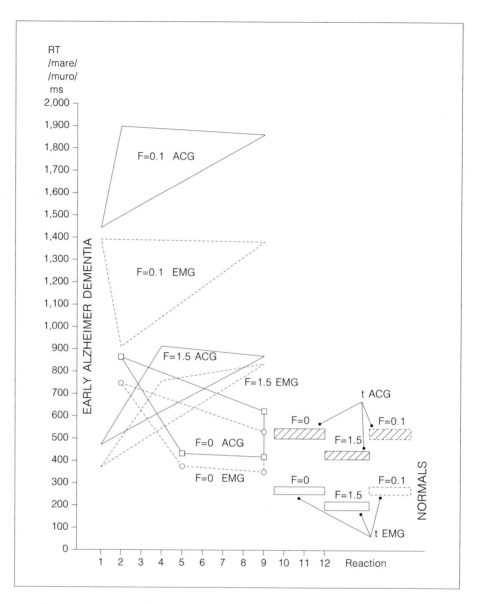

Fig. 116. Reaction times (RT) of /mare/ and /muro/ at different foreperiods (F). At a foreperiod of 0.1 s, blocking effect in early Alzheimer disease. On the left, distributions of ACG latencies (t) of 3 patients with early Alzheimer disease and impairment of short-term memory (intermediary process ratio >1) are shown, on the right the mean ACG latencies of 18 normal subjects.

In our investigations, very few patients with a moderate impairment of short-term memory showed an increase in the intermediary process ratio, and this happened also with the presentation of the word stimuli lasting during the whole foreperiod of the delayed reaction.

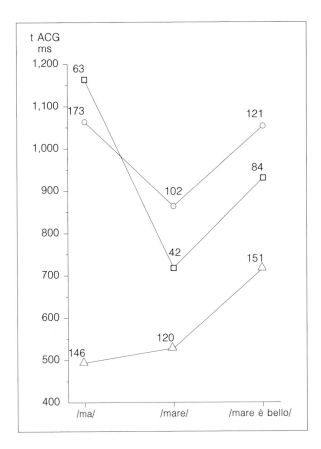

Fig. 117. ACG latencies (t) of patient A.E., female, 71 years old, with olivoponto-cerebellar disease. □ = FP$_0$; ○ = FP$_{0.1}$; △ = FP$_{1.5}$; figures near symbols indicate SD.

Before starting the analysis of our paradigmatic case, it seems right to recall some concepts of Baddeley [1985, 1992] of short-term and working memories, taking into account also the comment of Cornoldi [1995], which we quoted in 3.3.1.

Short-term memory is conceived as a system for the active maintenance of pieces of information that are necessary to psychic operations. This is the information on which the mind works, i.e. the information on the grounds of which, we think, understand, perceive, act, reason, decide, etc.

According to Baddeley [1992], the term 'working memory' implies a system for temporarily maintaining and handling information during the execution of different cognitive (and we can add psychomotor) tasks, as e.g. understanding, learning and reasoning (and we can add reading in delayed reactions).

Many investigations were carried out aiming to solve the problem whether the active short-term memory itself acts as working memory. The articulate model of working memory, as it has been elaborated after a decade of studies, provides for a central executive system requiring great attentive resources and numerous supporting systems that employ attentive resources sparingly and are committed to elaborate information related to specific modalities of perception and response. Two out of these systems have been particularly studied by Baddeley et al. [1984, 1986], i.e. the articulatory loop and the visuospatial 'sketch-pad', that are responsible for linguistic and visuospatial temporary maintenance.

Table 45. Patient C.A., female, 57 years old, with reversible ischaemic neurological deficit of the left cerebral hemisphere

	FP$_0$			FP$_{0.1}$		FP$_{1.5}$	
	EMG latency	ACG latency	ACG duration	EMG latency	ACG latency	EMG latency	ACG latency
After 1 month							
/mare/	354 ± 60	482 ± 64	381 ± 19	436 ± 60	548 ± 44	300 ± 52	431 ± 57
/muro/	311 ± 62	455 ± 53	369 ± 22	413 ± 102	550 ± 79	294 ± 132	479 ± 142
/vizio/	297 ± 47	583 ± 79	462 ± 79	342 ± 63	370 ± 120	293 ± 28	292 ± 86
/virtù/	303 ± 60	576 ± 84	496 ± 63	362 ± 78	665 ± 124	274 ± 33	555 ± 76
After 6 months							
/mare/	295 ± 36	468 ± 65	360 ± 21	408 ± 86	527 ± 104	228 ± 51	411 ± 39
/muro/	288 ± 41	449 ± 68	348 ± 27	374 ± 71	533 ± 92	232 ± 34	420 ± 46
/vizio/	257 ± 79	497 ± 69	441 ± 50	313 ± 104	581 ± 130	234 ± 56	484 ± 80
/virtù/	223 ± 77	490 ± 55	433 ± 69	278 ± 91	544 ± 103	221 ± 48	481 ± 63

Results are indicated in milliseconds.

The loop has been divided into a phonological store, committed to preserve information, and a reiterative active system (rehearsal) which assures the information to be maintained in the store. In this context, Logie and Reisberg [1992] have taken into consideration the occurrence of scanning sequential processes, in analogy with the eye scanning system.

The problem concerning the duration of short-term and working memories represents one of the most intricate points in Baddeley's model. The differentiations of what actually concerns the duration of traces in the passive store (that was calculated to be 1.5 or 2 s), echoic register and working memory were not clearly defined. Working memory is often interpreted as a trace-lengthening modality, a definition that is distorted by the wrong tendency to ignore the dynamic aspects of working memory (see Section 6).

Rehearsal processes were considered to occur in the passage to long-term memory, while their role in the facilitation of the executive module or facilitated neural assembly and the related time spent for it has been generally disregarded.

9.8.3
Cerebrovascular Lesions: Impairments of Abstract Word Reaction in Lesions of the Left Cerebral Hemisphere

In table 45, we report the findings of MDRV with reactions to /mare/, /muro/ and /vizio/, /virtù/ of a patient who suffered from a reversible ischaemic attack of the left (dominant) hemisphere. Signs of alteration in the territory of the frontoparietal branch of the left middle cerebral artery were detected by thermography and MRI. The patient had a right sensorimotor hemiparesis that regressed in the following 2 months.

MDRV was carried out 1 and 6 months after the attack.

A significant increase in ACG latency at FP$_0$ and, to a lower extent, at FP$_{0.1}$ and FP$_{1.5}$ was found in the first examination for the abstract word pair and particularly for /virtù/.

A Survey of Changes of the Intermediary Process Ratio in Psychiatric Patients

9.9.1
A Finding with Diagnostic Value for Schizophrenic Disorders

Clinical studies have analysed the cognitive impairment of severe psychiatric illness with particular regard to schizophrenia [Dunkley and Rogers, 1994]. As we have shown in the previous sections, we can today investigate the underlying neural dysfunctions. The most significant change ($p<0.0001$) emerging from our investigations with MDRV is the increase in ACG latency of 1.5-second delayed reactions in comparison with the immediate reaction ACG latency. This selective increase occurs in chronic schizophrenic patients and shows their inability to have normal access to the working memory making the programming commands available to the executive systems.

We have reported this change as an inversion of the intermediary process ratio. It appeared to be specific to these patients with the few exceptions of some cases with mild frontal impairment or alterations of short-term memory.

Also ACG latency in immediate reactions was increased in most chronic patients affected by schizophrenia, an increase that, as denominator, should diminish the value of the intermediary process ratio. In contrast, it increases in these patients in spite of the long ACG latency at FP_0, a finding that stresses even more its dependence on an impairment of intermediary processes.

The ACG latency increase at FP_0 represents a rather usual finding in neuropathological conditions and it is particularly marked in mental deterioration (see 9.8). This last condition is more specifically characterized by an increase in ACG latency at $FP_{0.1}$, with a consequent increase in the early process ratio, that may occur also in schizophrenics in the late chronic phase of the disease, but to a lower extent.

In young subjects affected by a positive schizophrenic syndrome for 6–19 months, the inversion of the intermediary process ratio occurred only with $FP_{0.5}$, with a normal early process ratio. This change was not reversed by antidopaminergic treatment but was masked by the administration of the Valium.

An exhaustive analysis of these findings implies to address some preliminary questions concerning their reliability and specificity.

9.9.2
Reliability of the Intermediary Process Index

As it has been noted by Sternberg [1969] and Van Lieshout et al. [1993], there is no doubt that the times of development of a reaction to an identical stimulus but under different conditions, like immediate and delayed reactions, do not necessarily belong to homogeneous processes. Consequently, differences and ratios between two of the related parameters cannot simply be assumed to indicate a well-defined entity or process. This criticism obviously calls for consistent caution in the evaluation of intermediary and early process ratios. However, at the present phase of MDRV research in the pathological domain, this does not absolutely imply that we must renounce a priori from these ratios. In fact, we could evaluate them as empirical indices, once we are aware of the limits of their meaning. The following criteria seem to offer reliable cues for validation.

(1) A semiological statistical criterion: if systematic research proves that the index is significantly different in a well-defined group of subjects, we can infer that it reveals a change or alteration in the events or processes that it depends upon. This is in fact the case of the inversion of intermediary process ratios in schizophrenics with respect to normals and the other pathological cases, once certain conditions are respected.

(2) A clinical integrative criterion: the evaluation of the indices must be integrated into the analysis of other variables that are related, with a different degree of valency, to the factors that influence the members of the differences or the ratios, like the intermediary process ratio. These integrating analyses may be carried out taking into consideration the principles of psychophysiology outlined in the previous chapters and reported also in Section 10.

9.9.3
The Specificity of the Inversion of the Intermediary Process Ratio

The main questions concerning the specificity of the inversion of the intermediary process ratio are: does it occur only in schizophrenics, i.e. does it have an absolute nosographic diagnostic specificity? Does it rather depend only upon a specific frontal functional impairment that may include not only the schizophrenic hypofrontality but also similar mild prefrontal impairments, i.e. does it have a second-order diagnostic functional specificity? Does it eventually depend on a frontal impairment of whichever origin, i.e. does it have a third-order physiopathogenetic specificity?

Further connected questions regard its constancy, i.e. whether it occurs in all schizophrenics.

The search for an answer to these questions requires a more detailed analysis of the results obtained from the different subgroups of patients.

9.9.3.1
Inversion of the Intermediary Process Ratio in Non-Schizophrenic Patients

We carried out a systematic study on the results of MDRV with a pair of disyllabic concrete words, with foreperiods of 1.5 or 3 s, with 98 normal subjects and 267 neuropsychiatric patients affected by heterogeneous degenerative and acquired diseases.

The values found in children and young adults up to 20 years of age have previously been reported in Section 7.

The intermediary process ratio never exceeded 0.9 [Pasetti et al., 1994] with few exceptions that were characterized by different changes of other parameters and/or well-defined specific conditions. Let us list these exceptions:

(1) Overtrained normal subjects with > 4 MDRV trials in few months can have intermediary process ratios of 1, but with very short ACG latencies at FP_0.

(2) Very few non-schizophrenic patients with increased intermediary process ratios (0.9–1) were characterized by an isolated impairment of short-term memory (see 9.8).

(3) Two non-schizophrenic patients with intermediary process ratios = 1 were one with Down syndrome and another young subject with limited prefrontal gliosis [Pinelli et al., 1994]. (On the contrary, 2 patients with Wilson disease and marked prefrontal demyelination had an intermediary process ratio <0.85.)

(4) The conditions that can lead to an increased intermediary process ratio in some parkinsonian patients have been analysed in 9.4.

9.9.3.2
Schizophrenic Patients Who Do Not Show any Increase in Intermediary Process Ratio

Values <0.9 have been found in only 2 out of 14 schizophrenics. They belonged to a group with negative syndromes, with residual schizophrenia lasting more than 15 years. In fact, ACG latency at $FP_{1.5}$ was significantly longer in these patients in comparison to normals, but ACG latency at FP_0 was markedly increased so that the respective ratio was lower than in the other patients.

(1) We wonder if possibly in these patients a sort of mental deterioration can develop and impair programming and intermediary processes, working memory included.

(2) On the other hand, the intermediary process ratio might be normalized in periods of remission, with behavioural improvement, and under treatment.

(3) Related research is still in progress, but, as far as treatments are concerned, we can even now observe that iatrogenic parkinsonian schizophrenic patients do not show any difference in intermediary process ratio in comparison to non-parkinsonian schizophrenics. On the other hand, a dissociation between behaviour and values of the intermediary process ratio has been noted and will be discussed in the following paragraphs.

9.9.4
Interpreting the Inversion of the Intermediary Process Ratio and Looking for New Physiopathogenetic Perspectives

We have previously pointed out that the increase in delayed reaction time found in schizophrenic patients can be attributed to a specific impairment of internal feedbacks of the intermediary processes. Delayed reactions are under the control of the prefrontal cortex. The inversion can thus be considered as the psychophysiological mark of the 'schizophrenic hypofrontality'.

In the search for a more detailed interpretation of these facts and speculations, we will now reconsider the contributions of neuro-imaging research.

Further investigations with multiple foreperiods will then be indicated.

9.9.4.1
Relationship with Fuster's Physiopathogenetic Perspectives

An important deficit of blood flow in the dorsolateral prefrontal cortex of schizo-phrenic patients has been detected especially when a cognitive test, such as performing the Wisconsin card sorting test, taxes short-term memory as well as other cognitive functions. A disruption of the prefrontal functions impairs memory and set, which, according to Fuster [1993], are critical for 'initiating and organizing actions'.

A more specific analysis of these functions and of the effects of their impairment, in line with the principles of psychophysiology outlined in this essay, could better define the role of the 'organizing' processes: intermediary processes seem in fact to organize the insertion of the initiating-programming impulses into the pre-executive neural assemblies.

We have previously emphasized that the inversion of the intermediary process ratio has many connections with these processes. A clearer definition of the modality and conditions of its occurrence can help interpreting the real nature of the functional disorders which it depends upon.

9.9.4.2
The Functional Impairments That Can Cause an Inversion of the Intermediary Process Ratio

The variables to be evaluated for the interpretation of the way by which a dysfunction of intermediary processes can produce an inversion of the intermediary process ratio emerged from the series of reactions with the triple task and multiple foreperiods of 0.1, 0.5, 1.5 and 4 s, taking into consideration the correlation between the increase in intermediary process ratio and duration of the foreperiods.

What we would particularly like to understand is the type of abnormalities that lead to an increase in the period of time required by the intermediary processes to effect their triggering task.

Four types of dysfunctions can be taken into consideration.

(1) A black-out of the reverberating circuits during the foreperiod: a rough interpretation of this abnormality could be given in psychological terms, as an *attention failure*. If it were so, the increase in the intermediary process ratio should be proportional to the duration of the foreperiod. This expected relation is contrary to the fact that young patients with recent positive schizophrenic syndrome show an increase in the intermediary process ratio only at a foreperiod of 0.5 s.

(2) A decrease in the triggering efficacy of reverberating circuits: the final task of the reverberating circuits is the activation of the hebbian neural assemblies that will produce the executive commands moving the articulatory mechanisms. If the triggering efficacy of the reverberating circuits decreased, the increase in the intermediary process ratio should be inversely proportional to the duration of the foreperiod. The 'weak' reverberating circuit could reach a triggering efficacy only in the long term. In fact, the cartesian curve of the ACG mean reaction time as a function of the foreperiod time is far from linear. This is clearly shown in the diagram of an 18-year-old patient affected by symptoms of withdrawal with delusions of persecution, somatic hallucinations and mnemic distortions for 6 months, reported in figure 118. In a case (male, 12 years old) affected by Friedreich-like syndrome due to familial degenerative periventricular gliosis, particularly marked in the frontal lobes (fig. 119), the

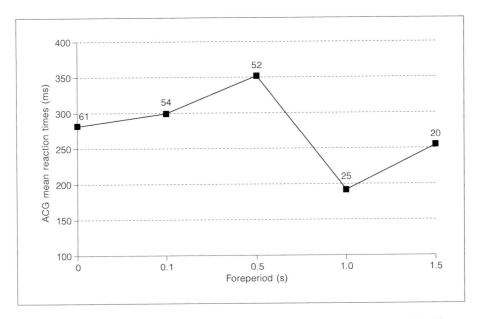

Fig. 118. ACG reaction times of patient N.W., 18 years old, with delusions of persecution. Figures near symbols indicate SD.

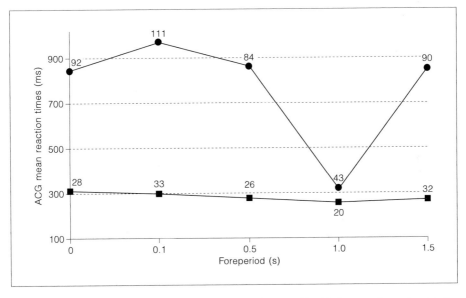

Fig. 119. ACG reaction times of patient C.C., male, 12 years old, with degenerative periventricular gliosis (○), and of normal subjects (■). Figures near symbols indicate SD.

curve of the ACG mean reaction time as a function of the foreperiod is just as irregular as that in figure 118, even though with higher absolute values.

(3) Slowing of reverberating circuit: a slowing of the single cyclic time of the reverberating circuit would produce an increase in the intermediary process ratio inversely proportional to the duration of the foreperiod. The measurement of the single reverberating circuit with the criteria outlined in Sections 2 and 7 could help differentiating this abnormality from that described for the previous type (point 2).

(4) Increase in threshold of the neural assembly: the synaptic efficacy of the neurons of the facilitated neural assemblies implied in the verbal reactions is produced by the phonological and the grammatical convertors that are known to possess a level of excitability modulated by genetic and epigenetic factors. At least two causes could give rise to an abnormally high threshold: (a) a developmental encephalopathy as it has been hypothesized to generate the schizophrenic disorder and/or (b) an early persistent misuse of the intermediary processes, in agreement with psychodynamic interpretations like that of the 'double message', could separate the neural assembly from the triggering patterns of the executive system.

9.9.4.3
The Heterochronism between Programming and Executive Processes:
Double Relation to Hypofrontality and Behavioural Disturbances

The impairments we inferred from the inversion of the intermediary process ratio may be seen as a dissociation between programming and executive processes. In this abnormal condition, the patterns of invariants elaborated by the sensorimotor activities and by the early CCP cannot be maintained to work in the period of time requested for an efficient adapting process. As a consequence, the invariants cannot be well and promptly adapted to the executive systems and to the neuromotor articulators, a function that is normally performed by afferent proprioceptive and by internal feedbacks [Perkell, 1991]. These are operating at three different levels of the control system to adjust the central commands, avoid errors and match the intended action to the actual executors.

With these concepts kept in our minds, we can analyse the sequence of processes leading from the stimulus to the responses in multiple delayed reactions, as it could be guessed to develop in the brain of schizophrenics.

Schematically we suggest the following temporal sequence to probably characterize the schizophrenic abnormality:

(1) the programming processes develop, as far as the tasks of MDRV can detect, in normal time, at least in the earliest phases of the disease;

(2) the intermediary processes are markedly slowed down, whichever is the causing factor: (a) slowed reverberating circuit, (b) increased threshold of the buffers or (c) mismatching between programming and executive processes; the common consequence is a longer time required by the intermediary processes to effect the triggering action;

(3) the initial reverberating circuits are not de-activated at the right moment; the longer the failure of de-activation, the longer the foreperiod at which the increase in the intermediary process ratio occurs.

From this scheme we can now outline the blueprint of the related dysfunctions.

The functional consequences of the heterochronism – between programming and intermediary processes and, in a more latent modality, between intermediary processes and executive performances – imply temporal changes, and these changes can be compensated by temporal delays in the executive processes.

On the other hand, the dysfunctions are partial and discontinuous because in these cases there is not only one threshold of the neural assembly: the model of the corresponding neural network must be conceived with several synaptic 'doors', and some among them 'remain open' in the schizophrenic disease.

Three different kinds of dysfunctions can be hypothesized.

(A) Under a condition of heterochronism, the programming processes undergo an overloading effect at the end of their pathway. They cannot continue at the next ring of the chain, when the intermediary processes lead to the adapted variants of the pre-executive system.

Hence a repercussion will run upwards in the programming processes themselves: they slow down gradually. On the other hand, at the new slowed level, the heterochronism is reduced. However, this sort of rebalancement is found to be a hard task for the brain. In previous Sections (1, 2, 7) we have mentioned the narrow limit of speed requested for human verbal communication [Lieberman, 1991]. We analysed how the demand for a high speed of speaking created the most suitable changes in the structure and functional organization of the vocal tract and brain representation centres. In the provisionally rebalanced schizophrenic brain, a natural tendency to re-assume the high speed of development of the programming processes will occur, in as much as the corresponding cortical circuits are in themselves normal. In fact, the genetic organic substrates contrast with an unnatural rearrangement at slowed brain functions.

(B) The invariants do not pass the intermediary phase. We can then have real blocks in the machinery with consequent negative syndromes. An alternative consequence could be an abnormal sequence of performances, an intermittent transmission, with more errors, long pauses and iterative outputs.

(C) Afferent feedbacks are abnormally delayed and interfere negatively with the earliest processes.

9.9.4.4
The Search for Correlations among Dysfunctions Related to Heterochronism, Changes of Intermediary Process Ratios and the Behavioural Level

The analysis of the negative consequences of heterochronism has been carried out in agreement with the principles of backward and upward overloading effects. A passage from the psychophysiological area to a behavioural level – as it would be wanted by the clinician – bring us a more speculative and hazardous and possibly tentative general working hypothesis.

The abnormal slowing in intermediary processes revealed by the inversion of the intermediary process ratio implies an impairment in the mental processes that we analysed and measured with reference to working-memory-like processes. Now the question is: which is the impact of this impairment on the mental activity and the behaviour of the subject affected by schizophrenia? We will consider as associated concausal factors aspecific brain injuries, like obstetric complications [McCreadie et al., 1992], and focus our attention on the functional cerebral impairment that is more strictly related to the endogenous vulnerability factor.

A point of reference in the study of this disease (as it is stated in DSM-IV) is represented by Bleuler's [1993] differentiation between primary and secondary mental disturbances. An impairment of the reverberatory circuits might represent the primary functional disorder responsible for the occurrence of gaps between the incoming patterns of impulses produced in the programming circuits and the adaptive processes taking place in the executive phase. A flow of non-programmed occasional internal feedbacks – from activated representations – could then be introduced through the gaps, and non-pertinent patterns of impulses might thus be included into the flow of the early normal impulses. The adaptation process that should take place between the programmed patterns and the peripheral constraints is hindered with the result of a distorted, contaminated ('dissociated') behaviour.

An equivalent process in the field of psychomotility might lead to the interference of abnormal psychogenic hyperkinetic movements and in the extreme case to a total failure of de-activation: catatonic symptoms could represent the extreme consequence.

On the other hand, a 'negative syndrome' could emerge, with apathy, lack of initiative and autistic withdrawal, when the following three events occur: slowing in intermediary processes is extended to long periods, no compensatory mechanism takes place, and overflow effects slow down and block initiation and programming activities.

In contrast, the 'positive syndrome' could correspond to abnormally persisting after-activity of reverberating circuits that occur independently of specific integrated purposeful actions.

These lines of interpretation could help monitoring the action of antidopaminergic treatments with MDRV, taking into account the changes in intermediary process ratios: iatrogenic parkinsonism and bradyphrenia could represent the collateral expression of the degree of slowing of the brain activities, rebuilding a certain degree of isochronism through a compensatory slowing in preserved normal functions.

9.9.5
Some Lines for Further Research

The application of MDRV has opened new windows on the temporal development of different brain processes, from initiation and programmation to executive coordinated actions, with interesting data on the intermediary processes linked to working-memory-like processes. Moreover, it has yielded new tools for the assessment of brain functions not only in the neurological but also in the psychiatric field.

The increase in the intermediary process ratio that seems specific for schizophrenia makes the study of this disease have a right of priority in psychophysiological research.

On the other hand, some peculiar changes in the intermediary process ratio, of opposite signs than in schizophrenia, have been found in obsessive-compulsive disorders: new perspectives, with new advanced methodologies, are then advisable for other psychiatric conditions.

Task stimuli specifically involving the dominant versus the non-dominant hemisphere can profitably be applied for the study of manic-depressive psychosis. On the other hand, the picture naming tests have shown some alterations prevailing in the non-dominant hemisphere in schizophrenic patients [Gruzelier et al., 1995].

On the basis of all these results and considerations, the place of MDRV seems warranted in the field of normal and applied psychophysiology. On the other hand, its further development and success will be guaranteed, if the fundamental clinical principles, however inctricate, are not neglected.

The plan of research and the evaluation criteria must cover all different factors that may influence the values of changes detected with MDRV: the phase of the disease, the primary or secondary nature of the symptoms under examination, the natural course of the alterations and the effects of drugs [McEvoy et al., 1991], beside the association of the effects of aging and mental deterioration [Goldstein et al., 1991]. The correlation with the changes of particular ratios as that of the intermediary processes must be studied at multiple foreperiods and with different tasks. All possible interfering factors like attention variations, effects of training and learning, and individual performance modalities linked to some specific 'ambiguous' stimuli must be taken into account.

This area of research is today investigated intensively with analogous methodologies of delayed reactions, and consistent results have been announced also in relatives of schizophrenics. We will report an abstract of these important and very promising data in Appendix 2.

10

Concluding Remarks

Main Cues Yielded by the Verbochronometric Tests

The multiparametric, multiforeperiod, verbal reaction methodology (MDRV), applied by us for the last 4 years, seems worth developing not only in the field of behavioural brain research but also in the clinical assessment of cerebral function maturation, mental deterioration of aging, neurological diseases and psychoses.

Besides being very cheap and well acceptable by the patients, who do not feel any discomfort and actually participate in a rather attractive task, it has the advantage of allowing a quantitative assessment, yielding original data on functional normal and physiopathological conditions. Moreover, I have provided, in the General Introduction and Section 1, both theoretical and experimental arguments demonstrating how the information gained on the motor control processes of the brain with our methodology might be extended well beyond the area of speech implying the task-independent processes.

Time values related to visuomotor transfer processes which activate internal circuits and internal feedbacks for verbomotor programmation can be measured as mean values of a series of 12 immediate and delayed verbal reactions (for reactions and indices, see Appendix 3).

As far as the mechanisms of utterance are concerned, the complexity of the CCP implied in word reading is not simpler than that required for the grammatical formulation. Word reading can be associated with picture naming with 2 or 3 alternatives. Further tasks of categorizations can thus extend the analysis to abstract computations.

But even with the simplest tasks of series of word pairs, a fundamental criterion concerns the frequency of use of those particular words. The consequent differences regard not only the total latency time but also the optimal latent time (that is the foreperiod) requested for the facilitation of the neural assemblies to be triggered at the appearance of the 'go' signal. Impairments of this latent immediate learning or preparatory anticipatory capacity have been observed in hand motor performances of parkinsonian patients. In contrast, we found that this is not the case in word reading reactions.

An essential procedure in our methodology remains the performance of delayed reactions with different foreperiods. We can thus identify three orders of cerebral internal circuits according to the phases of their occurrence and well-defined processes they fulfil in the cycle of speech control. In fact, these internal activities concern (1) programmation, (2) pre-activation corresponding to the so-called buffer and associated feedbacks of working memory and (3) executive activation.

A carefully detailed access to further differentiations of brain activities implied in the production and control of speech requires the inclusion of the tasks to be performed in both phonological and grammatical domains, each being characterized by its own rules. We have found that sentence reading requires in fact less time than syllable or word reading by normals but has less possibility to be further anticipated in latent immediate learning. This anticipation is normally maintained in akinetic parkinsonian patients, while it seems to be lost in schizophrenics.

···

Taking Advantage of the Intermediary Process Ratio as a Marker of the Schizophrenic Disorder

The inversion of the intermediary process ratio, found to represent a statistically highly significant index of schizophrenia, deserves a special comment.

The results of our investigations of schizophrenic patients versus normals, and versus neurological patients and non-schizophrenic psychiatric patients, entitle us to state that the inversion of intermediary process ratios is indeed a functional marker of schizophrenia and particularly of the positive syndrome. Negative findings in schizophrenics may rarely occur and have been observed in clinically normalized conditions under antidopaminergic treatment, in hyperkinetic syndromes and in negative syndrome in a very late stage (>15 years) of the disease. Positive findings in non-schizophrenic subjects occur also very rarely and are confined to cases with mild frontal impairment or with a specific impairment of short-term memory.

This functional marker should be used by the psychiatrist in order to plan a prophylactic treatment of subjects at risk, once they have made the proper tests at a premorbid phase. The rationale for this research project is outlined in the following points.

Scott Diehl together with Mars Eliot [1995] and Wang et al. [1995] have recently discovered that a link exists between gene locus 6p,22–25 and schizophrenia. A search for a correlation between this genetic alteration and the failure in working memory revealed by the inversion of intermediary process ratio could clarify the physiopathogenetic meaning of the genetic defect. As previously discussed in Section 9, the inversion of the intermediary process ratio may depend on an alteration of the prefrontal processes setting the performance of delayed reactions.

The application of MDRV to children (at 12–15 years of age) of families with the genetic alteration of chromosome 6 could detect an inversion of the intermediary process ratio. Further research is needed to better define the most sensitive foreperiod for the early phases of the schizophrenic alteration – preliminary researches seem to indicate the value of 0.5 s. We should also ascertain if there really are pseudo-negative and pseudo-positive findings with masking effects of some drugs like Valium at high doses and to which extent they occur.

Eventually, the evolution of the inversion of the intermediary process ratio in the course of the disease should be verified. Once these points have been determined, one could check the hypothesis that schizophrenia is the result of a developmental encephalopathy, involving mainly the prefrontal system.

The completion of this series of research with MDRV will prove the validity of the investigation of the temporal parameters of speech control by the brain in the neuropsychiatric field.

The psychomotor working-memory-like processes are a part or a specifically adapted function of the intermediary processes in the chain of the mental transfer activities. Our methodology offers new data on the functional state of these intermediary processes in some mental diseases. At the same time, it addresses new problems that call for a revision of current opinions and methods of measurement of the representations and processes involved in the latent mental activities that maintain the train of thought and master the delays in purposeful actions, allowing us to control our behaviour.

It seems reasonable to foresee that the prodigious acquisitions of PET and functional MRI will really help to solve the emerging problems of psychophysiology if they are specifically applied on the basis of more systematic current investigations in association with delayed reactions like MDRV.

··

A Blueprint for Further Research

A systematic series of investigations remains to be carried out to improve the precision of the measurements allowed by the methods applied and to obtain more selective recordings from the different oromandibular muscles through very small surface silver electrodes. Agonist, antagonist and synergistic muscle activities could thus be differentiated in neural disorders that impair the control of reciprocal innervation and coordination. Likewise, the recording of electroglottograms should be improved.

Spectrographic voice analysis should be added more systematically. Measurements of formant frequency can provide precise information on the response accuracy and on the state of the different sources of voice frequency harmonics.

The application in all tests of the warning stimulus and different degrees of pressure on the subject during his performances would certainly amplify the range of variables in the psychophysiological study.

Reference tables of mean values and SD of ACG latencies and durations as well as EMG and electroglottogram latencies must be provided in relation to age, level of education and the psychomotor traits analysed in the chapter on the kinetic factor in Section 8.

Learning effects on ACG latency and duration, with particular emphasis on SD, and on the intermediary process ratio (in relation to working memory) are to be investigated, in association with the effects of fatigue and, more generally, of prolonged activity.

The investigation into the effects of different times of delay of the word stimuli in MDRV on the multiple variables of verbochronometry should be carried out in studies planned to measure the maturation of cerebral functionality, in children under normal and pathological conditions and under pharmacological treatment. The effects of neurotoxic agents represent a further field of investigation.

Aging and mental deterioration should be analysed in line with the theoretical and experimental contributions of Myerson et al. [1990], Moskovitch et al. [1993] and Rastatter and McGuire [1990] to the structural-functional origin of information loss in the associative processes of the brain: MDRV adaptations let us differentiate short-term memory from working memory.

New phonological and grammatical tasks should be tested with suitable word stimuli of different frequencies of use and with pictures or sentences of well-defined semantic implications.

With these procedures we could further study still badly defined and partly overlapping processes like active short memory, memory of future, dynamic memory, working memory or working attention in different performances.

Maturation of cerebral speech control in children as well as age-dependent and pathological mental deterioration could be further investigated with the new task and recording systems, in relation to more clearly defined questions and more precisely measured variables.

The investigation of dominant versus non-dominant hemisphere functionality represents an important goal, particularly in relation to aging processes, different levels of education, focal cerebral lesions, depressive and pseudo-depressive disturbances. One current methodology may rely on the reactions to concrete target words like /mare/ and /-muro/ and abstract words like /male/ and /mito/.

Hemispheric presentations of target stimuli with tachistoscopic devices might represent a further development of this area of research. Moreover, one could investigate the interhemispheric callosal influences, of both facilitatory and inhibitory kinds, in normal aging and after injuries. The results obtained by Gruzelier et al. [1995] suggest to resume a more systematic application of picture naming tests, chosen with specific reference to dominant versus non-dominant hemisphere functions, in MDRV of schizophrenic patients.

Thanks to the new findings discovered in schizophrenia, the psychotherapist, taking care of the patient affected by this severe disease, should be invited to collaborate in specific systematic researches aiming to investigate the following groups of subjects:

(1) acute cases should be studied in the earliest phases, even before the period of 6 months requested to ascertain the diagnosis;
(2) drug-free patients should be investigated;
(3) patients with positive syndrome should be accurately analysed and differentiated from those with negative syndromes;
(4) longitudinal follow-up studies of patients with thorough clinical and psychological examinations, comparing the data of periods of improvement with those of worsening, could greatly enhance the meaning of the verbochronometric findings.

Apart from schizophrenia, another very interesting group of patients to be investigated with MDRV is represented by those affected by obsessive-compulsive disorders on one side and patients with capacitating anxiety on the other. Our preliminary investigations show significant differences in the findings of the two groups. A marked decrease in the intermediary process ratio was found only in patients with obsessive-compulsive disorders. To gather these and anxious psychotic patients into a single group – as some psychoneurosurgeons do – seems unjustified from a neurofunctional point of view.

Criteria of Evaluation and Principles of Functional Assessment

The repercussion of lower-level neural impairments on the higher-level processes must be borne in mind when evaluating top and backward effects.

The analysis of substituting mediations and of limitations in the speed of programming processes and executive mechanisms represents a fundamental procedure in the assessment and training plans of neurorehabilitation.

The very short foreperiod reading reactions (0.1 s), included in early processes, deserve further inquiries into pathological conditions, since the possibly prolonged first-order sensorimotor processes might extend the short foreperiod to values as long as 0.5 s.

The same consideration remains valid for the long foreperiod verbal reactions when the temporal course of the internal feedbacks is investigated under pathological conditions. The optimal foreperiod, particularly for unusual words, might be prolonged in relation to slower CCP at different levels.

The Actual Tools and Goals for the Future

On the grounds of previous considerations, we can state that multiple foreperiods of delayed reactions represent a valuable basic tool for the psychophysiologist intending to analyse how the brain controls speaking. In fact, the verbochronometric procedures described above allow us to gather data on the temporal flow of impulses running in the sensorial and motor channels and then of the early programming processes and the executive final performances. Accordingly, we will progressively lift the veil that still covers the internal feedbacks that keep the prepared representations active in the mind.

Phonological performances must be included in the reactions in order to determine the fundamental sensorimotor organization of the vocal organs; the grammatical convertor should be activated by the proper tasks, with reference to the innate genetic representations in the sense of Chomsky [1965] and Pinker [1995].

Reading should remain the prerequisite of the set of tests, since it represents the most recent cerebral acquisition and therefore the most vulnerable mental activity.

PET and functional MRI can then be associated with MDRV for crucial investigations in order to evaluate the metabolic activity of the brain during complex mental performances and particularly during reading phonological and grammatical tasks. Understanding the cerebral machinery involved in the different programming, rehearsal and executive processes could thus be greatly enhanced.

In the first Sections of this essay we outlined a general blueprint of the cerebral processes thought to be involved in the production of speech and more generally of purposeful sequential actions, i.e. in human behaviour.

As the goals proposed above were achieved, the blueprint could be revised in order to better specify the neural operative times, according to the best ways to substantiate the validity of the data collected with the most suitable recordings and the most precise measurements.

Anyway, I dare conclude that a platform has been created to develop the psychophysiological research on speech control by the brain with the aim of defining the general principles by which the human brain controls behaviour and the series of failures, repercussions, compensations and remapping occurring when it is impaired by congenital and acquired disorders.

Appendix

Reassembling Data for a Model of the Intermediary Recurrent Circuits

The multiple delayed verbochronometric tests (MDRV), which we have refined in the last 5 years in the neurophysiological and bio-engineering departments of the Institute for Research and Care of the Pavia Foundation of Professional Medicine in Veruno, enabled a new approach to the investigation of the higher nervous functions in clinical laboratories. It consists of a series of reading and naming, acousticographically and electromyographically recorded reactions. The methodology was developed in line with previous investigations on speech control carried out by Peters and collaborators at the Institutes of Speech Psychology and Phonetics of the University of Nijmegen.

The study started from the theoretical and technological acquisitions of *speech science,* particularly worked out by the systematic research of Gracco, Perkell and Levelt.

Aiming to apply and adapt the methodology to the field of clinical neurology and neurorehabilitation, we relied on *verbal reaction times* where the task and the response are specifically connected in an integrated natural chain between informative input and corresponding complex motor output. We are in fact dealing with a response represented by an actual action rather than with relatively indirect reactions.

Under these aspects, our procedure is substantially different from the most usual neuropsychological tests. In the classical reaction time experiments, the subject was asked to perform some mental task and to indicate the execution by pressing a key.

In MDRV, the sensorimotor formulation of the task by the subject and the motor performance are accomplished as naturally integrated brain functions. In this respect, we follow the general psychophysiological principle of Patricia Churchland: 'The brain is phylogenetically and ontogenetically formed to elaborate the most suitable and successful purposeful actions.'

Knowing the values of the verbal reaction times and of the response durations in different conditions, we have outlined some criteria to calculate the operative time of the mainly unconscious processes involved in the control and timing of behavioural performances.

In this way, we carry out a neurophysiologically oriented investigation of brain processes including the function of somatic distal executors. As these processes are studied in their natural development in the brain, psychological definitions become revisited and can be progressively replaced by more reliable models of neural networks and related representations and functions.

In fact, uttering a word is a complex, sequential purposeful action strictly related to uniquely human genetic and epigenetic substrates. For a current clinical investigation, very simple pertinent verbal tasks are chosen. Emotional concurrent prosodic factors are avoided in basal investigations in the so-called *neutral* condition.

The influence of emotional factors might be analysed in further experiments, particularly with picture naming.

In the most usual series of trials, the subject was requested to read some stimuli of both phonological and grammatical nature, with well-defined phonetic constraints and frequency of use. The subjects performed not only immediate but also delayed verbal reactions with different intervals (foreperiods) between stimulus presentation and 'go' signal, from very short (with the reaction cerebral activity still in progress) to long foreperiods chosen for the achievement of the shortest reaction time for that given specific task.

We could thus identify, among the times measured, those corresponding to four main neural processes. They are (1) a grammatical conceptually linked formulation, (2) the programming of the utterance, initiation and its whole sequence, (3) the neural timing process of the sequence and (4) the buffer coding (immediate memory) and its decoding.

A fundamental law to be applied in the evaluation of the results is the interdependence of the different neural processes with ensuing back-up effects.

The recent progress in the research on the cerebral substrates of the motor programmation, on the sensory-evoked cerebral potentials (P_{300}) and event-correlated potentials [Plum, 1993b], together with the study of the impairment of these processes in Parkinson disease and experimental Parkinson-like syndromes, provided valid criteria to effect the inverse operation, i.e. to go back from the differential reaction times to the time taken by the processes occurring in the corresponding cerebral systems.

It was possible to calculate the times of Hinton's internal feedbacks and, in a first approximation, corticocortical, corticogangliobasal and corticocerebellar processes, corresponding to the four previously listed functions.

A recent acquisition concerns the operative memory and the corresponding reverberatory circuits during the interval of the delayed verbal reactions and then the number of their repetitions during the long foreperiod tests allowing the shortest prepared reaction to be performed.

On the other hand, the very short foreperiod reactions open a valuable window on the PDP occurring in the initial sensorimotor elaborative phase. One can evaluate in the single subject whether there are parallel available channels or not, or whether facilitating stimuli may still operate.

The study of cases of multiple sclerosis with slowed conduction in the executive system and relatively better preserved central circuits showed specific conditions of heterochronism between the central and executive systems. On the other hand, in schizophrenia an impairment of the intermediary processes was found with a consequent heterochronism between the earliest brain processes of initiation and the intermediary working-memory-like processes.

A quite important, congenital or acquired, functional situation emerged from the study of hyperkinetic syndromes, which relates to a factor existing outside the cerebral processes under investigation but able to interfere with them. This is therefore a 'dirty factor' and we termed it *kinetic factor*. It is linked to a hyperexcitability of the motor output or a low threshold of the system involved in the executive functions, and it implies, for itself, a decrease in the final component of the reaction times. In the evaluation of the verbochronometric results, with respect to normal mean values, the kinetic factor must be estimated separately with suitable psychomotor tests and taken into account as a factor of correction in the analysis of the results. But it can be nullified when we rely on ratios of the results of comparative measurements of different tasks: ACG latencies of monosyllables to those of disyllabic words and sentences. Likewise the early and intermediary process ratios, with ACG latency at FP_0 at the denominator and at $FP_{0.1}$ and $FP_{>0.4}$, respectively, cancel the interfering influence of the kinetic factor, inasmuch as it occurs as a common factor in the two members of the ratios.

Therefore, for clinical investigations of brain functionality, we propose a series of *multiple tasks* of reading reactions with different stimuli (phonological vs. grammatical) and complexity (length and frequency of use). For simple routine tests we adopted a triple task: one syllable, one disyllabic word and a sentence, presented in random succession, 12 times each, in immediate reactions and with foreperiods of 0.1, 1.5, 0.5 and 4 s.

Discriminative quantitative data were obtained in infancy, aging, mental deterioration, akinesia, rigidity, central and peripheral paresis and schizophrenia.

In this way, we have actually created a 'clock window' on brain functions: the black box lets us listen to the time pulses of its functioning. Once the individual degree of fluency has been taken into account (the so-called kinetic factor), the speech velocity threshold, that is an absolute condition for the uniquely human language, is measured and analysed in its different components, from the central computational processes related to attention to the constraints of distal executors. Important data on the unconscious processes related to attention, programmation and operative memory under normal and pathological conditions have been obtained.

The semiological and physiopathogenetic aspects of this researches and the essential meaning of the emerging cues, in normal and pathological conditions, are summarized in the following tables 1–10.

Table 1. Brain control of speech (see Sections 2 and 3)

A.	Main parameters and their substrates 1. Latency time = operative processes occurring between the stimulus and the onset of the response 2. Duration = sequential processes from the onset to the end of the response
B.	Operative Processes 1. Preparatory activation: EMG onset 2. Reiterative circuits or internal feedbacks 3. Triggering neural assemblies for initiation, buffer coding, retrieval 4. Adaptation of invariants to variants
C.	Sequential processes Triple-order input and output channels

Table 2. Brain control of speech: Nature of the processes (see Sections 1, 2 and 4)

A.	Unconscious processes lose relation with psychological terms
B.	PDP imply overlapping processes with decrease in central ACG latency
C.	Parallel and serial processes with feedbacks imply intermediary matching with a stochastic modality of working

Table 3. Brain control of speech: Delayed reactions (see Section 5)

A.	Overlapping processes occur when: Time of the foreperiod < the initial cycle of brain sensorimotor processing
B.	Dynamic memory or temporal bridging repeatedly develops when: Time of the foreperiod > the initial cycle of CCP recurrent internal circuits

Table 4. Brain control of speech: General ratios (see Sections 6 and 8)

A.	Early process ratio = ACG latency at $FP_{0.1}$/ACG latency at FP_0
B.	Intermediary process ratio = ACG latency at $FP_{1.5}$/ACG latency at FP_0

Table 5. Brain control of speech: Phonological versus grammatical convertors (see Sections 5 and 6)

A.	The task: a monosyllabic word /ma/ a disyllabic word /mare/ a sentence /mare è bello/
B.	Grammatical threshold < phonological threshold
C.	The frequency law of decrease in ACG latency prevails over the word length law of increase in ACG latency
D.	Differential involvement of phonological versus grammatical reactions occurs in different intermediary processes

Table 6. Essence of brain functions in speech control: speaking as purposeful behaviour (see Section 6)

1.	Word reading and two-alternative picture naming tests, even in neutral contexts, even if they appear as 'amputated' performances with respect to spontaneous speech, develop in a communicative model where the subject understands his speech
2.	The speech-coordinated movements of word reading and picture naming develop as a purposeful meaningful action
3.	The communicative factor + the intentional commprehension + the purposeful character define a teleological dimension, corresponding to 'convergent correlations' [Sommerhoff, 1974] processed by the prefrontal network. It ensues that reading and naming cannot be considered as simple unintentional repetitions of verbal tasks but actually imply specific formulations as those that occur in spontaneous speech

Table 7. Brain functions in speech control: biological cycle and pathological conditions (see Sections 6, 7 and 8)

1.	Brain development from childhood to adult age and aging processes: PDP, myelination, synapsing and isochronism
2.	The pathological detectable alterations: mild functional disorders and secondary repercussions of gross pathological defects or impairments
3.	The parameters: early and intermediary process indices

Table 8. Brain dysfunctions in speech control: criteria of evaluation (see Section 8)

1.	Overloading and back-up effects from altered lower-level systems
2.	Heterochronism between CCP, intermediary processes and executive mechanisms
3.	Vulnerability of the invariant-to-variant adaptive systems, including reverberating internal circuits (dynamic memory)

Table 9. Brain dysfunctions in speech disorders (see Section 8)

A.	The assessment domain: dysarthria, spastic dysphonia, stuttering
B.	Dysfunction levels: (1) alterations of the executors; (2) upward repercussions; (3) compensating reactions
C.	Degree of reversibility: (1) functional reversible effects; (2) neuroplastic changes at vulnerable speech systems

Table 10. Brain dysfunctions in working memory alterations (see Sections 9 and 10)

A.	Working memory impairment with inversion of the intermediary process ratio: schizophrenia
B.	Working memory acceleration with decrease in the intermediary process ratio: obsessive-compulsive disorders

••

Risk Factors for Schizophrenia Evaluated in the Light of the Studies by Sohee Park

Thomas and Fraser's previous studies [1994] brought some evidence on an impairment of working memory in schizophrenia, but until recently, this claim has not been substantiated by systematic investigations to define its degree of specificity, its occurrence in the different schizophrenic syndromes and its meaning concerning the origin and physiopathogenesis of the disease.

A strong supporter of a 'dysfunction of working memory in schizophrenia' is Sohee Park [1991]. In his recent original article [Park, 1995] on spatial working memory deficits in the relatives of schizophrenic patients, along with Holtzman [1985; Holtzman et al., 1988, 1995] and Goldman-Rakic [1992], he claims that one of the 'cognitive deficits of schizophrenia is a dysfunction of working memory that leads to a breakdown of behaviours guided by internal representations'. Experimental neuro-anatomical and neurophysiological research carried out by Wilson et al. [1993] and Funuhashi et al. [1989, 1993] assign an important role to the prefrontal cortex in working memory deficits. In the rhesus monkey [Goldman and Rosvold, 1979; Goldman-Rakic, 1987], lesions in the dorsolateral prefrontal cortex, in particular the region of the principal sulcus, lead both to severe deficits in spatial working memory, as assessed by various delayed response tasks (DRT), and to some symptoms that resemble those of schizophrenia, such as distractibility and perseveration.

Since 1992, Park and his group [Park and Holtzman, 1992, 1993; Park and O'Driscoll, 1995; Park et al., 1995] have developed a human analogue of the oculomotor delayed response paradigm to test whether schizophrenic patients show spatial working memory deficits. They observed that schizophrenic in-patients were significantly impaired in a memory-guided DRT, whether the sensory modality was visual or haptic, but showed almost no impairment in a sensory-guided DRT. Bipolar in-patients, in contrast, showed no impairments in the memory-guided DRT. Park concluded that (1) schizophrenic in-patients have a deficit in the representational guidance of behaviour that is independent of the motor system itself and (2) this impairment is not restricted to the oculomotor system. The working memory deficit, as assessed by the memory-guided DRT, is consistent with evidence that implicates prefrontal dysfunction in schizophrenia. Schizophrenic out-patients in remission were also found to have deficits in the oculomotor DRT and percentage of errors [Park and Holtzman, 1993].

Since 1985, with research developed until 1991, several authors showed that some of the healthy relatives of schizophrenic patients show some traits related to schizophrenia. For example, a disorder of smooth-pursuit eye movements is present in nearly half of the first-degree relatives of schizophrenic patients in the absence of clinical symptoms of schizophrenia, whereas the prevalence of this eye dysfunction in the normal population is only about 8% [Holtzman, 1985; Levy et al., 1993]. Similarly, a significant elevation of thought disorder in about half of the first-degree relatives has also been reported [Shenton et al., 1989]. The existence of eye tracking dysfunction and thought disorder in a substantial proportion of these relatives cannot be attributed to medication effects, the effects of the illness itself or to a generalized deficit. If relatives of schizophrenic patients also show working memory deficits, it would suggest that these deficits are likely to reflect a behavioural trait rather than an effect of illness or its treatment.

A related approach is to study individuals with schizotypical personality characteristics [Lenzenweger, 1991]. Both the study of relatives of schizophrenic patients and the study of people with schizotypical traits address the additional issue of latent liability to schizophrenia, an issue that is relevant to genetic transmission [Matthysse et al., 1986; Holtzman et al., 1988].

Lastly, Park et al. [1995] showed that relatives of schizophrenic patients have significant changes of working memory in both oculomotor and visual-manual DRT, and they concluded that a delayed response paradigm may be used in elucidating the multidimensionality of the schizophrenic phenotype.

The methodology used by these authors is in many points different from the essential procedure of MDRV and has been developed according to some specific requirements of DRT. One main point to

Table 1. Impairment of intermediary processes

	n	ACG latency, ms			IR
		FP_0	$FP_{0.1}$	$FP_{1.5}$	
Normals	41	448	445	361	0.81*
Schizophrenics	18	587	606	732	1.21*
Residual schizophrenia	2	924	1,191	706	0.76
Frontal lesions					
or short-term memory impairment	4	656	898	712	1.08
Non-schizophrenic patients	43	601	728	484	0.80*

*$p < 0.001$. IR = Intermediary process ratio.

be stressed is the fundamental inclusion, in Park's methodology, of the short-term memory process that, according to our experience, could limit a differentiation between patients with short-term memory impairments and patients with pure schizophrenic mental disorder. In the visual-manual memory task of Park, a target appeared on the screen for 200 ms. Immediately after the target presentation, there was a 10-second delay period, during which the subject performed a category shift task (the distracter task). After the delay period, the fixation point and 8 'reference' circles (empty rather than black) appeared on the screen. Subjects were required to touch the screen at the remembered position of the target. If they touched the correct target position, the screen cleared and the next trial could begin. If the subject did not touch the correct position, the reference circles remained on the screen until the subject chose the correct position, or until 10 s had elapsed, whichever was sooner.

To control for the sensorimotor component of the visual-manual memory task, a sensory control task was conducted. The sensory control task was identical to the memory task except for one aspect: the target remained on the screen at all times. Subjects were required to touch the target itself after the delay period. This task, in Park's methodology type II, required no memory since the target was always present.

The methodology reported in our study (MDRV) allows us to measure the operative time of the brain processes involved in corticosubcortical recurrent internal feedbacks of the intermediary programming pre-executive phases of speech control. The intermediary operative time includes the time taken by the working memory defined according to Cornoldi [1995]. In a first series of investigation, during the test, a random sequence of two words was presented to the subject. The protocol consisted of an immediate reading task (the subject was requested to utter the word which appeared on a computer screen, immediately after its presentation) and a delayed reading task (the subject had to wait for a 'go' response signal before starting to speak) in which the foreperiod was randomly varied on the basis of two alternatives (0.1, 1.5 or 0.5 and 4 s).

In a first series, we investigated speech motor performance in a group of 14 schizophrenic patients and compared the results with the performance of an age-matched group of normal subjects (n = 17).

In order to represent an individual-education-independent index of the course of the intermediate processes, we computed the intermediary ratio defined as the ratio between mean reaction time in the 1.5-second foreperiod task and mean reaction time in the immediate task. It can be thought as an index of impairment in intermediary processes. In fact, the results reported in table 1 show that schizophrenic patients have a significantly higher intermediary process index ($p < 0.001$) than normals and non-schizophrenic patients (43 cases). (Mean ACG latencies at FP_0 are increased in comparison with normals, but this is an aspecific change, as it is evident from the FP_0 values of non-schizophrenic patients.)

Further research, including sentence tasks with foreperiods of 0.5 and 4 s and simple reactions, proved that in acute schizophrenia the intermediary process ratio is increased at $FP_{0.5}$.

Moreover, we confirmed the inversion of the intermediary process ratio to occur also in grammatical reactions, with few exceptions of schizophrenics with negative results and non-schizophrenic patients with positive results.

Schizophrenic patients with an intermediary process ratio <0.90 represent a small proportion (2 out of 9) of subjects affected by residual schizophrenia: they were under antidopaminergic therapeutic control, showed tardive dyskinesia and were rather old (>67 years). It is also important to note that the increase in ACG latency at FP_0 was greater in these cases (>5% compared to normals) than in schizophrenics with inverted intermediary process ratios.

Non-schizophrenic patients with an intermediary process ratio >0.90 were affected by heterogeneous disorders. We have recently studied 1 Wilson's disease and 1 Steele-Richardson syndrome with intermediary process ratios of 1.06 and 1.10, respectively, and a >50% increase in ACG latency at FP_0. The possibility to identify, with an easily available and cheap method, children and adolescents with a risk for schizophrenia – as it is detected by the inversion of the intermediary process ratio – may greatly help the psychiatrist to select the most appropriate psychotherapeutic treatment [Gabbard, 1992; Gabbard et al., 1993] in the most responsive period.

A Recording Chart of Verbochronometric Examinations

The Standard Verbochronometric Methodology

The standard verbochronometric examinations with reading reactions (MDRV) include three series of trials:

(1)   the simple reaction with a disyllabic word, e.g. /mare/;
(2)   the double task, e.g. with /mare/ and /muro/, with immediate and delayed reactions (with at least two foreperiods of 0.1 and 1.5 s but possibly also of 0.5 and 4 s);
(3)   the triple task with a monosyllable /ma/, the disyllabic word /mare/ and a sentence /mare è bello/ with immediate and delayed reactions.

The word stimulus /mare/ appears in all three trials.

The Reactions

Four series of reactions are considered:

R1 corresponds to the simple reaction.

R2 corresponds to the triple task choice reaction.

R3 and *R4* are double task choice reactions with a different persistence of the word stimulus on the PC monitor: during the whole foreperiod time or during 1.5 s of FP_4. The R3 set-up allows us to check short-term-memory-independent intermediary processes. On the contrary, the R4 set-up allows us to check a 1.5-second intermediary process dependent on short-term memory.

Picture naming reactions can also be carried out with simple, double and triple tasks (see Sections 7 and 8).

The Indices of Acousticogram Latencies

Index 1 corresponds to the latency time of the immediate reaction (x) – the latency time with a foreperiod of 1.5 s (y). Three subindices are calculated for the monosyllable, disyllabic word and for the sentence, respectively.

The index x – y (i.e. the subindices x – y_n, n being the foreperiod time) must be evaluated as percentage of the corresponding mean values of matched normal subjects.

Detailed criteria of interpretation may be applied to evaluate the different ratios of x and of y in relation to the tasks with /mare/, monosyllable, disyllable and sentence, triple reactions and to /mare/ in the double reactions.

The ratio of x and of y to the monosyllable gives us the ratio between the latency time of a one-syllable (/ma/) reading reaction and that of one word (/mare/). In fact, this specific Italian syllable could express an ambiguous meaning: the subject could perceive /ma/ as a nonsense syllable or as an adverb (in English 'but'). However, some comparative investigations carried out with simple reactions with /ba/ (a syllable that does not have any ambiguous meaning of being an adverb or whatever) did not show any significant difference in the mean reaction times of the two syllables /ma/ and /ba/.

A second question regards the modalities of lexical access and retrieval for /ma/ in the context of the other two stimuli, the disyllabic word and sentence. As a syllable without meaning, the stimulus /ma/ would have a high phonological congruity with /mare/ and should require a short retrieval from the /mare/ representation in the buffer. As adverb, its semantic congruity with /mare/ will be low, and a negative effect could occur in the passage from the monosyllable stimulus to the word stimulus. Nevertheless, the equal request for the articulatory performance of /MA/ and /MAre/ led us to adopt the test with /ma/ in spite of its phonological/semantic ambiguity. A further argument was the finding of equal values of the differences between EMG and ACG latencies for /ma/ and /mare/, respectively.

The evaluation of the ratio monosyllable to disyllabic word should be profitably associated with that of the ratio of ACG latency of /mare/ in the triple and in the double tasks. It might reflect the cross-effect (presumably facilitating) of the phonologically congruent stimuli like /ma/ versus /mare è bello/, at variance with the phonologically (and semantically) incongruent words /mare/ and /muro/.

Particular attention must be given to the ratio between the reaction time of a disyllabic word reading reaction and that of a sentence. The two brain performances imply two different convertors, the phonological and the grammatical ones. It could be objected that in a test of reading aloud, at variance with spontaneous speech, the subject is not mandatorily involved in the grammatical formulation of the sentence since this is offered to him in its complete form and he could then simply repeat it. However, our findings (see Section 5) of a dissociation of the reaction time taken to read the sentence as a function of the length of the task from the reaction time of the disyllabic word give evidence that the grammatical formulator is involved in reading a sentence.

The variable y may take different values in delayed reactions with different foreperiods. It ensues that we must measure separately $y_{0.1}$, $y_{0.5}$, $y_{1.5}$ and y_4. The lowest value of y will reflect the efficiency of the executive systems and of the vocal tract to produce ACG. Its meaning can be evaluated as percentage of the corresponding mean values of normals.

The variable $x - y$ gives us an important indication of the brain functionality mainly at the level of the intermediary processes. A negative difference can be found when the intermediary processes are markedly impaired.

Index 2 includes the latency time of the simple reaction, which we name u. Its value results from the time taken by automatic visuomotor processes and by the executive processes. Therefore the difference $x - u$ corresponds to the central computing processes (as defined in Sections 1 and 2).

Index 3 includes the value y_4 measured with the stimulus (a disyllabic word in choice reactions) presented on the PC screen for the whole foreperiod (R3) or with only a 1.5-second presentation (R4). Thus y_4 of R4 $- y_4$ of R3 gives us some indication about the factors dependent on short-term and working memories.

Index 4, i.e. $y - n$, differentiates between a focused discriminating visual attention, i.e. apperception (as it is required in choice reactions), and that of a simple perceptive process (as it is sufficient in simple reactions) plus the intermediary process (not occurring, at least in its completeness, in simple reactions).

Index 5 or the early process ratio is given by $y_{0.1}$ divided by x and represents an index of early programming process impairment. It exceeds the value of 1 in mental deterioration.

Index 6 or the intermediary process ratio is given by $y_{>0.4}$ divided by x and represents an index of intermediary process insufficiency. As discussed in Sections 2 and 3, the greatest advantage of the recourse to early and intermediary process ratios is their intrinsic meaning. The changes they can show with respect to the corresponding mean values of matched normal subjects are not significantly affected by individual constitutional and/or educational traits.

The results of the direct (FP_0) and delayed ($FP_{0.1}$, $FP_{1.5}$ and possibly $FP_{0.5}$ and FP_4) reactions to the stimuli monosyllabic /ma/, disyllabic /mare/ and the sentence /mare è bello/ are reported in the blueprint given below (table 1) with three subindices. Their values will enable a preliminary orientation towards temporal measurements of brain functions.

With the early process ratio, we can then evaluate the availability of open parallel channels and so get some data on mental deterioration.

With the intermediary process ratio and the indices 1–4 we may get some cues for a preliminary differentiation between normophrenia and bradyphrenia. The operative times taken by initiation and programmation, dynamic memory and related intermediary processes can be evaluated apart from the executive neuromotor processes.

Table 1. Reactions and indices

Reactions		
R1	d	simple reactions (to test mainly executive time)
R2	m, d, s	phonological and grammatical tasks
R3	d, d1	choice reaction to test working memory with $\Delta d = 0.5\text{--}4$ s
R4	d, d1	choice reaction to test short-term memory with $\Delta d = 1.5$ s at FP_4

tACG indices

Index 1 tACG at FP_0 – tACG at $FP_{1.5}$ for m, d and s of R2, testing central and intermediary processes

Index 2 tACG of d of R2 – tACG of d of R1 = CCP

Index 3 tACG of d of R4 – tACG of d of R3 = short-term memory – working memory

Index 4 Index 2 – Index 1 = apperception time + time of intermediary processes

Index 5 tACG at $FP_{0.1}$/tACG at FP_0, testing early central processes (or early process ratio)

Index 6 tACG at $FP_{1.5}$/tACG at FP_0, testing intermediary processes (or intermediary process ratio)

DACG indices

Indices 7–12 testing sequential timing processes and diadochokinetic mechanisms

d = Disyllabic word; d1 = disyllabic word in the simple task; m = monosyllable; s = sentence; Δ = persistence of the word stimulus on the PC screen; tACG = ACG latency; DACG = ACG duration.

Indices of Acousticogram Duration

The calculation of 6 indices for ACG duration in a similar modality than those of ACG latency previously reported may provide useful cues for the evaluation of the sequential brain processes (computed mainly as CCP by the brain) and the diadochokinetic mechanisms (worked out mainly by the co-ordinating feedbacks) responsible for the exact order of the uttered letters, syllables and words in the sentence.

Index 7 and *index 8*, similar to indices 1 and 2 of ACG latency, are particularly apt to detect impairments dependent on akinetic disorders. The slowest value of y is considered in relation to hypertonia and more generally to disorders of servo-mechanisms.

Index 9, similar to index 4 of ACG latency, may give useful data on impairments of short-term memory.

Index 11, i.e. the early process ratio, can help evaluate generalized mental deteriorations.

Index 10, similar to index 5 of ACG latency, in association with

Index 12, i.e. the intermediary process ratio, may provide supplementary information on impairments of working memory and other intermediary processes.

The occurrence of a 'busy-line' effect in delayed reactions must be borne in mind when ACG duration is abnormally increased. We must indeed add a basic index that has a great relevance also for the measurement of ACG latency in delayed reactions, particularly for $y_{>0.4}$. We might call it a *constraint index* (or the 13th index). It warns us to consider the value of ACG duration in relation to the value of the foreperiod of the delayed reaction during its course. If ACG duration exceeds the foreperiod, the corresponding descending commands from facilitated neural assemblies (see Sections 2 and 7) to the executive system may be blocked. The recurrent internal feedbacks that should deliver the triggering process develop in a time that matches the ACG duration since the adaptive processes (see 7.3 on the passage from the invariants to variants) follow a parallel course with the proprioceptive impulses coming from the articulators. We must also remember that these adaptive invariant-to-variant feedbacks modulating the adaptive processes take place, as Perkell's internal feedbacks, earlier than overt speech (Sections 1 and 2). As a consequence of all these factors, the invariants are not able to start working at the end of the foreperiod if ACG duration exceeds the foreperiod, the former representing a mirror of the preceding internal feedbacks.

As a consequence of this block, the value of y becomes artificially longer than the real reaction time in the delayed reaction. The results of case 3 with spastic dysphonia, reported in 9.2, can be re-examined as a paradigmatic example. In this condition, ACG latency at a foreperiod < ACG duration increases with an intermediary process ratio apparently > 1. As a counter-check, this artefactual increase in intermediary process ratio disappeared with a delayed reaction with foreperiod > ACG duration.

A Blueprint of Reactions and Resulting Indices

The whole set of reactions and indices is summarized in table 1 of this Appendix.

The percentage of errors should also be calculated, and the different kinds of omissions, mistakes, anticipations or time latency increases higher than 2 SD should be defined.

Equipment and Measurements

A personal computer (PC) is used as word images presenter (WIP) and a second one as signal acquisition system that manages the acquisition, elaboration and memorization of the biological signals and extracted parameters.

The WIP receives and interprets the commands sent from the signal acquisition system (through a serial interface) and visualizes a word (monosyllable, disyllabic word or sentence in random succession) during a 3-second period. In 30 presentations, the subjects must react (reading and pronouncing aloud the stimulus presented) immediately to what appears on the monitor. In the following 60 presentations, they must read the words immediately but wait to pronounce them aloud, until a light signal (the 'go' signal), represented by a row of yellow asterisks, appears above and below the word. The foreperiods with respect to the 'go' signal are 0.1 or 1.5 s (in random succession); in a second series of 60 presentations, they are 0.5 and 4 s.

The WIP monitor is placed at a distance of 80–100 cm from the subject under investigation. The word stimuli that are shown on the monitor measure about 7 cm and are generally of green colour on a black background. Each subject undergoes a preliminary complete ophthalmologic examination.

The intervals between presentations are hand regulated by the examiner in a range of 5–10 s.

An acoustic warning stimulus precedes each presentation for a period of 300 ms during which the subject continues breathing deeply.

Acquisition

This function is carried out by the signal acquisition system that manages also the elaboration and memorization of the following signals:

(1) The acoustic signal is transduced through a condensator microphone (Shire Prologue) that is placed before the mouth of the subject at a distance of about 20 cm. The ensuing microphonic signal is then amplified, filtered and recorded on the cathodic screen of an electromyograph (Medelec MS6), whose sweep is triggered by the appearance of the word stimuli in immediate reactions and by the appearance of the 'go' signal in the delayed reactions. The recordings can also be photographed on a tracing at the usual speed of 3 cm/s.

(2) The EMG signals from the orbicularis oris and digastric muscles are recorded with small surface electrodes (Dantec) also connected to the electromyograph.

(3) The movements of the vocal folds are recorded by two electrodes attached to the skin at the side of the larynx connected to an electroglottograph; this amplifies the impedance changes produced by the displacement of the vocal folds.

(4) Kinematics of the lips and jaws are transduced by skin electrodes that are attached to lips and jaws and fixed by means of a helmet. The transduced voltage variations are amplified by a system used by Perkell in the speech laboratory of the MIT and then recorded on the EMG. Internal vocal tract movements were recorded in a three-dimensional magnetic field by Schönle and Grone [1992] in Göttingen and with a magnetic resonance system at the Advanced Telecommunication Research Institute of Kyoto by Honda [1994].

Experimental research carried out in normals with combined EMG and kinesiologic recordings [Pinelli and Ceriani, 1992] showed that the primum movens for word stimuli (like /mare/) corresponds to the medial pterygoideus muscle that seems to act as a preparatory stabilizer. It is immediately followed by activation of the orbicularis oris muscle that precedes the onset of the electroglottogram in the speech chain.

(5) EMG of respiratory muscles was recorded in several investigations [Pinelli and Ceriani, 1992], but breathing movements can be more simply recorded with perithoracic bands with transducers connected to high time constant (or direct-current) amplifiers. Normal subjects are able to perform a long expiration and to utter about 10 syllables; with corticospinal lesions at the cortical or capsular level, the expiratory phase is shortened: one respiratory cycle is needed for each syllable [Pinelli and Ceriani, 1992]. It has been found that in many cases, a dysarthria is not simply an articulatory disorder but often associated with primary functional dyspnoea and more seldom with dysphonia.

Visualization and Measurement

Once acquisition and elaboration have been performed, the signals (ACG, EMG, electroglottograms, kinesiograms, pneumograms) are visualized on the screen of the signal acquisition system. A spectrographic analysis of the ACG signals was also performed with extraction of the fundamental frequency and harmonics of multiple orders. Reaction times and durations are signalled by means of a cursor moving directly on the wave shape, automatically counted and shown as a number at the end of each line of recording in the tracing.

The whole sequence of stimulation and reactions occurs in a dimly lighted environment without visual or acoustic interferences that might disturb the subject's attention.

Statistical Requirements, Neurophysiologically Oriented Interpretation and Routine versus Experimental Investigations

Owing to the intra-individual variability due to the trial-and-error operative system of the brain, at least 10–12 reactions are needed to obtain a reliable mean value. This variability and particularly the pathological changes cannot simply be ascribed to psychologically defined functions, namely to fluctuation in attention. Anyway, even attentive processes must be analysed with reference to underlying brain functions [Cohen, 1993].

In routine investigations, the main signals to be recorded are ACG and EMG. Particularly the association of orbicularis oris EMG with ACG is required because it allows us to investigate also the preparatory processes corresponding to the early period of the orbicularis oris EMG.

It precedes indeed the onset of the electroglottogram and is at least simultaneous with the onset of the expiration, measured as diaphragm EMG, and precedes the expiratory movement by 60 ms (corresponding to the EMG latency time).

The Origin of Multiple-Delayed-Reaction Verbochronometry, Areas of Application and Practical Benefits

The previously described methodology has been applied in the last 30 years by basic scientists and clinicians following two lines of study:

(a)　Basic investigation reached its full development in 1978 with the work of Sternberg but has been carried out mainly in three world-famous institutes, the Haskins Laboratories with Abbs [1973] and Gracco [1987], the New York Institute of Speech Control with Kelso et al. [1986] and the MIT Speech Laboratory with Perkell [1991]. A fundamental treatise based mainly on linguistic research was published in 1989 by Levelt of the Max Planck Institute for speech research in Nijmegen. On the same lines, with particular reference to the analysis of vocal tract movements, a large amount of detailed and precise data was collected by Saito et al. [1982], Saito [1992] and by Honda et al. [1994] at the International Institute of Advanced Telecommunication Research in Kyoto. Among the European contributions, that of Eimas [1974, 1975] and collaborators from the Language Institute of Paris must be cited as a good example of a neurophysiological approach to the study of speech in infants and that of Magno Caldonetto and Tonelli [1993] for the applications of electrophysiology in phonological and phonetic research. A fundamental book for clinical measurement of speech and voice was published by Baken [1987].

(b)　Applied clinical investigations were carried out by researchers working in the field of otorhinolaryngology with particular interest in stuttering.

Emphasis on neurological applications was claimed by neurologists and bio-engineers constructing sophisticated instruments for kinetic recording inside the vocal tract [Schönle et al., 1992]. In the last 10 years, systematic research was carried out by Peters et al. [1989, 1991] at the University of Nijmegen, while Pinelli and his group [Pinelli and Villani, 1984, 1986; Pinelli and Ceriani, 1993] at the Institute of Research and Care for Rehabilitation of Veruno started 12 years ago to extend and adapt the verbometric methodology in the field of aging and neuropathology. More recently, Dr. Ceriani applied these tests to the field of neuropaediatrics in the Paediatric Clinic of S. Paolo, Milan University Hospital. The investigations, carried out in large samples of normal people and patients with neurological and psychiatric diseases, yielded valuable new information on the effects that maturation and aging, brain lesions of different localization and nature, static encephalopathy and residual states exert on brain processes, concerning initiation, programming and particularly intermediary pre-executive activity.

The Neuropsychiatric Domain

Primary versus Secondary Increase in Intermediary Process Ratio

A correct interpretation of the increase in intermediary process ratio requires first of all a distinction of (1) direct primary alterations from (2) slowing effects exerted on the intermediary process ratio by heterogeneous impairments occurring at pre-intermediary or postintermediary processes.

Primary Increase. In a series of investigations carried out by Pinelli et al. [in press] in schizophrenics and non-schizophrenic patients, it appeared that only in schizophrenics does a statistically significant isolated increase in intermediary process ratios occur that may be thought to depend on a failure of prefrontal motor delayed setting.

Secondary Increase. On the contrary, in the few non-schizophrenic cases who may show an increase in intermediary process ratio, the primary abnormalities were represented by executor impairment with an increase in ACG duration, diminution of the difference between electroglottogram and ACG latencies, marked changes in EMG patterns and/or initial sensorimotor process impairment with a large increase in the early process ratio.

The Value of Verbometric Tests in Clinical Practice

Comparative Evaluation of Verbometric Tests among the Other Current Methodologies for Brain Function Assessment

Field of Investigation. Speech control processes must not be conceived as a limited sectoral area corresponding in pathology to the field of dysarthrias. In fact, not only task-dependent but also task-independent processes can be investigated.

The neurologist must be aware of the multifunctional availability of many cerebral structures. In fact, he should look at speech control as a general control of complex sequential purposeful actions, which are studied in the same way in behaviour sciences. Internal feedback circuits subserving PDP of sensorimotor translations and invariant-to-variant adaptation occur in the unconscious mental activity that corresponds to a series of psychologic events like attention, volitional acts, automatic activity and spatial and temporal programming implied in the brain's control of behaviour. Different intermediary and executive channels may be requested for the different types of actions, as they are for word reading and picture naming tests. However, in all tests, internal brain processes are activated at the highest level of brain organization. Thus, we study slowing and impairment of speech control, not so much as dysarthria (impairment of task-dependent processes) but also as impairment of task-independent processes, like e.g. mental deterioration, working memory impairments, akinesia, hemispheric functional asymmetries and heterochronism between the different phases of brain processes.

Degree of Test Sensitivity and Related Order of Impairment Severity to Be Investigated. Slowing of reading reactions reflects rather subtle impairments at a functional level. Primary alterations versus secondary upward and overloading effects are discriminated by preliminary semiological ascertainments that localize the impairments occurring in the whole chain of speech control.

In fact, gross structural alterations implying severe changes remain outside of the appropriate area of investigation with verbochronometry and rather represent the target of classical neuropsychological tests that detect errors, defects and failure more often than subtle functional changes.

Practical Advantages. In comparison to other current investigations of brain functionality, like those in neuropsychology, neurobiology and neuroimaging, the 'Veruno speech tests' offer three advantages:
(1) they are easily performed by the patient independently of his education;
(2) the patient participates actively in the tests without feeling judged by the examiner;
(3) they are inexpensive.

Reliability and Significance

The ratios of early and intermediary processes provide quantitative data on brain functionality that are independent of the subject's education and his actual attitude towards the environment.

The tests can be repeated in long-term longitudinal assessments, since in normal subjects the results remain constant in the range of ±8 % at 6-month intervals.

Which Specific Brain Functions Are Selectively Examined?

Early process ratios depend on the modular channels available in the sensorimotor translation and early programming.

Intermediary process ratios open a window on the intermediary processes including working memory, buffer coding and decoding at the level of phonological and grammatical operators. More discriminative cues can be obtained by adding further foreperiods from 0.5 to 4 s [Pinelli et al., in press].

Practical Benefits

Information about the course of primary impairments in internal brain circuits and adaptive processes, as well as retrograde upward effects of defects at the executive levels, is a fundamental requirement for neurorehabilitation and the neuropsychiatrists engaged in carrying out the optimal treatment and cure of their patients.

The assessment of psychomotor performances in complex disorders depending on both central and final process impairments, that is initiation and programming on the one side and reflex servo-mechanisms on the other, can be developed with suitable verbal immediate and delayed reactions (simple and choice, double and triple tasks). Eventually, one must not neglect the fact that the changes revealed by these tests concern the functional level and that there are rather high degrees of freedom in the relationship with the overt behaviour. Neuroplasticity, redundant anatomofunctional systems and neural re-organization at a lower level of complexity (Jacobson) are the important mechanism operations between the functional and behavioural levels.

One can thus find important cues as to the nature of the disease evolution, and one can analyse whether its variations are a matter of actual recovery or rather the results of compensation and remapping occurring in the normal systems of the brain.

References

Abbs JH: The influence of the gamma motor system in jaw movement during speech. J Speech Hear Res 1973;16:421–425.

Abbs JH, Cole KJ: Considerations of bulbar and suprabulbar afferent impulses upon speech motor coordination and programming; in Abbs JH (ed): Speech Motor Control. Oxford, Pergamon Press, 1982.

Abbs JH, Gracco VE, Cole KJ: Content of multimovement coordination: Sensorimotor mechanisms in speech motor programming. J Motor Behav 1984;16: 195–232.

Abbs JH, Hartman DE, Vishwanat B: Orofacial motor control impairment in Parkinson's disease. Neurology 1987;37:394–398.

Abbs JH, Hunter C, Barlow J: Differential speech motor subsystem impairments with suprabulbar lesions. Neurophysiological framework and supporting data; in Berry W (ed): Clinical Dysarthria. San Diego, College Hill Press, 1983, pp 21–56.

Adams MR: Fluency, nonfluency, and stuttering in children. J Fluency Disord 1982;7:171–185.

Adams MR: Voice onset and segment duration of normal speakers, and beginning stutterers. J Fluency Disord 1987;12:133–139.

Akbarian S: NOS-containing neurons in frontal lobes in schizophrenia. Arch Gen Psychiatry 1993a;50: 169–177.

Akbarian S: NOS-containing neurons in temporal lobes in schizophrenia. Arch Gen Psychiatry 1993b;50: 178–187.

Aldridge JW, Anderson RJ, Murphy JT: The role of the basal ganglia in controlling a movement initiated by a visually presented cue. Brain Res 1980;192:3–16.

Alexander GE, Crutcher MD: Functional architecture of basal ganglia circuits: Neural substrates of parallel processing. Trends Neurosci 1990;13: 266–271.

Alexander GE, Crutcher MD: Parallel processing in the basal ganglia up to a point. Trends Neurosci 1991; 14:56–58.

Alexander GE, Crutcher MD, De Long MR: Basal ganglia thalamo-cortical circuits: Parallel substrates for motor, oculomotor 'prefrontal' and 'limbic' functions. Prog Brain Res 1990;85:119–146.

Alexander GE, De Long MR, Strick PL: Parallel organization of functionally segregated circuits linking basal ganglia and cortex. Annu Rev Neurosci 1986;9: 357–381.

Alvisatos B: The role of the frontal cortex in the use of advance information in a mental rotation paradigm. Neuropsychologia 1992;30:145–159.

Andersen LR: Cognitive Psychology and Its Implications. San Francisco, Freeman, 1980.

Andreasen NC: Negative symptoms in schizophrenia: Definition and reliability. Arch Gen Psychiatry 1982;39:784–788.

Andreasen NC, Rezai K, Alliger R, et al: Hypofrontality in neuroleptic-naive patients and in patients with chronic schizophrenia: Assessment with xenon–133 single-photon emission computed tomography and the Tower of London. Arch Gen Psychiatry 1992; 49:943–958.

Arbib MA, Caplan D: Neurolinguistics must be computations. Behav Brain Sci 1979;2:449–483.

Asteggiano G, Bergamasco L, Zettin M, et al: Working memory: valutazione neurofisiologica e correlati neuropsicologici prima e dopo interventoneurochirurgico, in Moglia A, Marchese D (eds): Atti Soc Ital Neurofisiol Clin, National Meeting. Milano, Rozzano, 1995, p 143.

Atkinson JW: Motives in Phantasy, Action and Society. Princeton, Van Nostrand, 1954.

Atkinson JW, Feather KS: A theory of Achievement Motivation. New York, Wiley and Sons, 1966.

Baars BJ, Mothey MI, McKay D: Output editing for lexical status from artificially elicited slips of the tongue. Lang Speech 1979;22:201–211.

Baddeley A: Working Memory. Oxford, Oxford University Press, 1985.

Baddeley A: Working memory: The interface between memory and cognition. J Cogn Neurosci 1992;4: 281–288.

Baddeley AD, Lewis W, Vallar G: Exploring the articulatory loop. Q J Exp Psychol 1984;36A:19–22.

Baddeley A, Logil R, Bressi G: Dementia and working memory. Q J Exp Psychol 1986;38:603–618.

Baer T: Vocal jitter: A neuromuscular explanation; in Wemleny B (ed): Transcripts of the English Symposium on Care of the Professional Voice. New York, The Voice Foundation, 1979, pp 19–22.

Bajo MT: Semantic facilitation with pictures and words. J Exp Psychol Learn Mem Cogn 1988;14:579–589.

Baken RJ: Clinical Measurement of Speech and Voice. Boston, College Hill Press, 1987.

Baldissera F, Hultborn H, Illert M: Integration in spinal nervous system; in American Physiological Society (ed): Handbook of Physiology. Bethesda, American Physiological Society, 1981, vol 2, pp 509–595.

Banks G: Artificial Neural Networks. Boston, American Academy of Neurology, 1991.

Barlow SM, Muller EM: The relation between interangle span and in vivo resultant force in the perioral musculature. J Speech Ther Res 1991;34: 252–259.

Barnes RM: Motion and Times Studies, ed 6. New York, Wiley and Sons, 1968.

Barr WB, Bilder RM, Goldberg E, et al: The neuropsychology of schizophrenic speech. J Commun Disord 1989;22:327–409.

Barto A: From chemotaxis to cooperativity: Abstract exercises in neural learning strategies; in Durbin R, Barto A (eds): The Computing Neuron. Nottingham, Addison-Wesley, 1989.

Baum S, Blumstein S, Naeser M, Palumbo L: Temporal dimensions of consonant and vowel production: An acoustic and CT scan analysis of aphasic speech. Brain Lang 1990;39:33–56.

Beckett RL: Pitch perturbation as a function of subjective vocal constriction. Folia Phoniat 1969;21:416–425.

Beckman ME, Edwards T: Intonational categories and the articulatory control of duration; in Tokhura Y, Vatikiotis-Bateson E, Sagisaka Y (eds): Speech Perception, Production and Linguistic Structure. Amsterdam, IOS Press, 1992, vol 29, pp 359–376.

Bell-Berti F, Harris KS: A temporal model of speech production. Phonetica 1981;38:9–20.

Benes FM, McSparren J, Bird E, Sangiovanni J, Vincent S: Prefrontal cortex atrophy in schizophrenia. Arch Gen Psychiatry 1991;48:996–1001.

Berardelli A, Rothwell JC, Day BL, Marsden CD: Pathophysiology of blepharospasm and oromandibular dystonia. Brain 1985;108:593–668.

Berlucchi G, Crea F, Di Stefano M, Tassinari C: Influence of spatial stimulus-response compatibility on RT of ipsilateral and contralateral hand to lateralized light stimuli. J Exp Psychol 1977;3;505–517.

Bernstein J: Elektrobiologie. Braunschweig, Vieweg, 1912.

Bernstein NA: Human Motor Action: Bernstein Reassessed. Whiting, MTA, 1984.

Bertucelli Papi N: Che cos'è la pragmatica. Milano, Bompiani, 1993.

Bickerton D: The pace of syntactic acquisition; in Sutton LA, et al (eds): Proc 7th Annual Meeting of Berkeley Linguistic Society. Los Angeles, Berkeley Linguistic Society, 1992.

Bizzi R: Posture control and trajectory formation during arm movement. J Neurosci 1984;4:2738–2744.

Bleich A, Brown SL, Kahn R: The role of serotonin in schizophrenia. Schizophr Bull 1990;14:297–303.

Bleuler E: The Clinical Routes of the Schizophrenic Concept. Cambridge, Cambridge University Press, 1993.

Blumstein S, Cooper W, Goodglass H, Statlender S, Gottlieb J: Production deficits in aphasia: A voice onset time analysis. Brain Lang 1980;9:153–170.

Boshes B, Wachs H, Brumlik J, Mier M, Petrovick M: Studies of tone, tremor and speech in normal persons and parkinsonian patients. I. Methodology. Neurology 1960;10:805–811.

Bremer F: Nouvelles recherches sur le mécanisme du sommeil. CR Séances Soc Biol Filiales (Paris) 1936;122:460–464.

Brown J: The microstructure of action; in Brown J (ed): The Frontal Lobe Revisited. New York, IRBN Press, 1987, pp 250–272.

Brunner RL, Berry H: PKU and sustained attention: The continuous performance test. Int J Clin Neuropsychol 1987;2:68–70.

Capitani E, Laiacona M: Aging and psychometric diagnosis of intellectual impairment: Some considerations on test scores and their use. Dev Neuropsychol 1988;4:325–330.

Caplan D: Neurolinguistics and Linguistic Aphasiology. Cambridge, Cambridge University Press, 1987.

Caruso AJ, Conture EG, Colton RH: Selected temporal parameters of coordination associated with stuttering in children. J Fluency Disord 1988;13:57–82.

Cattell RB: The Scientific Analysis of Personality. Harmondsworth, Penguin, 1980.

Cavalli Sforza LL, Piazza A, Meuzzi P, Mountain J: Reconstruction of human evolution: Bringing together genetic, archeologic and linguistic data. Proc Natl Acad Sci USA 1988;85:6002–6006.

Ceriani F, Pasetti C, Pinelli P: Effetti dell'acinesi e della rigidità sulle prestazioni motorie dei parkinsoniani: valutazione quantitativa delle reazioni verbali. Atti XX Riunione LIMPE, Varese, 1993.

Ceriani F, Pinelli P: Multiple delayed reactions studied in children 4 to 12 years old. Mariani Found Meet, Milan, 1993. Berlin, Springer, 1994.

Chiodo LA, Bunney BS: Typical and atypical neuroleptics: Differential effects of chronic administration on the activity of A9 and A10 midbrain dopaminergic neurons. J Neurosci 1983;3:1607–1619.

Chomsky N: Aspects of the Theory of Syntax. Cambridge, MIT Press, 1965.

Churchland P: Neurophilosophy. Cambridge, MIT Press, 1986.

Cohen G: The Neuropsychology of Attention. New York, Plenum Press, 1993.

Cohen G: Faulkner D: Age differences in performance on two information processing tasks: Strategy selection and processing efficiency. J Gerontol 1983;38:447–454.

Collins AM, Quillian MR: Retrieval time from semantic memory. J Verbal Learn Verbal Behav 1969;8:244–247.

Colombo R, Parenzan R, Minuco G, Pinelli P: Metodologie di esame per lo studio dei processi della parola; in Pinelli P, Minuco G (eds): Il controllo della mano e della parola: teorie ed aplicazioni. Pavia, Fondazione Clinica del Lavoro, 1993, pp 155–168.

Connor NP, Abbs J, Cole KJ, Gracco VL: Parkinsonian deficits in serial multiarticulate movements for speech. Brain 1989;112:997–1009.

Cornoldi C: La memoria di lavoro visuo-spaziale; in Marucci FS (ed): Le immagini mentali. Roma, NIS, 1995, pp 145–181.

Cotterill R: No Ghost in the Machine. London, Heinemann, 1989.

Craft C, Gourovitch ML, Douton D, Swanson J, Bonforte S: Lateralized deficits in visual attention in early treated PKU: Neuropsychologia 1992;39:341–351.

Craggs MD, Carr AC: Neurophysiological aspect of psychiatry; in Weller, Eysenck HJ (eds): The Scientific Basis of Psychiatry, ed 2. London, Saunders, 1992.

Creutzfeld O: The neuronal generation of the EEG; Fessard A (ed): Handbook of EEG and Clinical Neurophysiology. Amsterdam, Elsevier, 1994, vol 2.

Crow TJ: Origin of psychosis and the evolution of human language and communication; in Langer SZ, Mendlewicz J, Racagni G (eds): New Generation of Antipsychotic Drugs: Novel Mechanisms of Action. Int Acad Biomed Drug Res. Basel, Karger, 1993, vol 4, pp 39–61.

Crow TJ, Johnstone EC, McClelland HA: The coincidence of schizophrenia and parkinsonism: Some neurochemical implications. Psychol Med 1976;6: 227–233.

Crucen G, Pauletti G, Agostino R, Berardelli A, Manfredi M: Masseter inhibitory reflex in movement disorders. EEG Clin Neurophysiol 1991;81:24–30.

Cummings JL: Frontal-subcortical circuits and human behavior. Arch Neurol 1993;50:873–880.

Curtiss Ch, Tallal P: On the nature of impairment in LLI children; in Miller JF (ed): Research on Child Language Disorders. Austin, PRO-ED, 1991, pp 189–210.

Daniels D, Plomin R: Origin of individual differences in infant shyness. Dev Psychol 1985;21:118–121.

Decetry J, Peram D, Jeannerod M, Bettinardi V, Tadary B, Woody R, Massiotta JC, Fasio F: Mapping vector representations and PET. Nature 1994;371: 600–602.

Dell GS, Juliano C: Connections approaches to the production of words; in Peters HF, Hulstijn W, Starkweather CW (eds): Speech Motor Control and Stuttering. Amsterdam, Elsevier, 1991, pp 11–35.

Dempsey EW, Morrison RS: The production of rhythmically recurrent cortical potentials after localised thalamic stimulation. Am J Physiol 1942;135: 293–300.

Denes PB, Puison EN: The Speech Chain: The Physics and Biology of Spoken Language. New York, Freeman, 1993.

Desmedt JE, Borenstein S: Trigeminal facial inhibitory reflexes; in Desmedt JE (ed): New Developments in EMG and Clinical Neurophysiology. Basel, Karger, 1973, vol 1, p 343.

Diehl S, cited in Wang et al [1995] and Eliot [1995].

Dietrich RB, Bradley WG, Zaragoza EJ, Otto RJ, Taira RK, Wilson GH, Kagarloo J: MR evaluation of early myelination patterns in normal and developmentally delayed infants. Am J Radiol 1988;150: 889–896.

Downes JJ, Roberts AC, Sahakian BJ, Eveden JL, Morris RG, Robbin TW: Impaired extradimensional shift performance in medicated and non-medicated Parkinson's disease: Evidence for a specific attentional dysfunction. Neuropsychologia 1989;27:1329–1343.

Dunkley G, Rogers D: The cognitive impairment of severe psychiatric illness: A clinical study; in David AS, Cutting JC (eds): The Neuropsychology of Schizophrenia. Hove, Erlbaum, 1994, pp 181–196.

Ebmeier K: Brain molecular resonance spectroscopy in schizophrenia. Cambridge Workshop Neurobiol Basis of Schizophrenia, Cambridge, March 1994 (reported by Winn [1994]).

Ebmeier KP, Blackwood DH, Murray C, et al: Single-photon emission computed tomography with 99mTc-exametazime in unmedicated schizophrenic patients. Biol Psychiatry 1993;33:487–495.

Eccles T: Evoluzione del cervello e creazione dell'io; in Eccles T (ed): Evolution of the Brain, Creation and the Self. Milano, Armando, 1990.

Edelman GM: Il passato presente. Milano, Rizzoli, 1991.

Edelman GM: Sulla materia della mente. Milano, Adelphi, 1992.

Eimas PD: Auditory and linguistic processing of cues for place of articulation by infants. Percept Psychophys 1974;16:513–521.

Eimas PD: Auditory and phonetics coding of the cues for speech: Discrimination of the (r-l) distinction by young infants. Percept Psychophys 1975;18: 341–347.

Einhauptl R, Schmidt A: Acta of Berlin European Meeting of Neurology, Berlin, 1993, p 401.

Eliot M: Dispute splits schizophrenia study. Science 1995;268:792–794.

Everitt BJ, Rawlins P, Robbins F: The control of reward-related responses. Cambridge Workshop Neurobiol Basis of Schizophrenia, Cambridge, March 1994 (reported by Winn [1994]).

Eysenck HJ: The Scientific Study of Personality. New York, Macmillan, 1954.

Eysenck HJ: The Structure of Human Personality. London, Methuen, 1970.

Feldman JA: Functional tuning of the NS with control of movement on maintenance of a steady posture. Biophysics 1966;11:556–578 and 766–775.

Fessard A: Brain potentials and rhythms: Introduction; in Field J (ed): Handbook of Physiology. Washington, American Physiological Society, 1959, vol 1.

Fioretti S, Leo T, Reale S: Modellistica matematica per l'analisi del movimento umano; in Leo T, Rizzolati G (eds): Bioingegneria della riabilitazione. Roma, Patron, CNR, Gruppo Nazionale Bioingegneria, 1990, pp 47–49.

Fitts PM: The information capacity of the human motor system in controlling the amplitude of movement. J Exp Psychol 1954;47:381–393.

Flanders M, Helms Tillery SJ, Soetching JF: Early stages in a sensorimotor transformation. Psychol Brain Sci 1992;15:309–362.

Fodor A: The Modularity of Mind. Cambridge, MIT Press, 1983.

Folkins JN, Brown CR: Upper lip, lower lip and jaw interactions in speech: Comments on evidence from repetition variability. J Acoust Soc Am 1987;82: 1919–1924.

Fowler CA: Coarticulation and theories of extrinsic timing control. J Phonet 1980;8:118–138.

Frakowiak RST: Functional mapping of verbal memory and language. Trends Neurosci 1994;17:109–115.

Franke P, Maier W, Hain C, Klinger T: Wisconsin card sorting test: An indicator of vulnerability to schizophrenia? Psychiatr Res 1994;54:251–272.

Frith CD: The Cognitive Neuropsychology of Schizophrenia. Hove, Erlbaum, 1992.

Frith CD: The value of PET in psychiatry. Eur J Neurol 1995;2:125–126.

Fromkin V, Ladefoged P: EMG in speech research. Phonetica 1966;15:219–242.

Funuhashi S, Bruce CJ, Goldman-Rakic PS: Mnemonic coding of visual cortex in monkey's dorsolateral prefrontal cortex. J Neurophysiol 1989;61:331–348.

Funuhashi S, Bruce CJ, Goldman-Rakic PS: Dorsolateral prefrontal lesions and oculomotor delayed response performance: Evidence for mnemonic scotomas. J Neurosci 1993;13:1479–1497.

Fuster J: Frontal lobes. Curr Opin Neurobiol 1993;3: 160–165.

Gabbard G: Psychodynamic psychiatry in the decade of the brain. Am J Psychiatry 1992;149:991–998.

Gabbard G: Lazar S, Hersh E: Cost-offset studies show value of psychotherapy. Psychiatr Times 1993, p 21.

Galderini S: Evidenze neuropsicologiche di una disfunzione dei sistemi fronto-sottocorticali in pazienti ossessivo-compulsivi. Atti VI Congr Soc Ital Neurosci, Milano, June 1995.

Garber SR, Siegel GM: Feedback and motor control in stuttering; in Routh DK (ed): Learning, Speech and the Complex Effects of Punishment. New York, Plenum Press, 1982, pp 93–123.

Gardner RA, Gardner BT: Prelinguistic development of children and chimpanzees; in Wind J, Chiarelli B, Bichakjian B, Nocentini A, Jonker A (eds): Language Origin: A Multidisciplinary Approach. Proc NATO ASILO, Cortona, 1988. Dordrecht, Kluwer, 1992.

Gay T, Harris K: Some recent developments in the use of EMG in speech research. J Speech Hear Res 1971;14:242–246.

Gayfield GJ: Excerpta international. Meeting on Parkinson, Rome, March 1994.

Gentil M: Variability of motor strategies. Brain Lang 1992;42:30–37.

George M, Costa D, Kouris K: Cerebral blood flow abnormalities in adults with autism. J Ment Nerv Dis 1992;188:413–417.

Georgopoulos A, Kolaska J, Massey J: Spatial trajectories and reaction times of aimed movements: Effects of practice, uncertainty and change in targeted location. J Neurophysiol 1981;46:725–743.

Gigley H: HOPE-AL and the dynamic process of language behavior. Cogn Brain Theory 1983;6:39–88.

Glaser WR, Düngelhoff F: The time course of picture-word interference. J Exp Psychol Hum Percept Perform 1984;10:640–654.

Goldman PS, Rosvold HE: Localization of function within the dorsolateral prefrontal cortex of the rhesus monkey. Exp Neurol 1979,20:221–226.

Goldman-Rakic PS: Circuitry of primate prefrontal cortex and regulation of behavior by representational knowledge; in Plum F, Mountcasle V (eds): Handbook of Physiology: The Nervous System. Bethesda, American Physiological Society, 1987, vol V, pp 373–417.

Goldman-Rakic PS: Prefrontal cortical dysfunction in schizophrenia: The relevance of working memory; in Carrol S (ed): Psychopathology and the Brain. New York, Raven Press, 1992, pp 1–23.

Goldstein G, Zubin DA, Pogue-Geikle MF: Hospitalization and the cognitive deficits of schizophrenia: The influences of age and education. J Nerv Ment Dis 1991;179.202–206.

Goodschalk M, Lennon R, Nijs M, Kuypers M: Behaviour of neurons in monkey periarcuate and precentral cortex before and during visually guided arm and hand movements. Exp Brain Res 1981;44:44–103.

Gourovitch ML, Craft S, Dowton SB, Ambrose P, Sparta S: Interhemispheric transfer in children with early treated PKU. J Clin Exp Neuropsychol 1994; 16:393–404.

Goyette CH, Conners CK, Ulrich RF: Normative data for the revised Conner's Parent and Teacher Rating Scales. J Abnorm Child Psychol 1978;6: 221–236.

Gracco VL: Multilevel control model for speech motor activity; in Peters HF, Hulstijn W (eds): Speech Motor Dynamics in Stuttering. New York, Springer, 1987.

Gracco VL: Sensorimotor mechanisms in speech motor control; in Peters HF, Hulstijn W, Starkweather CW (eds): Speech Motor Control in Stuttering. Amsterdam, Elsevier, 1991, pp 53–76.

Gracco VL, Abbs JH: Dynamic control of the perioral system during speech: Kinematic analyses of autogenic and nonautogenic sensorimotor processes. J Neurophysiol 1985;54:418–432.

Gracco VL, Abbs JH: Variant and invariant characteristics of speech movements. Exp Brain Res 1986;65: 158–199.

Gracco VL, Abbs JH: Central patterning of speech movements. Exp Brain Res 1988;71:515–526.

Granit R: Receptors and Sensory Perception. New Haven, Yale University Press, 1955.

Gray JA: Modèle général du système limbique et des ganglions de la base: application à la schizophrénie et aux comportements compulsifs d'allure obsessionelle. Rev Neurol (Paris) 1994;150:605–613.

Gray JA: Dopamine release in the nucleus accumbens: The perspective from aberrations of consciousness in schizophrenia. Neuropsychologia 1995;33: 1143–1153.

Greenfield P: Language, Tools, Brain. Behav Brain Sci 1991;14:540–575.

Gruzelier J, Liddiard D, Davis L, Wilson L: Topographical EEG differences between schizophrenics and controls. J Psychophysiol 1995;8:275–282.

Gur RE, Skolnick BR, Gur BC: Brain function in schizophrenic disorders: Regional blood flow in medicated schizophrenics. Arch Gen Psychiatry 1983; 40:1250–1254.

Guy W: Abnormal involuntary movement scale (AIMS); in Goetz CG (ed): ECD EU Assessment Manual for Psychopharmacology. Bethesda, US Department of Health, Education and Welfare, 1976, pp 534–537.

Hacking, 1975, cited by Pinelli and Ceriani [1992].

Halsband V, Passingham R: The role of premotor and parietal cortex in the direction of action. Brain Res 1982;37:340–368.

Hardcastle WJ: EPG and acoustic study of some connected speech processes. Proc ICSL, Edinburgh, 1994, vol 2, pp 515–518.

Harris KS: EMG as a technique for laryngeal investigation; in Harris KS (ed): Proceedings of the Conference on Assessment of Vocal Pathology. Rockville, American Speech-Language-Hearing Association, 1981.

Harvey P, Earle-Boyer EA, Wielgus-MS, et al: Encoding, memory and thought disorder in schizophrenia and mania. Schizophr Bull 1986;12: 252–261.

Hausch EC, Syndulko K, Cohen SN, Golberg ZI, Potvin AR, Tourtelotte WW: Cognition in patients with Parkinson's disease: An event-related potential perspective. Ann Neurol 1982;11:599–607.

Hawkins T: Word Order Universals. New York, Academic Press, 1983.

Hebb DO: The Organization of Behaviour. New York, Wiley, 1949.

Hecker MHL, Kreul EJ: Description of the speech of patients with cancer of the vocal folds. I. Measures of fundamental frequency. J Acoust Soc Am 1971;49: 1275–1282.

Heiss WD: Positron emission tomography: Present and future; in Pedotti A, Rabischong P (eds): Third European Conference on Engineering and Medicine. Firence, Gnocchi, 1995, p 11.

Hellerstein D, Bickford RG: The electrical activity of the brain; in Critenley (ed): Scientific Formulations of Neurology. Edinburgh, Churchill Livingstone, 1974.

Henneman E, Somien G, Carpenter DO: Functional significance of cell size in spinal motoneurons. Neurophysiology 1965;28:560–580.

Hinton GE, Plaw D, Shallice T: Simulatingbrain damage. Adults with brain damage make some bizarre errors when reading words. If a network of simulated neurons is trained to read and then is damaged, it produces strikingly similar behavior. Sci Am 1993; 269:58–67.

Hinton GE, Shallice T: Lesioning an attractor network: Investigations of acquired dyslexia. Psychol Rev 1991;98:711–795.

Hockett CF, Altman SA: A note on design features; in Sebeck TA (ed): Animal Communication. Bloomington, Indiana University Press, 1968.

Hoehn MN, Yahar MD: Parkinsonism: Onset, progression and mortality. Neurology 1967;17:427–442.

Hoffman RE, Sledge W: An analysis of grammatical deviance occurring in spontaneous schizophrenic speech. J Neurolinguist 1988;3:89–101.

Hoffman RE, Stopek S, Andreasen NC: A comparative study of manic versus schizophrenic speech disorganization. Arch Gen Psychiatry 1986;43:831–838.

Hofstadter DR: Godel, Escher, Bach: Un'eterna ghirlanda brillante. Milano, Adelphi, 1991 (from Basic Books 1979), chapt 18: Il calcolo proposizionale.

Holmes G: The Croonian lectures on the clinical symptoms of cerebellar disease and their interpretation. Lancet 1922;i:1177–1231 and ii:59–111.

Holtzman PS: Eye movements dysfunction and psychosis. Int Rev Neurobiol 1985;27:179–205.

Holtzman PS, Coleman M, Lenzenweger MF, et al: Working memory deficits, antisaccades, and thought disorder in relation to perceptual aberration; in Raine A, et al (eds): Schizotypical Personality. New York, Cambridge University Press, 1995.

Holtzman PS, Kringlen E, Matthysse S, et al: A single dominant gene can account for eye tracking dysfunctions and schizophrenia in offsprings of discordant twins. Arch Gen Psychiatry 1988;45: 641–647.

Honda K: Organization of tongue articulation for vowels. J Phonet (special issue for the 2nd ACCOR workshop), 1994, pp 1–20.

Honda K, Hirai H, Kurosawa N: Modeling vocal tract organs based on MRI and EMG observations and its implication on brain function. Annu Bull RILP (Kyoto) 1994;27:37–39.

Horack FB, Anderson ME: Influence of globus pallidus on arm movements in monkeys. J Neurophysiol 1984;52:290–304, 305–322.

Horiui Y: Jitter and shimmer in sustained vocal phonation. Folia Phoniat 1985;37:81–86.

Hughlings-Jacksons J: Croonian lectures on the evolution and dissolution of the nervous system. Lancet 1884;i:555–558, 649–652, 739–744.

Ingvar D: Memory of the future: An essay on the temporal organization of conscious awareness. Hum Neurobiol 1985;45:127–136.

Ito M: The Cerebellum and Neural Control. New York, Raven Press, 1984.

Iwata S, von Leden M: Pitch perturbations in normal and pathological voices. Folia Phoniat 1970;22:412–424.

Jacobs F: Evolution and tinkering. Science 1977;196: 1161–1166.

Jeannerod M, Arbib MA, Rizzolatti G, Sakata H: Grasping objects: The cortical mechanisms of visuomotor transformation. Trends Neurol Sci 1995;18: 314–320.

Jerry, 1995, cited by Cornoldi [1995].

Johnson, 1983, cited by Lieberman [1991].

Joseph R: The Neurological Fundaments of Psychiatry. Harmondsworth, Penguin, 1993.

Karniol R: Stuttering, language and cognition: A review and a model of stuttering as suprasegmental sentence plan alignment. Psychol Bull 1995;117: 104–124.

Keele SW: Behavioural analysis of movement; in Brooks V (ed): Handbook of Physiology: The Nervous System. Bethesda, American Physiological Society, 1981, vol 2: Motor Control.

Keele SW: Learning and control of coordinated motor patterns: The programming perspective; in Scott Kelso JA (ed): Human Motor Behaviour, an Introduction. Hillsdale, Erlbaum, 1982.

Kelso JAS, Tuller B: The timing of articulatory gesture: Evidence for relational invariants. J Acoust Soc Am 1984;76:1030–1036.

Kelso JAS, Tuller B, Harris KS: A dynamic pattern perspective in the control and coordination of movement; in MacNeilage RF (ed): The Production of Speech. New York, Springer, 1983.

Kelso JAS, Tuller B, Harris KS: A theoretical note on speech timing; in Perkell JS, Klatt DK (eds): Invariance and Variability in Speech Processes. Hillsdale, Erlbaum, 1986.

Kempen C, Huybers P: The localization process in sentence production and naming. Cognition 1983;14: 185–209.

Kennedy JC, Abbs JH: Anatomic studies of the perioral motor system: Foundations for studies in speech physiology; in: Speech and Language: Advances in Basic Research and Practice. New York, Academic Press, 1979, vol I.

Kent RD, Rosenbeck TC: Prosodic disturbances and neurologic lesion. Brain Lang 1982;15:259–291.

Klapp ST: Syllable dependent pronunciation latencies in number naming: A replication. J Exp Psychol 1974;102:1138–1140.

Klapp ST, Anderson WG, Berrian RW: Implicit speech in reading, reconsidered. J Exp Psychol 1973;102: 368–374.

Klapp ST, Wyatt EP: Motor programming with a sequence of responses. J Motor Behav 1976;8:19–26.

Klimidis N, Stuart GW, Minas IH: Positive and negative symptoms in the psychoses: A re-analysis of published SAPS and SANS global ratings. Schizophr Res 1993;9:11–18.

Kornbrot PE: Organization of keying skills: The effect of motor complexity and number of units. Acta Psychol 1989;70:19–41.

Kornhuber HH, Deecke L: Hirnpotentialänderungen bei Willkürbewegungen und passiven Bewegungen des Menschen. Pflügers Arch Physiol 1965; 284:1–17.

Koshino Y, Madokoro S, Ito T: A survey of tardive dyskinesia in psychiatric inpatients in Japan. Clin Neuropharmacol 1992;15:34–43.

Kowalska D, Bachevaijer J, Mishkin M; The role of inferior prefrontal convexity in performance of delayed nonmatching-to-sample. Neuropsychologia 1991;29: 583–600.

Kroll JF, Smith S: Naming pictures and words in categories. 1st Annu Meet Am Psychol Soc, Alexandria, 1989.

Kuhl KP: Methods in the study of infant speech perception; in Gottlieb G, Krasnegor N (eds): Measurements of Audition and Vision in the First Year of Postnatal Life: A Methodological Overview. Norwood, Ablex, 1985, pp 223–251.

Kuhl KP: Speech prototypes; in Tokhura Y, Vatikiotis-Bateson E, Sagisaka Y (eds): Speech Perception and Production and Linguistic Structure. Amsterdam, IOS, 1992, pp 239–264.

Kutas M, Van Patten C, Besson M: Event-related potential asymmetries during the reading of sentence. EEG Clin Neurophysiol 1988;69:218–233.

Lacquaniti F, Soetching JF: Coordination of arm and wrist motor during a reaching task. J Neurosci 1982; 4:394–408.

Lacquaniti F, Soetching JF, Terzuolo CA: Path constraints on point-to-point arm movements in three-dimensional space. Neuroscience 1986;17: 313–324.

Lashley KS: Basic neural mechanisms in behaviour. Psychol Rev 1930;37:1–21.

Lashley KS: The problem of serial order in behavior; in Lashley KS (ed): Cerebral Mechanisms in Behavior. New York, Interscience, 1951.

Lashley KS: Search of the quantitation effect of cerebral lesions; in Lashley KS (ed): Psychological Mechanisms in Animal Behavior. Soc Exp Biol Symp. London, Cambridge University Press, 1980, vol 24.

Lechner BK: Effects of delayed auditory feedback and masking on the fundamental frequency of stutterers and nonstutterers. Speech Hear Res 1979;22:343–353.

Lee YW: Statistical Theory of Communication. New York, Wiley, 1960.

Lenzenweger MF: Confirming schizotypic personality configurations in hypothetically psychosis-prone university students. Psychiatr Res 1991;37:81–96.

Leo T: Sliding space and sliding subspaces in manual prehension. Abstr 3rd Meet Soc Eng Med, Ancona, September 1993.

Levelt WJM: Speaking from Intention to Articulation. London, MIT Press, 1989.

Levelt WJM: Lexical access in speech production: Stages versus cascading; in Peters HF, Hulstijn W, Starkweather CW (eds): Speech Motor Control and Stuttering. Amsterdam, Elsevier, 1991, pp 2–7.

Levelt WJM: Lexical Access in Speech Production. Cambridge, Blackwell, 1993.

Levy DL, Holzman PS, Matthisse S, Mendell NR: Eye tracking dysfunction and schizophrenia: A critical perspective. Schizophr Bull 1993;19:461–536.

Libet B: Cortical activation and unconscious experience. Perspect Biol Med 1965a;9:77–86.

Libet B: Neuronal versus subjective timing for a conscious sensory experience; in Bauser PA (ed): Cerebral Correlates of Conscious Experience. Amsterdam, North-Holland, 1965b, pp 69–82.

Libet B: Chronometry in unconscious and conscious performance. Behav Brain Sci 1985;8:13–21.

Libet B, Pearl DK, Morledge DE, Gleason CA, Hosobuchi I, Barbaro MM: Control of the transition from sensory detection to sensory awareness in man by the duration of a thalamic stimulus. Brain 1991;114: 1731–1797.

Liddle PF, Morris DL: Schizophrenic syndromes and frontal lobe performance. Br J Psychiatry. 1991; 158:340–345.

Lieberman P: Perturbations in vocal pitch. J Acoust Soc Am 1961;33:597–603.

Lieberman P: Uniquely Human: The Evolution of Speech, Thought and Selfless Behaviour. Cambridge, Harvard University Press, 1991.

Lieberman P, Crelin ES: The speech of Neanderthal man. Linguist Inquiry 1991;11:203–222.

Van Lieshout P, Alfonso PJ, Hulstijn W, Peters HFM: I. Significance of relative timing towards an interpretation of articulatory sequencing. II. RT across word size and task complexity: Cognitive, linguistic and motor determinants. Annu Conv ASHA, Anaheim, November 1993.

Van Lieshout P, Hulstijn W, Peters MFM: Word size and word complexity: Differences in speech reaction time between stutterers and non-stutterers in a picture and word naming task; in Peters HF, Hulstijn W, Starkweather CW (eds): Speech Motor Control and Stuttering. Amsterdam, Elsevier, 1991, pp 311–324.

Linden D: Long-term synaptic depression in the mammalian brain. Neuron 1994;12:457–472.

De Lisi L: Malattie del sistema extrapiramidale; in Ceconi A, Michele F (eds): Medicina interna, ed 2. Torino, Utet, 1940, vol IV, pp 437–458.

Loesner A, Alavi A, Lewandowski KV, Mosley P, Sonder E, Gur R: Qualitative analysis of regional cerebral functions with PET in healthy volunteers: Changes with age and normal patterns. Abstracts 1993 Meet EFN Sci, Berlin, December 1993.

Logie RH, Reisberg D: Inner eyes and inner scribes: A partnership in visual working memory. Abstracts on Imagery and Cognition, Tenerife, 1992, pp 167–169.

De Long MR: Primate models of movement disorders of basal ganglia. Trends Neurosci 1990;13:281–285.

De Long MR: Models of Movement Disorders in Parkinson Disease. International Meeting on Parkinson, Rome, March 1994. Amsterdam, Elsevier, 1994.

De Long MR, Alexander GE, Georgopoulos AP, Crutchler MD, Mitchell SJ, Richardson RT: Role of basal ganglia in limb movements. Hum Neurobiol 1984;2: 235–244.

Lorente de No R: Analysis of the chains of internuncial neurons. J Neurophysiol 1938;1:207–244.

Ludlow, 1991, cited by Levelt [1993].

Lyberg B: Some observations on the timing of Swedish utterances. J Phonet 1977;5:49–59.

McClelland JL: The organization of memory: A parallel distributed processing perspective. Rev Neurol (Paris) 1994;150:570–579.

McCreadie RG, Hall D, Berry IJ, et al: The Nithdale schizophrenia surveys: Obstetric complication, family history and abnormal movements. Br J Psychiatry 1992;160:799–805.

McDowell FH, Lee JE, Sweet RD: Extrapyramidal disease; in Baker AB, Joiynt RJ (eds): Clinical Neurology. Philadelphia, Harper & Row, 1986, vol 3, pp 24–26.

McEvoy JP, Hogarty GE, Steingerd S: Optimal dose of neuroleptic in acute schizophrenia: A controlled study of the neuroleptical threshold and higher haloperidol dose. Arch Gen Psychiatry 1991;48: 739–745.

McGrath J: Ordering thoughts on thought disorders. Br J Psychiatry 1991;158:307–316.

MacKay DG: Constraints on theories of sequencing and timing in language perception and production; in Allport SL, et al (eds): Language perception and Function. London, Academic Press, 1987.

McKay DM: Cerebral organization and the conscious control of action. Pont Ac Sci VIII Semin, Rome 1965, pp 627–655.

McKay DO: The Organization of Perception and Action: A theory for Language and Other Cognitive Skills. New York, Springer, 1987.

McLean MD: Lip muscle EMG response to oral pressure stimulation. J Speech Hear Res 1991;34: 248–251.

MacNeilage PF: The Production of Speech. New York, Springer, 1983.

Magno Caldonetto E, Tonelli L: Organizzazione ed accesso lessicale; in Laudania A, Burano C (eds): Il lessico: processo e rappresentazioni. Padova, La Nuova Italia Scientifica, 1993.

Maier W, Franke G, Hain Ch, Kopp B, Rist F: Neuropsychological indicators of vulnerability to schizophrenia. Prog Neuropsychopharmacol Biol Psychiatry 1992;18:703–718.

Marie P: Révision de la question de l'aphasie. Semaine Méd 1906;21:241–247, 493–506, 565–571.

Markowitsch HJ: Anatomical basis of memory disorders; in Gassaniga MS (ed): The Cognitive Neurosciences. Cambridge, MIT Press, 1995, pp 665–679.

Marsden CD: The pathophysiology of movement disorders. Neurol Clin 1984;2:435–459.

Marsden CD: Which motor disorder in Parkinson's disease indicates the time motor function of the basal ganglia? in Evererd D, O'Connor M (eds): Functions of the Basal Ganglia. London, Pitman, 1988, pp 225–236.

Martin JG: Rhythmic (hierarchical) versus serial structures in speech and other behaviour. Psychol Rev 1972;79:487–509.

Masataka N, Symmes D: Effect of isolation. Am J Primatol 1986;10:271–278.

Matthysse S, Holzman PS, Lange K: The genetic transmission of schizophrenia: Application of mendelian latent structure analysis to eye tracking dysfunctions in schizophrenia and affective disorder. J Psychiatr Res 1986;20:57–66.

Mehler J, Christophe A: Speech processing and segmentation in Romance languages; in Tokhura Y, Vatikiotis-Bateson E, Sagisaka Y (eds): Speech Perception, Production and Linguistic Structures. Amsterdam, IOS, 1992.

Mehler J, Dommergues JY, Frauenfelder U, Segui J: The syllable's role in speech segmentation. Verbal Learn Verbal Behav 1981;20:298–305.

Mehler J, Dupoux E, Segui J: Constraining models of lexical access: The onset of word recognition; in Altmann G (ed): Cognitive Models of Speech Processing: Psycholinguistic and Computation Perspectives. Cambridge, MIT Press, 1991.

Miller LG, Jankovic J: Drug-induced movement disorders: An overview; in Joseph AB, Young RR (eds): Movement Disorders in Neurology and Neuropsychiatry. Oxford, Blackwell Scientific Publications, 1992.

Mindus P, Nyman H: Normalization of personality characteristics in patients with incapacitating anxiety disorders after capsulotomy. Acta Psychiatr Scand 1991; 83:283–291.

Mindus P, Nyman H, Mogard Y, et al: Frontal lobe and basal ganglia metabolism studied with PET in patients with incapacitating obsessive-compulsive disorder undergoing capsulotomy. Nord Psykiatr Tidskr 1990;44:309–312.

Mingazzini P: Anatomia clinica del sistema nervoso; quoted by Gozzano M (ed): Trattato delle Malattie Nervose VIII. Padova, Nuova Libraria Piccin, 1981, p 158.

Model JG, Mounts JM, Curtis GC, Greden JF: Neurophysiologic dysfunction in basal ganglia limbic striatal and thalamocortical circuits as a pathogenetic mechanism of obsessive-compulsive disorders. J Neuropsychiatry 1989;1:27–36.

Molt LF: Selected acoustic and physiologic measures of speech motor coordination in stuttering and nonstuttering children; in Peter HF, Hulstijn W, Starkweather W (eds): Speech Motor Control and Stuttering. Amsterdam, Elsevier, 1991, pp 433–439.

Moore W: Some effects of progressively lowering electromyographic levels with feedback proceeders on the frequency of stutterers' verbal behaviors. J Fluency Disord 1978;3:127–138.

Morice R: Beyond language: Speculations on pre-frontal cortex and schizophrenia. Aust NZ J Psychiatry 1986;20:7–10.

Moruzzi G, Magoun HW: Brain stem RF and activation of EEG. EEG Clin Neurophysiol 1949;1:455–473.

Moskovitch M, Vriezen E, Goshen-Gottstein Y: Implicit tests of memory in patients with focal lesions or degenerative brain disorders; in Bollert, Grafman (eds): Handbook of Neuropsychology. Amsterdam, Elsevier, 1993, vol 8, pp 133–173.

Munhall KM, Flanagan JR, Ostry DJ: Sensorimotor transformation and control strategies in speech; in Tokhura Y, Vatikiotis-Bateson E, Sagisaka Y (eds): Speech Perception and Production and Linguistic Structure. Amsterdam, IOS, 1992, pp 329–340.

Murdock BE: Speech and language skills in children with early treated PKU. Am J Ment Retard 1990;94: 625–632.

Murri L: Electroencephalographic mapping. Curr Opin Neurol Neurosurg 1991;4:788–792.

Myerson J, Hale S, Wagstaff D, Poon WL, Smith GA: The information loss model: A mathematical theory to age-related cognitive slowing. Psychol Rev 1990; 97:475–487.

Nakamura Y: Neural basis of rhythm generation of jaw movements. Prog Neural Res 1986;30:237–250.

Neely, 1977, cited by Spicer et al. [1994].

Netsell R, Daniel B, Celesia GG: Acceleration and weakness in parkinsonian dysarthria. J Speech Hear Disord 1975;40:170–178.

Nudelmann HB, Herbrich KE, Hoyt BD, Rosenfiels DB: A neuroscience model of stuttering. J Fluency Disord 1989;14:399–427.

Occam, cited by Pinelli and Ceriani [1992].

Oldfield RC, Wingfield A: Response latencies in naming objects. Q J Exp Psychol 1965;17:273–281.

Owens DGC, Johnstone EC, Frith CD: Spontaneous involuntary disorders of movement: Their prevalence, severity and distribution in chronic schizophrenics with and without treatment with neuroleptics. Arch Gen Psychiatry 1982;39:452–461.

Pallman SE, Watts R, Juncos JL, Sanes JN: Movement amplitude and choice reaction time performances in Parkinson's disease may be independent of dopaminergic status. J Neurol Neurosurg Psychiatry 1990;53:279–283.

Park S: The Role of the Prefrontal Cortex in Spatial Working Memory Deficits of Schizophrenic Patients; thesis Harvard University, 1991.

Park S: Working memory function in schizophrenic patients; in Spitzer M, Maher BA (eds): Experimental Psychopathology. New York, Cambridge University Press, 1995.

Park S, Holtzman PS: Schizophrenics show spatial working memory deficits. Arch Gen Psychiatry 1992;49:975–982.

Park S, Holtzman PS: Association of working memory deficit and eye tracking dysfunction in schizophrenia. Schizophr Res 1993;11:55–61.

Park S, Holtzman PS, Lenzenweger MF: Individual differences in spatial working memory in relation to schizotypy. J Abnorm Psychol 1995;104:355–363.

Park S, O'Driscoll G: Components of working memory deficit in schizophrenic patients; in Matthysse S (eds): Psychopathology: Evolution of a New Science. New York, Cambridge University Press, 1995.

Pasetti C, Conti R, Terazzi M, Colombo R, Pinelli P: Analisi verbocronometrica in soggetti con M. di Parkinson idiopatico e parkinsonismo iatrogeno. Atti XXII Riunione LIMPE, Palermo, 1994.

Paulesu E, Frith CD, Bottini G, Frakowiak RSJ: Functional anatomy of working memory: Articulatory loop. J Neurol Sci 1993a; suppl 141: 37.

Paulesu E, Frith CD, Frakowiak RSJ: Functional anatomy of verbal components of short-term memory. Nature 1993b;362:342–345.

Penfield W, Roberts S: Speech and Brain Mechanisms. Princeton, Princeton University Press, 1959.

Perkell JS: Phonetic features and the physiology of speech production; in Perkell JS (ed): Language Production. London, Academic Press, 1980, vol I: Speech and Talk.

Perkell JS: Testing theories of speech production: Implications of some detailed analysis of variable articulatory data; in Perkell JS (ed): Speech Production and Speech Modeling. Dordrecht, Kluwer, 1991.

Perkell JS, Oka D: Use of an alternating magnetic field device to track midsagittal plane movements of multiple points inside the vocal tract. J Acoust Soc Am 1980;67:92–93.

Peters HFM, Hulstijn W, Starkweather CW: Acoustic and physiological reaction times of stutterers and nonstutterers. J Speech Hear Res 1989;32:668–680.

Peters HF, Hulstijn W, Starkweather CW: Speech Motor Control and Stuttering. Amsterdam, Elsevier, 1991.

Petersen JE, et al: PET studies of the cortical anatomy of single-word processing. Nature 1988;331:585–589.

Petrides M, Alvisatos B, Meyer F, Evans AC: Maintenance of visuospatial verbal information for short periods of time in the dorsal prefrontal cortex. Proc Natl Acad Sci USA 1993;90:878–882.

Pfaff DW: The Physiologic Mechanisms of Motivation. New York, Springer, 1981.

Pinelli P: Contributo EMG alla fisiopatologia dei riflessi, in particolare di un riflesso dell'arto superiore paragonabile al Babinki. Acta Neurol Atti XI Congr SIN, Napoli, 1952, pp 553–564.

Pinelli P: Interessi attuali dello studio del 'riflesso preparato' di Exner-Cattel e della reazione di rilassamento. Riv Sper Freniatria 1964;88:426–439.

Pinelli P: Schemi, motori e iniziativa psicomotoria. Totus Homo, Ist Psico-Sintesi Scientifica, Milano, 1970, vol 2, pp 1–5.

Pinelli P: L'ipotesi dei circuiti centrali interni di programmazione in neuropsichiatria. Boll Atti Accad Med, Roma, 1970–1971, pp 59–72.

Pinelli P: Logica del cervello vivente e neurologia comportamentale. Milano, De Angeli, 1977.

Pinelli P: Sulle strutture e funzioni del sistema verbofasico; in Macchi G (ed): Neurologia e scienze di base. Milano, Vita e Pensiero, 1989.

Pinelli P: Valutazione della fatica muscolare e neuronale in varie condizioni cliniche; in Antonetto G (ed): La fatica muscolare e neuronale. Milano, Pytagora Press, 1991, pp 1–15.

Pinelli P: Neurophysiology in the science of speech. Curr Opin Neurol Neurosurg 1992;5:744–755.

Pinelli P: From the neurophysiological assessment to neurorehabilitation. Atti Congr AEI, Ancona, 1993, vol VI.

Pinelli P: Errori e correzioni nel controllo cerebrale del comportamento. Milano, Ambrosiana, in press.

Pinelli P, Ceriani F: Rappresentazioni e processi del parlare. Milano, Ambrosiana, 1992.

Pinelli P, Ceriani F: Motor firing and serial reactions: Functional changes during repetitive activity; in Pedotti A (ed): Electrophysiological Kinesiology. Amsterdam, IOS Press, 1993.

Pinelli P, Ceriani F, Poloni P: Modificazioni specifiche dei tempi di reazione verbale di scelta nelle pseudodemenze. Arch Neurol Psicol Psichiat 1994;62:114–129.

Pinelli P, Ceriani F, Pasetti E: Verbal delayed reactions are impaired in schizophrenics. Neurol Neurosurg Psychiatry, in press.

Pinelli P, Valle M: Studio fisiopatologico dei reflessi muscolari nelle paresi spastiche. Arch Sci Med 1960;11:128–234.

Pinelli P, Villani A: The Neurophysiological Assessment of Motor Function. Padova, Liviana, 1984.

Pinelli P, Villani A: Plasticity of Spinal Cord Servomechanisms. Padova, Liviana, 1986.

Pinelli P Jr, Baroni L, Pellegrino F: La verbocronometria nei pazienti con trauma cranico; in Ferri R (ed): Atti IV Congresso Psicofisiologia. Troina, Oasi, 1995, pp 53–54.

Pinker St: The Language as Instinct. New York, Penguin, 1995.

Pivetau J: L'apparition de l'homme. Paris, OEIL, 1986.

Plate et al, 1987, cited in Levelt [1991].

Plomin R: Behavioural genetics and personality; in Liebert RM, Wicks-Nelson R (eds): Developmental Psychology. Englewood Cliffs, Prentice-Hall, 1987.

Plum F: Focal unconsciousness in neurological disease (honorary lecture). Meet EFNS, Berlin, December 1993a.

Plum F: Neurological processes and consciousness (lecture). WFN Congr, Vancouver, 1993b.

Popper KR: The place of mind in nature; in Elvee RQ (ed): Mind in Nature. Nobel Conference XVII. San Francisco, Harper and Row, 1982, pp 31–59.

Posner MI, Dehane S: Attentional networks. Trends Neurosci 1994;17:75–79.

Posner MI, Mitchell RF: Chronometric analysis of conscious actions. Psychol Rev 1967; 74:392–409.

Posner MI, Snyder CRR: Attentional and cognition control; in Solso RL (ed): Information Processing and Cognition. Hillsdale, Erlbaum, 1975, pp 55–85.

Potvin A, Syndulko K, Tourtelotte WW, Golberg Z, Potvin JK, Hanoch FC: Quantitative evaluation of normal age related changes in neurologic function; in Maletta P, Pirozolo E (eds): Advances in Neurogerontology. New York, Praeger, 1981, vol 2.

Potvin A, Tourtelotte WW: Quantitative Examination of Neurologic Functions. Boca Raton, CRC Press, 1985, vol II, pp 98–99.

Pullman SE, Watts RL, Juncos J, Sanes JN: Movement amplitude choice reaction time in Parkinson's disease may be independent of dopaminergic status. J Neurol Neurosurg Psychiatry 1990;53:279–283.

Rafal RD, Posner MI, Walker JA, Friedrich FJ: Cognition and the basal ganglia: Separating mental and motor components of performance in Parkinson's disease. Brain 1984;107:1083–1094.

Raja M: Neurological diagnoses in psychiatric patients. Ital J Neurol Sci 1995;16:153–158.

Rapaport H, Wise SP: Obsessive-compulsive disorder evidence for basal ganglia dysfunction. Psychopharmacol Bull 1988;24:380–384.

Rappelsberger P, Weiss S: EEG-coherence analyses deficit functional relations during cognitive processing; in Pedotti A, Rabishong P (eds): Third European Congress on Engineering and Medicine. Milano, Gnocchi, 1995, p 36.

Rastatter M, McGuire RA: Some effects of advanced aging on the left and right hemispheres: Evidence from unilateral tachystoscopic viewing. J Speech Hear Res 1990;33:134–140.

Rawlins JNP: Latent inhibition and attentional processes in animals and men. Cambridge Workshop Neurobiol Basis Schizophrenia, Cambridge, March 1991 (reported by Winn [1994]).

Rey A: L'examen clinique en psychologie. Paris, Presse Universitaire de France, 1964.

Rizzolati G, Scandolara C, Maselli M, Gentilucci M: Afferent properties of periarcuate neurons in macaque monkeys. Behav Brain Res 1981;2:12–146.

Rocca P: Correlati biologici del disturbo ossessivo-compulsivo. Atti VI Congr Soc Ital Neurosci, Milano, June 1995.

Rochester SR: Are language disorders in acute schizophrenia actually information processing problems? J Psychiatr Res 1978;14:275–283.

Roelofs A: A spreading activation theory of lemma retrieval in speaking; in Levelt WJM (ed): Lexical Access in Speech Production. Cambridge, Blackwell, 1992, pp 107–142.

Ron MA, Harvey I: The brain in schizophrenia. J Neurol Neurosurg Psychiatry 1990;53:725–729.

Rosenbaum DA: Successive approximations to a model of human motor programming. Psychol Learn Motiv 1987;21:153–182.

Rosenbaum DA, Gordon M, Stillings NA, Feinstein MH: Stimulus response compatibility in the programmation of speech. Mem Cogn 1987;15:217–224.

Rosenfeld J: The FDP Network and Cortico-Ganglio-Basal System. New York, New York Review of Books, 1993.

Rothwell JC: Control of Human Voluntary Movement. Beckenham, Croom Helm, 1987.

Rourke BP: The syndrome of nonverbal learning disabilities: Developmental manifestations in neurological disease, disorders and dysfunctions. J Clin Exp Psychol 1988;2:293–330.

Rourke BP: Nonverbal Learning Disabilities: The Syndrome and the Model. New York, Guilford Press, 1989.

Rugg MD: Memory and consciousness: A selective review of issues and data. Neuropsychologia 1995; 33:1131–1141.

Saito S: Speech, Science and Technology. Amsterdam, IOS, 1992, vol II.

Saito S, et al: Speech, Science and Technology. Amsterdam, IOS, 1982, vol I.

Salthouse TA: A Theory of Cognitive Aging. Amsterdam, North-Holland, 1985.

Salthouse TA: Romberg B: Time accuracy relationships in young and old adults. J Gerontol 1982;37:349–353.

Saltzman EL, Kelso JAS: Skilled actions: A task dynamic approach. Psychol Rev 1987;94:84–105.

Saltzman EL, Munhall KG: A dynamical approach to gestural patterning in speech production. Ecol Psychol 1989;2:333–382.

Schieppati M, Di Francesco G, Nardone A: Patterns of activity of perioral facial muscles during mastication in man. Exp Brain Res 1985;77:103–112.

Schmidt RA: Motor Control and Learning, a Behavioural Emphasis. Champagne, Human Kinetic Publishing, 1988.

Schönle PW, Grone BF: Analysis of tongue movements in dysiatric and aphasic patients. Brain Lang 1992;42: 40–44.

Schönle PW, Grone BF, Roche G: Electromyographic articulography: A new method to simultaneously track multiple points in the articulators outside and inside the vocal tract. Third Advanced Course of Neurorehabilitation, Gargnano (Milan University), May 1992. Pavia, Fondazione Medicina di Lavoro, 1992.

Schriefers W, Meyer AS, Levelt WJM: Exploring the time course of lexical access in production: Picture-word interference studies. J Mem Lang 1990;29:86–102.

Scott DF: Understanding EEG. London, Duckworth, 1976.

Seashore RH: Stanford motor skills unit; in Miles H, Stark S (eds): University of Iowa Studies in Psychology. Univ Iowa Psychol Monogr. Iowa City, University of Iowa, 1928, vol 5, pp 39–82.

Serratrice G, Habib S: The Processes of Writing in Normals and Neurological Patients. Marseille, Marseille University Press, 1993.

Shallice T: From Neuropsychology to a Mental Structure. Cambridge, Cambridge University Press, 1988.

Shenton ME, Solovay MR, Holzman PS: Thought disorder in the relatives of psychotic patients. Arch Gen Psychiatry 1989;46:897–901.

Sherrington CS: The Integrative Action of the Nervous System, ed 2. New Haven, Yale University Press, 1947.

Simon C: The variability of consecutive wave-lengths in vocal and instrumental sounds. Psychol Monogr 1927;36:87–91.

Simone R: Fondamenti di linguistica. Bari, Laterza, 1990.

Smith MC, Maggie LT: Tracing the time course of picture-word processing. J Exp Psychol Gen 1986;109: 373–392.

Snyder SH: Dopamine receptors, neuroleptics, and schizophrenia. Am J Psychiatry 1981;138:460–464.

Soetching JF, Ranish NA, Palminteri R, Terzuolo CA: Changes in motor pattern following cerebellar and olivary lesions in squirrel monkeys. Brain Res 1976; 105:21–44.

Sommerhoff G: Logic of the Living Brain. London, Wiley, 1974.

Sorensen D, Ord Y: Directional perturbation factors for jitter and shimmer. J Commun Disord 1984;17: 143–151.

Sperry R: Consciousness, personal identity and the divided brain. Neuropsychologia 1984;22:661–673.

Spicer KB, Brown GG, Gorell J: Lexical decision in Parkinson's disease: Lack of evidence for generalized bradyphrenia. J Clin Neuropsychol 1994;16: 457–471.

Sternberg S: High speed scanning in human memory. Science 1966;153:652–654.

Sternberg S: Memory scanning: Mental processes revealed by reaction time experiments. Am Sci 1969; 57: 21–457.

Sternberg P, Monsell S, Knoll RL, Wright CE: The latency and duration of rapid movements sequences: Comparisons of speech and typewriting; in Stelmach GE (ed): Information in Motor Control and Learning. New York, Academic Press, 1978.

Sutako K: Speech Production and Perception. Kyoto, Rilpo, 1992.

Swash M, Kennard C: Scientific Basis of Clinical Neurology. Edinburgh, Churchill Livingstone, 1985.

Tamminga CA, Thaker GK, Buchanan R, et al: Limbic system abnormalities identified in schizophrenia using PET with fluorodeoxyglucose and neocortical alterations with deficit syndrome. Arch Gen Psychiatry 1992;49:522–530.

Thomas P, Fraser W: Linguistics, human communication and psychiatry. Br J Psychiatry 1994;165:585–592.

Thomas P, King K, Fraser W: Linguistic performance in schizophrenia: A comparison of acute and chronic patients. Br J Psychiatry 1991;156:204–210.

Thomas P, Leudar I, Johnston EM: Syntactic processing in the written language output of first onset psychotics. J Commun Disord 1993;26:209–230.

Titze IR: A model for neurologic sources of aperiodicity in vocal fold vibration. J Speech Hear Res 1991; 34:460–472.

Tobias PV: L'évolution du cerveau humain. Recherche 1980;109:282–292.

Tokhura Y, Vatikiotis-Bateson E, Sagisaka Y (eds): Speech Perception and Production and Linguistic Structure. Amsterdam, IOS, 1992.

Tononi E: Cerebral re-entry processes; in Ferri E (ed): Proceedings of the 3rd International Meeting of Psychophysiology – Troina (Italy). Troina, OASI Press, 1995, pp 63–64.

Walter GG: The Living Brain. London, Duckworth, 1953.

Wang SB, Sun CE, Walerath CA, Ziegler JS, Kipps BR, Lynn R, Goldin G, Diehl S: Evidence for a susceptibility locus for schizophrenia on chromosome 6-pter–p22. Nat Genet 1995;36:41–46.

Webster DD: Clinical analysis of the disability in patients with Parkinson disease. Mod Treat 1968;5: 257–282.

Webster WG: Neuropsychologic models of stuttering. I. Representations of sequential response mechanisms. Neuropsychologia 1985;23:263–267.

Weinberger DR: Implications of normal brain development for the pathogenesis of schizophrenia. Arch Gen Psychiatry 1987;44:660–670.

Weinberger DR, Berman KF, Daniel DG: Mesoprefrontal cortical dopaminergic activity and prefrontal hypofunctions in schizophrenia. Clin Neuropharmacol 1992;15(suppl 1):568–569.

Weinberger DR, Berman KF, Illowsky BP: Physiological dysfunction of dorsolateral prefrontal cortex in schizophrenia. III. A new cohort and evidence for a monoaminergic mechanism. Arch Gen Psychiatry 1988;45:609–615.

Weinberger DR, Berman KF, Suddath R, Torrey EF: Evidence of dysfunctions of a prefrontal-limbic network in schizophrenia: A magnetic resonance imaging and regional cerebral blood flow study of discordant monozygotic twins. Am J Psychiatry 1992;149: 890–897.

Wejner, 1991, cited by Tokhura et al. [1992].

Welford AT: Reaction Times. London, Academic Press, 1980.

Welsch MC, Pennington BF, Rouse B, McCabe ERB: Neuropsychology of early treated PKU: Specific executive function deficits. Child Dev 1990;61: 1697–1713.

White FJ, Wang RY: Differential effects of classic and atypical antipsychotic drugs on A9 and A10 dopamine neurons. Science 1983;221:1054–1057.

Wiesendanger M, Wiesendanger R: The SMA in light of recent investigations. Exp Brain Res 1984;9: 382–392.

Williams JM, Watts FN, Macleod G, Mathews A: Cognitive Psychology and Emotional Disorders. Chichester, Wiley, 1988.

Wilson FAS, Scalaidhe O, Goldman-Rackic PS: Dissociation of object and spatial processing domains in primate prefrontal cortex. Science 1993;260: 1955–1958.

Wind J, Chiarelli B, Bichakijan B, Nocentini A, Jonker A: Language Origin: A Multidisciplinary Approach. Proc NATO ASILO, Cortona, 1988. Dordrecht, Kluwer, 1992.

Winn PH: Schizophrenia research moves to the prefrontal cortex. Trends Neurosci 1994;17:265–268.

Woody CD: Memory Learning and Higher Functions: A Cellular View. New York, Springer, 1982.

Yairi E, Ambrose N: A longitudinal study of stuttering in children: A preliminary report. J Speech Res 1992;35: 755–760.

Yairi E, Ambrose N, Nierman R: The early month of stuttering: A developmental study. J Speech Hear Res 1993;36:521–528.

Yaniv SD, Meyer DE, Gordon PC, Muff CA, Sevald CA: Vowel similarity, connectioning models, and syllable structure in motor programming of speech. P Mem Lang 1990;29:1–26.

Yoshida Y, Honda K, Kakita Y: Noninvasive EMG measurement of laryngeal muscles and physiological mechanism of prosody control. ATR Tech Rep 1993; 3:1–12.

Zimmerman G: Articulatory dynamics of fluent utterances of stutterers and nonstutterers. J Speech Hear Res 1980;23:95–107.

Zipser et al, 1993, cited by Fuster [1993].

Zovato S: Ricerche di fonetica. Quaderni CNR. Padova, Progetto, 1994, vol 13.

Zvarich C, Magno-Caldognetto E, Wagges K: La balbuzie come disturbo della produzione articolatoria. Acta Phonet Lat 1994;16:157–183.

Subject Index

Acoustic masking, effect on testing 145
Acousticogram, *see also* Word acousticogram
    duration
        aging effects 152–154, 155
        busy-line effect 203, 204
        indices 319, 320
        neuroplastic effects 205
        pathological effects 197, 198
        short-term memory loss effects 198
    formant analysis 17
    latency times, *see also* Early process ratio,
        Intermediary process ratio
        aging effects 147, 148, 151–154, 166–171,
           184–187
        central time 161
        correction factor in initial aging process
           187, 188
        developmental changes 215, 216
        executive time 161
        factors affecting 133–138
        grammatical formulator and latency 140,
           142–144
        indices 317, 318
        measurements 2, 5, 48
        obsessive-compulsive disorder 278–280
        Parkinson disease 243, 244, 246–258
        schizophrenia 268–271, 273, 275–277
        sentences vs words 39
        stutterers 230, 231, 233, 235, 237, 239–241
        working memory evaluation 63, 64
    spastic dysphonia 224–228
Active memory
    delayed reactions 120, 121
    multiple-delayed-reaction verbochronometry
        of impairment 286–290
Adaptation
    executors in psychomotor control 13
    variables in testing
        attention span 97, 98
        eye movement 98
        respiratory cycle 98
Aging effects
    acousticogram
        duration 154, 155
        latency times
           children 147

        middle-aged subjects 148, 151
        old people 152–154, 166–171
        teenagers 148, 151
    delayed reaction preservation 171–173, 175,
        176
    early process ratio 196, 218–220
    intermediary process ratio 200–203, 218–220
    parallel diffuse processes 155, 156
Akinesia, *see* Parkinson disease
Articulation variability, overcoming in speech
    testing 95, 96
Attention
    deficit and hyperactivity disorder, multiple-
        delayed-reaction verbochronometry 216,
        217
    definition 100
    span, variability in testing 97, 98
    stochastic function relationship 102, 103

Body schema, *see* Schema
Botulinum, spastic dysphonia treatment 222, 224
Bradyphrenia, *see* Parkinson disease
Broca's area
    damage and delayed-reaction measurement
        90
    speech production role 45, 46
Buffer, definition 179

Central cerebral processes, *see also*
    Reverberating circuits
    aging effects 155, 168–170, 183
    commands 103, 104
    duration and cyclic repetitions 59, 60
    intrinsic variability 105, 106
    measurement at different foreperiods 89, 90,
        184, 185
    preparatory processes 51, 52
    types 52, 53
Corpus callosum, development and linguistic
    communication 20

Decoding-triggering processes, delay in reading
    reaction 121
Delayed reaction time
    chain of events 119–121
    preservation in old subjects 171–173, 175, 176

P$_{300}$, working memory measurement 61
Parallel diffuse processes
    aging effects 155, 156
    artificial neural networks 38
    efficiency 195
    functional probes 3
    network connections 10
    sentence processing 33, 40, 42
Parkinson disease
    akinesia 242
    basal ganglia impairment 92, 242
    hypertonia 242
    multiple-delayed-reaction verbochronometry
        akinesia effects 248, 249, 257
        bradyphrenia effects 255–257
        central and distal slowing, measurement
            249, 250, 255
        statistical evaluation of ratios 258
        tremor effects 243, 244, 246–248
Pauses, classification 145
Phenylketonuria, multiple-delayed-reaction
    verbochronometry 216, 217
Phonological unit
    definition 53
    extraction from grammatical unit 144
    programmation from pre-invariants 53
Picture naming tests, see also Nijmegen test,
    Veruno test
    speech control maturation in children 205,
        211–215
Pontine proper nuclei, speech production role 44
Positron emission tomography
    functional imaging 1, 4, 102
    multiple-delayed-reaction verbochronometry
        co-testing 308
Prefrontal cortex, role in delayed reactions 162
Process
    definition 177, 178
    reading vs speech 179–181
Programmation phase, functions 52
Psychomotor control
    adaptation of executors 13
    phases in speech 38, 39
    starting process 10
    topographical distribution of innervation 12
    translation of sensory signals 11, 13, 50
    tuning of mechanisms 12
    vocalization 18
    voice amplitude 14

Representation, definition 178, 179
Respiratory cycle, variability in testing 98
Reverberating circuits, see also Central cerebral
    processes
    formulator activation 123

internal circuits 123, 124
    measurement 124, 125

Schema, analysis at brain organization level 107
Schizophrenia
    dysfunctions in healthy relatives 314
    eye tracking dysfunction 262, 314
    genetics 303
    hypofrontality 261–264
    intermediary process impairment 89, 261, 262
    multiple-delayed-reaction verbochronometry
        chronic disease 265, 268–271
        controls 269
        discovery of delayed reactions 264
        intermediary process ratio 270, 271, 273,
            291, 293, 298, 299, 303, 304, 315, 316
        recent disease 271, 273, 275–277
        valium effects 271, 273, 277
    neurophysiological model 264
    positron emission tomography 263, 304
Sentence
    organization 37, 38
    processing 36, 37, 40
    time latency 39
Short-term memory
    differentiation from working memory
        287–290
    multiple-delayed-reaction verbochronometry
        of impairment 286–290
    processes 56
    reaction time 61
Spastic dysphonia, intra-individual variation of
    verbochronometric parameters 127, 128
    multiple-delayed-reaction verbochronometry
        224–228
    pathogenesis 224
    treatment 222, 224
Spectrography
    formant frequency 82
    Fourier analysis 81
    fundamental frequency 82
    jitter measurement 111
Speed of speech
    neural velocity 33, 42
    tachyphemic threshold, overloading effects
        and cyclic time 41–43
Standard deviation
    heuristic value in foreperiod reactions 113,
        114
    interpretation 112, 113
Stimulus onset asynchrony, expected retrieval
    latency derivation 121, 122
Stochastic function
    attentional process relationship 102, 103
    definition 102

Stochastic function (continued)
    degrees of freedom in speech control 107, 108
    interpretation 100, 102
    variability
        genesis 104, 105
        trial-and-error functions 103
Stroke, multiple-delayed-reaction verbochrono-
    metry findings 290
Stuttering
    mechanism 43, 229, 230
    multiple-delayed-reaction verbochronometry
        comparison with dysarthric disorder 237,
            239
        heterogeneous cases 233, 235
        increase in acousticogram latency 239, 241
        neural impairment analysis 237, 239, 240
        paradigmatic cases 230, 231, 233

Tachyphemic threshold
    development 23
    overloading effects and cyclic time 41–43
Trigeminal reflex, speech 108–110

Utterance, length 39

Valium, effects in schizophrenia 271, 273, 277
Velocity, *see* Speed of speech
Verbophasic system, definition 45
Veruno test, protocol 131
Visual perception
    duration of process 59
    input sequence 68
Vocal tract
    cortical representations 46
    phylogenetic modification 16, 20–22
Vocalization
    anatomofunctional bases in brain 33, 34
    children
        chimpanzee 17
        glottis descent 20–22
        grammar explosion 26, 27

        linguistic communication development
           19, 20
        motor control 17, 47
        object handling and early speech control
           23–25
        phases of verbal development 25, 26
        phonetic mechanisms 18, 19
    motor control 17, 18
    phonetic mechanisms 18, 19
Voice jitter, *see* Jitter

Wernicke's neural assembly
    damage and delayed-reaction measurement
        90
    speech production role 45, 46
Word
    acousticogram, *see also* Electromyogram
        disyllabic word pairs 74
        duration
            factors affecting 81, 154, 155
            standard deviation 79, 81
        five-letter mono- and disyllabic words 73
        heuristic value 70, 72
        latency time
            factors affecting 81
            standard deviation of mean values
                74, 78
        non-word pairs 73
    artificial word and latency time 134, 136, 180,
        181
    cerebral control 37, 38
    frequency of use 39, 134
    length and latency time 135–138
    processing 36, 37, 41
    time latency 39
Working memory
    differentiation from short-term memory
        287–290
    psychomotor evaluation 63
    reaction time 56, 61
    schizophrenia deficits 314